Osteopathic Medicine

PHILOSOPHY, PRINCIPLES AND PRACTICE

T0213382

The book is dedicated to the Weimar Kraskas.

Osteopathic Medicine
PHILOSOPHY, PRINCIPLES AND PRACTICE

Walter Llewellyn McKone DO

Introduction by W. Podmore

**Blackwell
Science**

© 2001 by
Blackwell Science Ltd
Editorial Offices:
Osney Mead, Oxford OX2 0EL
25 John Street, London WC1N 2BS
23 Ainslie Place, Edinburgh EH3 6AJ
350 Main Street, Malden
  MA 02148 5018, USA
54 University Street, Carlton
  Victoria 3053, Australia
10, rue Casimir Delavigne
  75006 Paris, France

Other Editorial Offices:
Blackwell Wissenschafts-Verlag GmbH
Kurfürstendamm 57
10707 Berlin, Germany

Blackwell Science KK
MG Kodenmacho Building
7–10 Kodenmacho Nihombashi
Chuo-ku, Tokyo 104, Japan

Iowa State University Press
A Blackwell Science Company
2121 S. State Avenue
Ames, Iowa 50014-8300, USA

The right of the Author to be identified as the Author of this Work has been asserted in accordance with the Copyright, Designs and Patents Act 1988.

All rights reserved. No part of this publication may be reproduced, stored in a retrieval system, or transmitted, in any form or by any means, electronic, mechanical, photocopying, recording or otherwise, except as permitted by the UK Copyright, Designs and Patents Act 1988, without the prior permission of the publisher.

First published 2001

The Blackwell Science logo is a trade mark of Blackwell Science Ltd, registered at the United Kingdom Trade Marks Registry

DISTRIBUTORS

Marston Book Services Ltd
PO Box 269
Abingdon, Oxon OX14 4YN
(Orders: Tel: 01235 465500
             Fax: 01235 465555)

USA
Blackwell Science, Inc.
Commerce Place
350 Main Street
Malden, MA 02148 5018
(Orders: Tel: 800 759 6102
             781 388 8250
             Fax: 781 388 8255)

Canada
Login Brothers Book Company
324 Saulteaux Crescent
Winnipeg, Manitoba R3J 3T2
(Orders: Tel: 204 837-2987
             Fax: 204 837-3116)

Australia
Blackwell Science Pty Ltd
54 University Street
Carlton, Victoria 3053
(Orders: Tel: 3 9347 0300
             Fax: 3 9347 5001)

A catalogue record for this title is available from the British Library

ISBN 0-632-05263-5

Library of Congress
Cataloging-in-publication Data
McKone, W. Llewellyn.
  Osteopathic medicine: philosophy, principles, and practice/Walter Llewellyn McKone; introduction by W. Podmore.
    p. cm.
  Includes bibliographical references and index.
  ISBN 0-632-05263-5 (alk. paper)
  1. Osteopathic medicine. 2. Osteopathic medicine—Philosophy. I. Title.
  [DNLM: 1. Osteopathic Medicine.
WB 940 M479oa 2001]
  RZ341.M35 2001
  615.5′33—dc21

                                00-048550

For further information on
Blackwell Science, visit our website:
www.blackwell-science.com

Contents

Foreword

I have known Walter since he was a boy and would like to think that I had some influence in his becoming an osteopath. I encouraged and helped Walter with his studies and his manipulation techniques and it was wonderful to see him develop into a brilliant student with a craving for furthering his knowledge.

I think that Walter felt that most osteopathic textbooks did not cover all the aspects of the origin of disease (osteopathic theory), the philosophy and mechanical principles originated by Andrew Taylor Still. These needed more clarification, research and development. He felt he needed to remind us of these principles we have neglected and bring them into a modern context.

Walter has spent many years collecting material and facts about Andrew Taylor Still and Johann Wolfgang von Goethe giving us a broad view of the scientific philosophy of wholeness in relation to nineteenth century ideas of health and disease. Students and practitioners alike will find this collection of ideas, facts and theories on osteopathic philosophy, principles and practice fascinating.

Even after nearly fifty years as a practitioner the thoughts, principles and ideas in this book excite me. I am nearing the end of my career and if the future of osteopathy is in the hands of excellent young men like Walter then I am content.

Kenneth Underhill
August 2000

Preface

'We have wanted someone to bridge the gap between the biology of present day text books and the biology of Dr Still, someone with sufficient vision to interpret Dr Still's words and to uncover the meaning hidden in his vague language.'

H.P. Frost, DO, 1918

On 24 May 1998, while walking in Goethe Park, Weimar, in the former East Germany, it struck me that I had it within me to write something timeless, like osteopathy itself. Weimar itself is an important link in this book's development and a direct inspiration for the book's style. As Europe's City of Culture in 1999, it boasts many inspirational residents – Nietzsche, Mann, Schweitzer, Liszt, Schiller and, most significantly, Goethe.

Goethe showed that mankind had developed to become dominated by a mathematical style of consciousness or thinking. Although he was not wrong, his organic style removes 'something' between a phenomenon and us. The mathematical style is ingrained everywhere, in our language, philosophy, education, economy, and habits. Goethe realised that at the other end of the style spectrum lies an organic mode of consciousness, subjective and open to phenomena, recognising the presence of the observer in that event.

Today's evidence based practice can be seen as detrimental to osteopathic medicine, if it is allowed to become dominant. The problem is not that of evidence based practice itself, but the delusion that it is the only evidence that counts in modern medical science. Osteopathic medical knowledge is characteristically different from allopathic medical knowledge. 'Scientia' (or science) is more than an accumulation of 'knowledge', more correctly it is defined as 'coming into knowledge'. Osteopathic medicine is a continual coming into knowing that does not resolve itself in either knowing or holding onto certainty as a consciousness. At its purest form, osteopathy only exists whilst it is being performed, as it demands the mechanism of the patient's body and the osteopath at the same time.

Osteopathy is spontaneous, and it is only our inherent mathematical mode of Cartesian–Newtonian consciousness that keeps us analysing and looking for certainty.

For osteopathy to reach its potential it should, as much as possible, redress the balance of the 'science' that is reductionist, positivist and associated with the medical model.

This book is my first attempt at redressing some of this imbalance and reintroducing the consciousness of osteopathy at the beginning of the twenty-first century. My aim is to introduce into all osteopathic education and practice an osteopathic consciousness that will flow through all osteopathic colleges and schools throughout the world. I have tried to meet Frost's request in trying to 'uncover the meaning hidden in his (Still's) vague language.' Luckily I have found that Still's language was not vague, it was organic and poetic in the style similar to that of Goethe. Once Still's thinking is understood then all his work literally jumps out of the page and becomes manifest in the patient. Understanding this osteopathic consciousness will make all osteopathic education and practice a distinct system of health care.

I now understand why Still had trouble explaining osteopathy to other people: he had to use language. He was not a highly educated academician. The father of osteopathy was essentially a hillbilly farmer with an increasing interest in self-taught rural medicine. As a man who worked in harmony with nature he was blessed with a simple organic consciousness, only believing what his eyes and hands told him. Consequently his work and teachings have been both misunderstood by latter day osteopaths and written off as quackery by the over-educated medical establishment. So much so that these so-called educated medical minds, constrained by their mathematical style of consciousness, systematically applied academic subversion – resulting in the eventual disempowerment and contamination of osteopathy.

Finding the right style for this book was difficult and so was the order, because philosophy, principles and practice happen together in osteopathy. On numerous occasions I repeat myself; this is intentional. I also reproduce a number of papers that demonstrate a style of thinking in the earliest part of the twentieth century. Still demonstrates that the agent of osteopathy is the osteopath. There should be nothing between the practitioner and the phenomenon – miracle of nature – known as the patient.

'Too often biologists cannot bring themselves to make a sufficiently serious study of the structural aspects of their problems. Yet there can be no reason to assume that, while Nature uses methods of infinite subtlety in her chemistry and control mechanisms, her structural approach should be a crude one.'
J.E. Gordon, *Structures or Why Things Don't Fall Down*

I would like to thank the following people for believing in me: William Podmore, Henri Bortoft, Jonathan Curtis-Lake, Martin Collins, Kenneth and Evelyn

Underhill, the Rasmussen family, Brigitte Kraska, Katharina Kraska, Maxillian McKone, Colin M. Jarman, David Worton, Duncan Bowles, Alan Clark (BSO patient), my patients for having patience, my students and colleagues at the British School of Osteopathy (for keeping my feet on the ground and not taking me seriously), Donna Smith, Lisa Gilbert, Elsworth Wray (for keeping me alive), Peter Dunleavy, and Nedialka Penner.

Walter Llewellyn McKone
London

Introduction

Walter McKone is playing a leading role in the current renaissance of osteopathic thought. In his extraordinary new book, he pioneers the attempt to place osteopathy's creation and development in its social and intellectual context. This is a quite original contribution to the history of ideas.

Walter shows that Andrew Taylor Still, who first 'unfurled the banner of osteopathy to the wind', did not develop his ideas in a vacuum. The great thinkers of the European Enlightenment, particularly Goethe[1] and Hegel, proposed the ideas of organic form and interrelatedness that inspired osteopathy. They had moved beyond the dualism of René Descartes, who divided matter from ideas and body from mind. The poet and educator Samuel Taylor Coleridge[2] popularised this tradition of German philosophy in Britain in the nineteenth century, as Ralph Waldo Emerson did in America.

In particular, Goethe, who played the part in Germany's culture that Shakespeare did in Britain's and Dante in Italy's, also made enormous contributions to scientific thinking. Goethe's universalism showed not just in his poetry, dramas, travel writing and autobiography (surely one of the greatest books ever written about the development of a mind), but also in his scientific writings on anatomy, botany and physics.

Walter combines an unusually wide-ranging outlook with a detailed study of the workings of the body. He also shows us that the relationship between the

---

[1] See Nicholas Boyle's biography: *Goethe the poet and the age*, Volume 1: *The poetry of desire* (1749–90), and Volume 2: *Revolution and renunciation* (1790–1805), Oxford University Press, 1991 and 2000.

[2] See Richard Holmes' magnificent biography of Coleridge, *Coleridge: early visions* (1989) Hodder & Stoughton; and *Coleridge: darker reflections* (1998) HarperCollins.

osteopath and the patient is the heart of osteopathy and explains why osteopathy works so well.

William Podmore
August 2000

CHAPTER 1

Origins and Development

'All writing is subjective, and consequently liable to error and personal bias, so that the historian, who is himself subject to prejudice and capable of mistaken interpretations, has to attempt to assess the value of each piece of his raw material and fit it into his general picture of the age he is describing. It is essentially his picture, and the reader is free to accept or reject it according to his own preconceptions and knowledge of the period.'

> J.J. Bagley, *Historical Interpretation: Sources of English Medieval History, 1066–1540* (1965)

'There is nothing more difficult than a beginning.'

> Byron

The influences involved in the development of any 'science' are multifaceted and complex. Each arises from the legacies of the past, the impressions of the present and our dreams for the future. So, for osteopathy, no single factor determined its development, and no single person, including its founder Dr. Andrew Taylor Still, could direct its future. Dr. Still, like so many men of science, possessed characteristics and interests that the modern researcher would find easy to fault. Too often, people and societies abstract what they value and ignore the remaining material or use it to criticise a particular individual, for example singling out Sir Isaac Newton's physics, and using his alchemy studies against him. If there seems to be nothing of value, then it may be ignored; this is dangerous, as values and needs change with time. We will begin with some key people and times in the development of medicine, continue into the nineteenth century with the development of osteopathy, and then look at the beginning of the twentieth century.

Prehistoric medicine

On a wall of the Trois Frères cave in the Pyrenees is possibly the oldest drawing of a 'medical man', thought to be drawn by someone of the Aurignacian period in about 15 000 BC. Some of the earliest medically intentional procedures included *trepanning* or *trephining*, the surgical operation in which a hole is bored into the skull. Even in the beginning of the twentieth century there were still islands in the South Pacific where this operation was performed for relief from epilepsy, headache or psychiatric illness. This procedure was always supported by the administration of plants used for their pain killing and antibiotic properties. Also, early forms of massage have been noted in drawings and in cultures in many different remote areas of the world.

The first medical people

Well after the prehistoric period, there arose cultures that shared signs of some degree of organisation and an attempt at understanding and treatment of disease. The earliest of these was the Babylonian society under the rule of Hammurabi (1948–1905 BC). As organised as this culture was, there was still an easily recognisable sign of 'magic' and the existence of many amateur physicians. This was due to the custom of laying the sick in the street and insisting that nobody could pass by without attempting to administer some kind of help. It is possible that these early physicians were mainly priests – a trend, or influence, that would continue into our modern times.

Early Greek and Egyptian medicine

The philosopher–physicians of ancient Greece mark a significant change in the rationale for the causes and reasons of disease. Obviously, little is really known in any great detail about the lives of these philosopher–physicians.

We will begin with Pythagoras of Samos (580–498 BC), who was known to have been a traveller at some time and spent a significant part of his life in Croton in Southern Italy. Pythagoras is famous for his discovery of a theory of numbers; he believed that the earth was a sphere, an opinion resulting possibly from his extensive travelling. Alcmaeon of Croton (about 500 BC), a pupil of Pythagoras, dissected animals and described the Eustachian tubes; unfortunately he also put forward the theory that goats breathed through their ears. He was able to make the distinction between arteries and veins, even if the arteries did contain air, due to their being empty after death.

Women had a significant role as physicians in the early history of medicine. Of particular interest are the classical Egyptian schools at Heliopolis and Sais. In Homer's *Iliad*, 'Agamede of the golden hair', was a skilled physician. Philista (372–318 BC) was an ancient Greek physician who apparently was so popular, due to her beauty, that she had to lecture from behind a closed curtain. Not much has survived about women physicians because most surviving information was written by and about men. Early physicians began to appear in Homer's *Iliad* and the *Odyssey*, although due to the style of writing it was difficult to distinguish between the gods and mortals. In the *Iliad* there were surgeons: 'wounded is Odysseus, spearman renowned, and Agamemnon; and smitten is Eurypylos on the thigh with an arrow. And about them the leeches skilled in medicine are busy, healing their wounds'.

Hippocrates was born about 470 BC in Chios (now Khios), Greece, and died about 410 BC. He was a contemporary of Socrates, known as the father of medicine and medical ethics, and was the first to treat the body (person) as a whole. His principle was *primum non-nocere*: 'first do no harm'. On the island of Cos there is the Hippocratic tree where, it is said, Hippocrates would sit for shade from the sun. Hippocrates had a view of medicine that has been translated into many languages; he was known for his well documented description of diseases. In his book on *The Sacred Disease*, which is thought to be epilepsy, he wrote 'every disease has its own nature and arises from external causes, from cold, from sun, or from changing winds'. He was one of the first physicians to realise the effects of food, occupation and climate in causing diseases. Unlike many before, and even fewer after him, he believed in the *Vis Medicatrix Naturae*, 'the healing power of nature'. Hippocrates wrote 'Our natures are the physicians of our diseases'.

Aristotle (384–322 BC), a pupil of Plato, was known as the father of science. He proposed that reality can be classified and categorised, and believed that truth is discovered through perception; reality includes the perception of being whereby the distinction between 'soul' and 'body' is meaningless. He was close behind Hippocrates with his basic understanding of comparative anatomy and embryology.

Galen (*c*. 131–201 AD) was born at Pergamos in Asia Minor and advocated the balance of the humours as essential to wellbeing. Like Hippocrates, he believed the body was composed of four fundamental humours: blood, phlegm, yellow bile and black bile. In addition he considered the four fundamental elements: air, fire, earth and water; and the four fundamental qualities: heat and cold, dryness and moisture.

The development of the modern scientific movement

'The history of science is science itself.'

Johann Wolfgang von Goethe

Contrary to popular belief, modern science did not begin at a certain point in time when people suddenly became aware of their surroundings and senses. We can begin to understand the origins of the modern scientific movement with the work of Copernicus (1473–1543). Copernicus, known as the father of modern astronomy, asserted that science was firmly grounded in the belief that any experience you had involved your senses and was therefore an illusion. Science would then become a system of getting behind the illusion of your senses by forming mathematical relationships with these experiences; these mathematical relations are known in modern physics as the Laws of Nature.

Through his astronomical writings Copernicus maintained that the entire world as we experience it is an illusion. This was the first major step in the externalising of our consciousness and our relationship with solid objects. His writings reflected the Renaissance aesthetic ideal with which people were already acquainted in architecture, painting and sculpture. This developed from his understanding of symmetry, order and harmony in the universe. Copernicus proposed that we should never trust our senses and we must develop ways of thinking to substitute our so-called sense of reality. The main method of thinking was to develop an analytical mathematical mode.

Paramount to this mode of thinking was the fundamental construct of Neo-platonism. Part of this mode of thinking represents the Sun as God making it the centre, and our movement around it as the creator of our illusions. Hence the substitution of sense perception by mathematics, something stable with numerical and geometrical relationships.

This is an example of the cultural–historical development present in all 'sciences'. The Copernican example of substitution is a major part of the development of science that is regularly left out. We are otherwise led to believe that the development of science is through objective experimentation or new observations, but this is far from the case. Scientific experiments are but demonstrations of a particular style or mode of consciousness. In the case of Copernicus there are no new observations or experimental constructs in any of his work. But still this form of science dominates primarily because of its internal historical dimensions. As will be seen later, a science cannot develop outside the cultural–religious–social context within which the thoughts are developed.

Osteopathy is no exception to the rule that the development of any 'science' is the result of a cultural, religious and historical interaction. Cultural, religious and historical factors determine the forms of the sciences used within a society. Science is not an autonomous activity; it never was and never will be. Unfortunately modern or positivist science has become more reductionist in its attempts to become autonomous and acquire 'pure knowledge'. The fewer and more specialised the people involved in a branch of science, the more the field develops its own style of thinking, which is a direct result of the meaning placed in it by the few involved in it. This does not affect the truth of the science and again osteopathy is no exception.

To understand the origin and development of osteopathy we have to give some time to the culture in which osteopathy developed. Areas of interest include the effect of enlightenment and reformation before and into the nineteenth century, the industrial revolution, religion, social organisation, capitalism and war. Obviously there will be a reciprocal influence in all these areas.

Reformation and enlightenment

During the fourteenth to sixteenth centuries the ideas of citizenship developed within a dynamic new social structure generating new forms of awareness. Between the sixteenth to eighteenth centuries massive changes in civilisation posed an ever increasing challenge to the role of the Roman Catholic church. The beginnings of the scientific thinking and method, world trade and travel brought a new light to European society. Control and order were beginning to grow and the idea of natural creation began to replace that of divine creation. Mathematics, instead of the senses and independent imagination, was the new language, with analysis and experimentation as the proof of truth.

Martin Luther (1483–1546), Ulrich Zwingli (1484–1531) and John Calvin (1509–64) were three singleminded people who influenced the fundamental aspects of culture in Europe by developing a Protestant ethic. This ethic promoted wealth as a duty and profit as virtuous. In the early 1500s King Henry VIII (1491–1547) adopted Protestantism so this implementation has been interpreted as for political rather than for religious reasons. Of Luther, Zwingli and Calvin, Calvin was probably the most important in changing, or speeding up changes in, Western culture. He was originally a lawyer and his impression on American culture was such that native Americans have been called *Calvinist* in the way they think and act. Like Zwingli, he advocated an exact following of the Christian scriptures to the letter. What was not in them could not be done and if it was in them it had to be done. Calvin and Zwingli believed that the whole structure of politics, society and religion should be based on these scriptures. Naturally if this meant roasting a few people, on the way, then that is what had to happen.

Of even greater direct impact on the structure of science, especially medicine, are the combined contributions of René Descartes (1596–1650) and Sir Isaac Newton (1642–1727) with their analytical mode of scientific consciousness and Johann Wolfgang von Goethe (1749–1832) with his organic mode of scientific consciousness in understanding nature. These states of consciousness are complementary, not opposing. Western culture adopted the theory and practices of Descartes and Newton during its cultural development: this had a profound effect on today's medical science. Due to the constructs of our culture the analytical system has become predominant and is now beginning to show its limitations, especially in areas of physics and medicine. We tend not to use the organic scientific approach due to its lack of development and the discomfort caused by a paradigm shift. We would have to turn everything inside out.

René Descartes was a French mathematician, philosopher and physiologist who was famous for his quote *cogito ergo sum* (I am thinking, therefore I exist). He produced the first systematic account of the difference between mind and body, the separation of which gave his theories the name of Cartesian dualism. Descartes would never get up before midday, spending the time in bed engaged in a kind of meditation and 'pure thought'. In 1617 he joined the army, as did all gentlemen, of Prince Maurice of Orange, in Holland, and still managed not to get up before midday. Descartes was a successful teacher of science and was invited to tutor the Queen of Sweden in 1647. Unfortunately for Descartes, she was a very early riser and the change did not suit him. He died from bronchitis a few months later.

Sir Isaac Newton was born in Woolsthorpe, England in the year that Galileo died. Newton was considered primarily a mathematician and his contribution to science cannot be underestimated. He furthered Descartes' laws of motion, developed the optical telescope and expanded other laws predicting the actions of nature. It is now becoming apparent that most of his written work and time was spent engrossed in alchemy, a form of occult chemistry. The *Newtonian–Cartesian* combination is the essential developmental root of modern medicine. At the beginning of the twentieth century western culture was dominated by physics, while at the beginning of this twenty-first century our culture is marked by progress in genetics.

Johann Wolfgang von Goethe was born in Frankfurt and is remembered more for his poetry and plays, particularly *Faust*, than for his contribution to science. His major scientific contributions included his *Theory of Colour* (giving an alternative to Newton's theory) and the discovery of the premaxillary bone in the upper jaw of man, thus making the first link between man and animals. Goethe recognised that the history of science is science itself and began an in-depth study of the history of science, which lasted his entire life. Unfortunately his scientific work was also interpreted as poetic until recently. Due to our Newtonian–Cartesian mode of thinking it has only been in the last few years that we have discovered Goethean science as organic, in the form of an awareness of nature in all phenomena. Goethe died in Weimar.

The origins and development of osteopathy

Education and communication on a mass level began to emerge in the nineteenth century, which made change even faster. The so-called *peasant characteristics*, contemplation, wholeness, fatalism and a non-domination of nature, were changing. As no science is autonomous in its origins, certain cultural aspects have to be considered before, during and after the official date of the beginning of osteopathy in the USA. The aspects we shall consider will be the following:

- the industrial revolution
- religion
- culture and social organisation
- the American Civil War
- nineteenth century medicine.

The industrial revolution

It was between the American Civil War and the First World War that the greatest changes in industry occurred in the United States These were the years of the presidents Buchanan, Lincoln, Johnson, Grant, Hayes, Garfield, Arthur, Cleveland, Harrison, McKinley, Roosevelt, Taft and Wilson. The ruralism of America had become urban, and the frontier by the 1920s had all but disappeared. After the Civil War America was a country of production with steel mills, railroads and agriculture covering vast areas of land. This was the usual post-war phenomenon since wars need mass production, and the Civil War was no exception. Many of the products used for the war effort found a commercial avenue for their survival, especially pharmaceuticals. Drugs production, administration and self medication grew with the industrial revolution to such a degree that there was a real threat of the American population becoming a nation of cocaine addicts by the beginning of the 1900s.

During the nineteenth century, although the industrial revolution was well under way, agriculture was still the USA's main source of income. The number of farms grew three-fold between 1860 and 1910. In addition the harvests of wheat, corn and cotton between 1860 and 1890 were the best in the history of farming. Things were getting easier for the people with the hardest jobs and the United States was entering the era of mass production. There was movement towards the West and new machines in farming freed the farmer from the backbreaking use of the hand sickle. These machines included potato planters, cutters, sowers, threshers etc. In 1840, a farmer, Cyrus McCormick, cut two and two-and-a-half hectares a day, a miracle. Science, or rather technology, was here to save and prosper. This anticipation of an easier more productive life would have a profound effect on the public's perception and trust in modern medicine.

The outlook of the developing modern industrial society has been becoming rational, analytical, quantitative and materialistic, ever since the fourteenth century. Using their new technology, people had an even greater desire to manipulate nature. Instead we have only excelled in the manipulation of matter at a particle level with little or no understanding of nature. It was a science of materials and matter with increasing specialisation within the professions.

Religion

Historically, religion moved from tribal (supernatural), to agricultural (organised religion with codes of conduct), to industrial (becoming a personal sense). Complementary aspects of religion and science express themselves through the culture of the day. The main religious influence from the seventeenth century was Protestantism in which, since that time, there have been four major sects: Calvinism, as we have seen above; Pietism; Methodism and the various branches of the Baptist movement. It becomes apparent that none of these sects can be independent since they grew from the same base. As we will see in more detail it was Methodism as a sect of Protestantism that had an influence on the origin of osteopathy. The least known of these branches is Pietism, which was a breakaway group from the Calvinists in England.

Of particular interest in the development of osteopathy is Methodism. John Wesley, an ordained clergyman in the Anglican church founded this religious movement in Britain in 1739. Two other ordained clergymen were prominent in its beginning, Charles Wesley (brother of John), a hymn writer, and George Whitefield, a preacher and revivalist. The Wesley brothers were born in Epworth, Lincolnshire. In Oxford on 22 November 1729, John joined a small group of students organised by his brother with the objective of deeper study of the scriptures and carrying out their religious duties. John Wesley would in the future name his entire group the 'Perfectionists' but other students referred to them in derogatory terms; two used were 'the holy club' and 'the Methodists.' This was the origin of the movement's name.

The development of Methodism in the United States had nothing to do directly with the Wesley brothers or their visit to Georgia in 1735. In 1766 in New York a local preacher, Philip Embury, was asked to deliver a sermon for a Mrs Barbara Heck. Both were natives of Ireland who had moved to America in 1760. Over the years the sermons continued, and the attendance increased especially after the involvement of Captain Thomas Webb, another preacher. With his motivation, St George's Methodist Church, the first in America, was erected in Philadelphia. At almost the same time, Methodism was being introduced in Maryland. It then began to spread along a route from Philadelphia, via New Jersey and onto Virginia.

These itinerant preachers would have a circuit to serve of around 20 to 40 appointments or societies. Methodist Francis Asbury developed 'circuit riding' as a way of visiting the districts where one or more appointments were served. Methodists became split over the issue of slavery, which sent waves throughout the movement. Many clashes took place in the early nineteenth century with slave owners, reaching a peak in the middle of the nineteenth century when the Methodists split with their southern delegates over this issue.

John Wesley studied medicine and developed his brand of prevention and treatment consistent with Methodist principles. His system was that of a unifying concept of body and soul, with disease as obviously a discontinuity of this harmony. With his experience he wrote the *Primitive Physick*. As with Methodism he advocated the simple life and a natural way of prevention and treatment with exercise and control over eating and drinking. Methodists definitely did not tolerate the drinking of alcohol.

There is no area where Protestant ethics and theology had more impact than in the development of psychology and its various branches. As we shall see, in the section on psychology, the original name for psychology was moral philosophy, the way to conduct your life. The original word for mind was soul, which could not be in your body so was placed in the head and the narrative of psychology therapy is very similar to confession.

Culture and social organisation

In the 1990 census more Americans claimed German ancestry or ethnic origin than any other group: 57.9 million (23%). Among other significantly large groups 38.7 million (15.6%) claimed Irish ancestry, 33.7 million (13.1%) English, 23.8 million (9.6%) Afro-American, and 14.7 million (5.9%) Italian. Lack of previous information in relation to association with Germany was due to the atrocities of the First and Second World Wars. Mass immigration by Europeans to the United States was most notable after the Napoleonic wars in 1815, with the largest European group being around 20 000 from Germany. In 1854 the first major influx of 220 000 immigrants arrived and were registered at American ports; the highest number was 250 000 in 1882. With this movement to the United States came the culture of Germany. Among these men and women were thousands of intellectuals who successfully promoted ethical, moral and material welfare and whose influence was strong, as we shall see.

Most German immigrants in the eighteenth and nineteenth centuries were skilled craftsmen and farmers. German farmers were more business-like than other farmers and were less likely to succumb to 'speculative fever'. They tended to try to purchase more land in their area for their families. One of the biggest areas of German farm land was in Missouri. In 1868, a German farmer in Missouri described the opposite attitude of other ethnic groups:

'There are people here who are forever moving around. They buy themselves a piece of land, live on it a while, work like a dog, and then, when they do not end up rich in a few short years, they curse the area, sell everything for a song, and move on to spots where they finish up worse off than they left. Sometimes they return and would be delighted if only they could buy back their original land. In this way they frequently move five or six times before they finally come to their senses and admit that wealth does not fly into every mouth that opens.'

Kamphoefner (1987)

Over the period of the nineteenth century, the vast majority of Germans settled in a quadrangle encompassing the states from Ohio to Missouri on the south quadrant, and from Michigan to North Dakota and down to Nebraska on the north and west quadrants. Many emigrants of certain occupations were advised not to leave Germany. An emigrant handbook of 1859 advises that

'...a sloppy student would end up a fanatic Methodist preacher; a discarded lieutenant would end up splitting wood or boiling soap; a proud baron would end up driving a team of oxen; a Catholic priest might end up with a wife and child, happily farming; but a clever stable hand is now in charge of one of the largest business places in St. Louis.'

Adams (1999)

Professor Willi Paul Adams at the John. F. Kennedy Institut für Nordamerika Studien at the Freie Universität, Berlin, goes on to write that 'during the century preceding the First World War, a pluralistic German-language culture existed in America; as late as 1910 an estimated nine million people in the United States still spoke German as their mother tongue.'

A short German-American cultural chronology

1850   Levi Strauss produces his first jeans.

1853   Heinrich Steinweg created the Steinway piano in New York (*weg* means way).

1859   Abraham Lincoln acquired the *Illinois Staatsanzeiger* paper even though he struggled with German.

1861   During the Civil War German–American militia safeguarded Missouri for the Union.

1865   Of the 5000 German born volunteers in the Union army, 41 held the rank of Major General.

1888   Over 800 German language publications represented more than 50% of America's foreign language press.

1928   Herbert Hoover (Huber) was elected as president, the first with German ancestry.

1942   General D. Eisenhower commanded US Forces in Europe. His original family name was Eisenhauer.

The effect of the German culture can be seen in the early osteopathic texts. John Martin Littlejohn's books, *Physiology* and *Psycho-physiology*, 1899, have their chapter and subsection titles in German style fonts, with the 'ö' appearing occasionally in early osteopathic texts. Ralph Waldo Emerson wrote *Representative Men* in 1849, writing, 'hence almost all the valuable distinctions which are current in higher conversations have been derived to us from Germany'. Of the Germans whose philosophical influence on America was possibly the most important Emerson chose Goethe, as the following excerpt shows.

'Every word was carved before his eyes into the earth and the sky; and the sun and stars were only letters of the same purport and of no more necessity. But how can he be honoured when he does not honour himself; when he loses himself in a crown; when he is no longer the lawgiver, but the sycophant, ducking to the giddy opinion of a reckless public; when he must sustain with shameless advocacy some bad government, or must bark, all year round, in opposition; or write conventional criticism, or profligate novels, or at any rate write without thought, and without recurrence by day and by night to the sources of inspiration? Some reply to these questions may be furnished by looking over the list of men of literary genius in our age. Among these no more instructive name occurs than that of Goethe to represent the powers and duties of scholar or writer. The man cooperates. He loves to communicate; and that which is for to say lies as a load on his heart until it is delivered.'

From a broader aspect urbanisation meant that people started being subjected to behavioural cues far more than they realised, or realise today. The industrial revolution affected our social organisation in a way that people started to become *individuated*. Individuated persons describe themselves in terms of their acts, ideas, and possessions. It is now recognised that the more you become individuated, the more you become 'two' or more people: the real you and the acted-out you as a reflection of how you want others to see you. Our social structure began to move from very personal family relationships to an increasing level of relations with strangers. Wealth and abundance become increasingly important, affecting people's relationships to each other and their ability to travel. During this developing revolution the effects of society were brought to the conscious level by the writings of Max Weber (1864–1920). Disliking the class analysis in the work of Karl Marx (1818–83), he founded the methodology of the ideal type, proposed the elective affinity of causal relationships and held that there was no universal law of society.

Society began to experience these achievements through doing and the building of 'character' through work. There was an ever-increasing need to achieve an order to the world around us through moves towards democratic principles, progress, new concepts and the Protestant work ethic. Everyday language was changing, as words such as success, opportunity, time, change, growth and free enterprise were becoming more commonplace. Lastly, the map of the United States of America was different to that of today and was changing at an unprecedented rate.

The American Civil War

Abraham Lincoln was first inaugurated on 4 March 1861. On 12 April there was an attack on Fort Sumter; by 15 April Lincoln had called for 75 000 volunteers to suppress the uprising. It was in this same year that Andrew Taylor Still enlisted in the 9th Kansas Cavalry of the Union army. The Emancipation Proclamation was issued on 1 January 1863. Abraham Lincoln was well aware that this was not a war just over the issue of slavery. The aim of the Emancipation Proclamation was to release slaves into the rebel territory as a weapon of war recognising there were areas controlled by the rebels which were 'then, thence forward, and forever free'. This proclamation only applied to slaves in areas not under Federal control. Of note during the Civil War was the work of the Massachusetts abolitionist Governor John A. Andrews who organised an African–American unit between January and May 1863. This unit was the 54th Massachusetts Regiment and consisted of black solders with white officers. Under the command of Colonel Robert Gould Shaw this Union regiment of mostly black educated soldiers led the attack on Battery Wagner in the South Carolina sea islands on 18 July 1863. Even though the attack failed it motivated the African–American community and subsequently nearly 179 000 enlisted in the Union army. Abraham Lincoln apparently said that this single act of the 54th Massachusetts made a major contribution to the Union success in the Civil War. The story of this regiment was dramatised in the film *Glory*.

The practice of medicine during the Civil War was straightforward. Diarrhoea was checked with sulphate of magnesia; quinine (with or without whiskey) was administered for practically anything including malaria, and morphine, which was rubbed or dusted into the wound, was the most important painkiller. There were no antibiotics, no antiseptic protocols and there was ignorance of opiate addiction. This was the last war where there was no knowledge of the germ theory. Due to overuse of opiates many soldiers returned home as addicts, augmenting the continuing opiate self-medication in American society. All good druggists could supply opiates as painkillers.

At the beginning of the Civil War there were fewer than 100 surgeons and assistant surgeons. All medical personnel were called surgeons in those days. There were no physicians as we know today, hence the term 'bloodless surgeon' used in the early days of the development and practice of osteopathy and the influence of the technical approach used by Still. The most common procedure was amputation: it was estimated that three out of four surgical procedures were amputations. This was due to the effect of the Minie ball shot used in firearms which would shatter bone or at least leave it in splinters. Due to the number of casualties the science of embalming was making leaps and bounds. Families wanted to bury their own relatives and friends. During the war the concept of medical neutrality developed: medical personnel could not be shot at or taken prisoner.

Disease and illness during the American Civil War has been called the 'third army'. Death from disease was immense, about 275 000 deaths in the 2.2 million Union solders, and around 164 000 deaths of the 750 000 in the Confederate camp. In the Union camp, pneumonia, including influenza and bronchitis, accounted for 1 765 000 episodes of illness and 45 000 deaths; typhoid for 149 000 episodes and 35 000 deaths; diarrhoea/dysentery for 360 000 episodes and 21 000 deaths; and malaria for 1 316 000 episodes and 10 000 deaths. Full details of the Confederate suffering and deaths were lost when Richmond was taken and the records were destroyed (Sartin, 1993).

Union spirits were generally high. The most popular and first professional songwriter in American history, Stephen Collins Foster (1826–64) made his contribution to Union army morale. It was Robert E. Lee who said, 'without music there could be no war'. Foster was extremely upset by the outbreak of the Civil War and this inspired him to write *That's What's the Matter*.

We live in hard and stirring times,
Too sad for mirth, too rough for rhymes;
For songs of peace have lost their chimes,
And that's what's the matter!
The men we held as brothers true,
Have turn'd into rebel crew;
So now we have to put them thro',
And that's what's the matter!

Chorus:
That's what's the matter,
The rebels have to scatter;
We'll make them flee,
By land and sea,
And that's what's the matter!

Foster's works influenced America, at that time, and his works are still influential today. His more popular compositions included *Beautiful Dreamer* (posthumously published in 1864), *Jeanie with the Light Brown Hair* (1854), *Oh! Susanna* (1848) and *Gwine to Run all Night* or *De Camptown Races* (1850).

Nineteenth-century medicine

The beginning of the nineteenth century was not a particularly good time for regular allopathic physicians in the United States of America. They were not unified in their approach, and being fewer in number were generally outnumbered by other therapists and scarcely available to the public. There were at least four groups of therapists.

(1) The allopaths themselves, generally originating from William Cullen (1710–90) and continuing with his two pupils Benjamin Rush (1745–1813) and John Brown (1735–88).
(2) Indian doctors, also called herb doctors, who obtained their knowledge from American Indians.
(3) The Thomsonians founded by Samuel Thomson (1779–1843), who preferred to use steam baths, Native American Indian emetics and the lobelia root, also known as Indian tobacco.

(4)   The homeopaths, who used the medicating system developed by the German physician Samuel Hahnemann (1755–1843).

The heroic dosing of the allopathic system was rationalised by the diagnosis developed by Cullen, Rush and Brown. It was based on the excitability of the patient due to outside influences. If you gave in to external factors this was a *sthenic* disease and if you showed little giving in to external influences this led to *asthenic* disease. Most diseases were described as asthenic and presented, for example, as exhaustion due to excessive excitability. Naturally different diseases needed different treatment. For the sthenic disease the treatment regime was generally bloodletting, emetics and cathartics. In the case of the more popular asthenic disease the treatment was opium and alcohol. Benjamin Rush made his own contribution to diagnosis and pathology, discovering that all disease was due to preternatural tension in the arteries, and could only be cured with massive bloodletting by use of the lancet and the 'sheet-anchor' of medical practice, calomel (mercurous chloride, $Hg_2 Cl_2$).

What were the effects of their actions? The following item appeared in the *Botanical and Eclectic Medical Journal*, 1849, and describes the effects of the heroic administration of calomel and other medications to children in the nineteenth century:

'A lad named Rout, sixteen years of age, died at Covington Ky., last week from the effects of mercury, administrated ten weeks ago by a physician, to alleviate typhoid fever. The Commercial says: "In a few weeks purple spots made their appearance on each side of the face, followed by mortification and sloughing of the parts, the usual result of mercurial poisoning when thus manifested. For several weeks the poor sufferer lay thus, the poison gradually augmenting its awful work, until the whole jaw, with the exception of a small portion of the chin, was exposed to view from loss of surrounding flesh. The upper and lower lips were entirely gone, and the appearance was presented of a skull covered with flesh, excepting the teeth and jaws – a most pitiable sight. On the right side of the face the mortification extended to the eye, scalp, and ear, and had the youthful sufferer lived a few days longer, he would have lost his right eye, ear, and all the flesh on the side of the face and head. But fortunately for himself and friends, death kindly came to his aid and relieved him of his misery. It is impossible for words to convey an impression of the loathsome, sickening spectacle presented above."'

The joining of medicine at the end of the nineteenth century with modern science sealed the trust of the public in a new medicine. Science produced harvesting machines which brought prosperity to farmers, so obviously it would work if combined with medicine. Symbolically the white coat was the final sign of the 'marriage' of medicine and science. Initially adopted in hospitals, it would be quickly adopted at the beginning of the twentieth century as a symbol of medicine becoming a science.

Andrew Taylor Still

Andrew Taylor Still, the founder of osteopathy, was born on 6 August 1828 in Lee County, Virginia. As a young man he must have seen and witnessed the impact of science in the form of mechanisation helping the farmers and the community in ways they could not have previously imagined. Agriculture at this time was developing into the basic breadwinner for the nation, but even with the leaps in mechanisation the real effect would be some years ahead. Major historical events took place before Still was born that would affect his life, notably the declaration of the United States constitution in September 1788, the Louisiana Purchase by President Jefferson for $15 million in 1804 and the prohibition by Congress of the importation of slaves in January 1808.

It is believed to be of great significance that Still's father, Abram Still, was a Methodist preacher and 'physik of the people'. He was a fire and brimstone preacher, of hell and damnation, the judgement day and a 'son of thunder'. His Methodist faith allowed him to exercise his hatred of slavery and alcohol. In 1834 the Still family moved to Newmarket, East Tennessee; this was a year after the formation of the American Anti-slavery Society. As early as the age of ten Still came across what he called 'his first discovery in the science of osteopathy'. He had a headache and for some reason thought it might help if he lowered a rope that was swung between two trees, which he had been using as a swing, to just above ground level. He lay down with the back of his head on the rope and fell asleep. When he awoke his headache was gone.

As a child he was fascinated by nature and would collect small insects and animals for his 'practical laboratory'. He took up examining animals that he had caught through hunting and shooting. Still enjoyed studying the muscles and nerves and the 'hard names' of the bones. He had no formal education, very few people did, and this 'peasant' unstructured education would have a significance to the development of osteopathy. He developed a sense of unity with the parts of natural life, a 'oneness in wholeness'. As with most of America he grew fascinated by mechanics and would describe nature as a 'natural mechanic'. In 1837 the family moved once again, this time to Bloomington, Macon County, Missouri.

Still began to show an interest in medicine, to the disgust of his father, even though he still served his apprenticeship with him. He read many medical books and served an apprenticeship as was the educational way of many physicians at the time. The law for official attendance at medical school would not come into force until the years 1870 to 1880, and even then most schools did not have written exams. In 1849 Still married Mary Margaret Vaughan while serving his apprenticeship for a medical education; obviously he used the heroic approach of medicine. Still and his father would even attend to Indians of particular note during 1853, with a combination of heroic and Indian remedies. This year marked another family move, this time to the Wakarusa Mission in Kansas. It was in 1854 that Kansas was put on the map due to the proslavery–abolitionist conflict of that year. The following year he joined the abolitionist movement, being introduced to Major J.B. Abbott, John Brown and Jim Lane. It was around the middle 1800s that Still showed the early signs of discontent with the heroic system of medicine and started to question its usefulness. A further meeting with Major Abbott, an inventor, naturalist and abolitionist from New York, may have started Still's disillusionment with heroic medicine. Abbott informed Still 'that something would come forward to take the place of allopathy and homeopathy'. In 1855 one of Still's children died in infancy. In 1859 another child died and his wife a month later. The following year he married Mary Elvira Turner, a schoolteacher.

On his return from the American Civil War it took a terrible personal loss for Still to make the biggest change and greatest contribution in health. During the spring of 1864 there was an epidemic of spinal meningitis which fatally infected three of his children. With as many as four physicians at their bedside they still died and so it was in 1864 that Still, regarding medicine as a failure, 'set out on the path to find the meaning of life and death; health and disease'. He had by this time developed a distrust for heroic medicine, alcohol and homeopathy. After this tragedy he moved to Baldwin City Missouri and began his investigations into all modes of treatment. His second wife was involved with other therapists including mesmerists, phrenologists and spiritualists. With the combination of his wife and Major Abbott he had a good introduction into the world of non-heroic therapies.

During the middle of the 1800s the industrial revolution was starting to take hold and like many others Still was impressed and took an interest in machines. His interest led to instruction in the workings and use of harvesting and milling machines. He even invented machines and improved upon already popular farming designs, but he did not patent these and many were taken up by man-ufacturing companies. It was in 1871 that he developed and made working butter churns and actually received a certificate that allowed him freedom to market the churn in 1874. The mechanical frame of mind was now well developed.

Still began to regard the body as a machine in which both structure and form were reciprocal with function. And it was his Methodist beliefs that led him to surmise that the 'first great master mechanic left nothing unfinished in the machinery of his masterpiece'.

To further his studies he exhumed the bodies of dead Indians for dissection to 're-learn his anatomy'. This went on for over a year in which he would pains-takingly chart all his findings and cover the walls of his home in anatomical drawings. During this time, the 1870s, he was advertising as a magnetic healer, probably being introduced to this therapy by his wife and Major Abbott, which brought some money into the house.

After years of study he wrote in his autobiography '[w]ho discovered osteopathy? On 22 of June at 10.00 a.m., I saw a small light in the horizon of truth. It was put into my hand, as I understood by the God of nature. God is the father of osteopathy. Osteopathy is God's Law'. Still 'unfurled the banner of osteopathy to the wind' in 1874 and enrolled as a physician and surgeon in Macon County, Missouri.

Still met a like-minded critical Scottish physician by the name of John M. Neal in that same year. When Dr Neal returned to Britain he sent Still a copy of the work of the evolutionist Herbert Spencer (1820–1903) whose work was popular in the US during the 1870s. Spencer wrote the *First Principles* in 1862, emphasising the reciprocity of structure and function and applying his evolutionary approach to all branches of knowledge, specifically biology, sociology and ethics. It was Spencer who coined the phrase *'survival of the fittest'*. As a social Darwinist he believed that there was a constant struggle between and within the species and the strongest survived while the weaker perished. Spencer's mechanistic and scientific views of small homogenous groups evolving into more complex groups as in a society was attractive to Still. The educational structure proposed and implemented by Spencer has left its mark in today's structured educational curricula.

During a walk with a friend in Macon Still saw a child who was suffering with the flux (fever and bloody diarrhoea). Still had encountered this condition many times before, not least in himself some time earlier. The child's mother had heard of Still and on examination he found the child's back to be hot and the abdomen was cold. We now know this to be a reflex autonomic vascular shift due to contraction of the intestines. Gentle manipulation relieved the child's complaint. Unfortunately his popularity was not long lived and the regular physicians managed to give Still a bad name in Macon. Due to his label as a sinner and quack he moved on to Kirksville, Missouri. By 1875 Still had began to be known as a magnetic healer and a rather eccentric quack doctor.

Between 1876 and 1877 Still suffered from typhoid and this may have been one of the reasons why by the latter end of the 1870s he did not seem to be involved in any form of therapeutic practice. After this period he began to lecture on the ethics and morals of 'Man's Lost Centre', as times were becoming very tough. His brothers and sisters did not want to know him and due to his poverty he found he had to find money selling hair oil door to door.

By 1883 he added bone setting to his magnetic healing: there survives today an old business card of his with the words 'lightening [sic] bonesetter'. This combination of bone setting, magnetic healing and anatomy led Still to form the idea that displaced joints would obstruct 'the free flow of blood' blocking circulation and leading to disease. He came to the conclusion that 'the rule of the artery is absolute, universal – it must be unobstructed or disease will result'.

Still believed that 'all diseases are mere effects, the cause being a partial or complete failure of the nerves to properly conduct the fluids of life' and propounded 'the law of the freedom of the nutrient nervous system'. He then developed osteopathy as an independent system of healing that involved surgery. Because Still was opposed to the heroic dosing of the lethal medications of the time he became known as a 'drugless practitioner'. Still did recognise certain drugs in his every day practice. In an affidavit dated 4 April 1940, Dr Charles E. Still stated 'that he personally witnessed his father, the said Andrew Taylor Still, personally perform a large number of surgical operations and administer anaesthetics and narcotics in connection therewith, all of which the said Andrew Taylor Still believed to be and expressed to be an integral part of osteopathy' (Siehl, 1984).

Still's travelling led to some degree of financial security and he established an infirmary at Kirksville in Missouri. Over the years so many patients attended the infirmary that a special train service was organised, and guesthouses for people to stay during the time of their treatment sprang up in the area. Still then developed the idea of a school, being aware that he would have to train his students to be in competition with the heroic allopathic system. This institution would require special facilities such as a large building with enough space for classes, clinical services and, he hoped, a laboratory and dissection programme (Still, 1991). On 10 May 1892, Still received a charter from the Missouri State capital granting him the right to teach the science of osteopathy. On 14 May 1892, the certificate of incorporation was filed in the office of the secretary of state. The purpose and object of the American School of Osteopathy (ASO) was:

'to improve our systems of surgery, midwifery and treatment of diseases in which the adjustment of the bones is the leading feature of this school of pathology. Also to instruct and qualify students that they may lawfully practice the science of osteopathy as taught and practiced by A.T. Still.'

Chila (1990)

Still's intention was that osteopathy was not meant to be an alternative or separate profession to allopathic medicine, but a reformation of the allopathic system of the time. The ASO was opened on 1 November 1892 with ten students, five of whom were Still's children and five were women. The first degrees were awarded in 1894 and the town committee helped raise money for a new three-storey building which was erected in 1895 and gave around 30 000 treatments a year. Here the 'rich were kept waiting while the poor were treated'.

Following the ASO, other colleges of osteopathic medicine and surgery, of various standards, began to spread across America. At one point there were as many as 37 colleges in the United States, a number of these institutions being correspondence courses or 'diploma mills'. The damage to the profession in America and in Europe caused by these poorly trained practitioners has led to a misconception of what osteopathy really is, leading the public, especially in Europe, to perceive osteopathy as a backbone therapy. This meant more people sought this kind of treatment, reinforcing their beliefs and eventually being referred more and more on the backbone basis, so filling an osteopath's practice with back-pain patients.

By 1906 Still's health began to fail; he was urged to write his autobiography, which he published in 1907. In 1914 he suffered a stroke from which he never fully recovered and he died in 1917. His last recorded words to the osteopathic profession were, 'keep it pure, boys, keep it pure'.

How osteopathy got its name

The following is taken from Booth's *History of Osteopathy: Twentieth-Century Medical Practice* (1924).

'Many criticisms have been offered as to the appropriateness of the term osteopathy to designate a system of medical practice, in its broad sense. No one word has been found that would more aptly express the ideas involved in the principles and practices of the science. The term was never used in the sense of a diseased bone, neither was it employed to indicate a bone-setting treatment.

The following explanation of the origin of the name osteopathy is given by Dr. Still in the catalogue of the American School of Osteopathy for 1902–3:

"I had worked and tried to reason that a body that was perfectly normal in structure could keep a man in the full enjoyment of health just as long as the body was perfectly normal. On that conclusion I worked, first, to know what was normal in form and what was not normal; then I compared the two in disease and health. I found by hard study and experimenting that no human body was normal in bone form whilst harboring any disease, either acute or chronic. I got good results in adjusting these bodies to such a degree that people began to ask what I was going to call my new science.

I listened to all who thought I ought to name my science, so I began to think over names, such as allopathy, hydropathy, homeopathy, and other names, and as I was in Kansas when the name Osawatomie was coined, by taking the first part of the word Osage, and the last part of Pattawattamie, and the new word coined represented two tribes of Indians, I concluded I would start out with the word os (bone) and the word pathology, and press them into one word – osteopathy.

I wanted to call my science osteopathy, and I did not care what Greek scholars said about it." '

The Flexner report

No single person accelerated changes in the system of American medicine more than Abraham Flexner, even though changes were already taking place albeit slowly (Banta, 1971). In 1910 he had published the *Flexner Report* for restructuring the basic curriculum of medical training. Flexner was born in 1866 to a German–Jewish family in Louisville, Kentucky. By the age of 17 he was sent to college at Johns Hopkins where he stayed for two years earning a Bachelor's degree in medicine. In 1886 Flexner returned to Louisville and by 1890, aged 23, he had opened his own private school. The educational standard was high enough for him to be able to send his brother Jacob to Johns Hopkins. By 1906 he had spent a year at Harvard and was about to spend the next two years in Germany. This is significant, as it brought the influence of German medicine to bear on the future of American medicine. The custom at the time was to travel to Germany for post-graduate education. On returning he was invited to assess the standard of medical education in the United States for the Carnegie Foundation. Flexner initially thought they must have confused him with his brother Simon, a physician. With his knowledge and a model of the Johns Hopkins system he began visiting schools from 1909. Schools cooperated willingly, knowing that he was from the Carnegie Foundation, possibly hoping some money was on the way. His major finding was that the 'schools' were small affairs, where only a small number of students could actually write, let alone read. After the publication of the report in 1910, Flexner went on to work in Europe, especially in Great Britain.

Due to the Flexner investigation the comparative educational curricula of medicine and osteopathy were published (see Table 1.1). In Booth's *History of Osteopathy: Twentieth-Century Medical Practice* (1924) the average hours in each subject and the average totals in medical and osteopathic educational programmes were compared. These were from the medical schools of Johns Hopkins, University of Pennsylvania, Cornell, Harvard University, University of California and the University of Illinois. The osteopathic schools were the American School of Osteopathy, Chicago College, Des Moines Still College, Massachusetts College and the Philadelphia College.

Mark Twain's support for osteopathy

Around about 1900 Mark Twain wrote in his *Notebook*: 'To ask a doctor's opinion of osteopathy is equivalent to going to Satan for information about Christianity.'

Twain developed an interest in osteopathy after coming into contact with it in his hometown of Hannibal, Missouri. Dr Still had an office in Hannibal for some months late in 1889 before setting up the American School of Osteopathy. In mid-1899 the Twain family took a trip to Europe. A little while before they left, Twain's second daughter, Jean Clemens, developed epilepsy. While in London a friend urged Twain to seek the help of a Dr Henrik Kellgren in Sweden. They continued on to Sweden, finally ending in Senna where Jean had treatment

Table 1.1 Comparative medical and osteopathic curricula.

Fundamental sciences	Medical	Osteopathic
Histology	171	188
Anatomy	489	696
Physiology	329	279
Embryology	72	52
Chemistry	284	288
Pathology	405	342
Bacteriology	157	154
Diagnosis	146	201
Hygiene	66	119
Gynaecology	131	135
Genito-urinary	42	48
Surgery	549	489
Obstetrics	196	172
Jurisprudence	13	25
Eye, Ear, Nose & Throat	187	154
Paediatrics	123	60
Dermatology	41	50
Orthopaedics	71	62
Psychiatry	160	155
Symptomatology	531	653
TOTAL	4163	4322

between July and October in 1899. The treatments were beneficial and on their return to London they continued treatment at a branch of the Kellgren system.

On his return to America Twain was wintering in New York and his enthusiasm for osteopathy was growing. In 1901 he appeared before the Assembly Committee, New York, supporting the Seymour bill for the legalisation of osteopathy. He went on to say:

'[I] was born in the Banner State, and by "Banner State" I mean Missouri. Osteopathy was born in the same State, and both of us are getting along reasonably well. At a time during my younger days my attention was attracted to a picture which bore the inscription "Christ Disputing with the Doctors". I could attach no other meaning to it than that Christ was actually quarrelling with the doctors. So I asked an old slave, who was a sort of herb doctor in a small way – unlicensed, of course – what the meaning of the picture was. "What has he done?" I asked. And the coloured man replied: "Humph, he ain't got no license."'

(Cited in Brashear, 1973.)

The beginnings of osteopathy in Britain

John Martin Littlejohn was born on 15 February 1865 in Glasgow. At the age of 18, in 1881, he attended Glasgow University to study arts, Hebrew and oriental languages, necessary for a career in the church. In 1885 he moved to Ireland to study theology in Belfast and was ordained in 1886. On returning to Glasgow University, in 1889, he received an MA in classical languages and in 1892 he studied law leading to a first class degree in legal science. He also received the William Hunter Gold Medal in Forensic Medicine.

Due to health problems in his neck and throat, he was advised to move to somewhere warmer. At 27 years of age, in 1892, he moved to New York, enrolling at Columbia University for a PhD, which he finished in one year after special permission from the University. In 1893 he was ill again and spent time in Philadelphia and Wisconsin; while recovering he took up a research programme in psychology in Chicago, becoming a Research Fellow of the National University. Due to his outstanding work he secured a post as President of Amity College, College Springs, Iowa, in 1894, making him, at 29, one of the youngest college presidents in the US.

With his health giving him problems once again he was forced to resign his post at Amity College in 1898. It was then that he heard of Dr Andrew Taylor Still in Kirksville. To improve the chances of recovery he moved to Kirksville and was so impressed with the treatment that he decided to stay and study osteopathic medicine at the American School of Osteopathy.

In July 1898, Littlejohn travelled to London to address the Society of Science, Letters and the Arts on 'Osteopathy in Line of Apostolic Succession to Medicine'. The following year saw the publication of one of his most important books, *Psycho-physiology*, the first book on the lectures given in the previous years at the ASO on osteopathic psychology. In the early part of 1900 he moved to Chicago with his brothers and formed the American (Chicago) College of Osteopathic Medicine and Surgery and the Chicago Osteopathic Hospital.

In 1913 Littlejohn returned to England and lived at Badger Hall, Thundersley, Essex. This was the beginning of his contribution to osteopathy in the UK. From here he opened clinics in Thundersley, Enfield and London (at 69, Piccadilly, W1). On 7 March 1917 he founded the British School of Osteopathy, London with Francis Joseph Horn. It was not until 1921 that the curriculum for a four-year course had been completed which excluded surgery and the materia medica. By 1925 Littlejohn had become the President of the British Osteopathic Association.

During the Second World War, Littlejohn kept the school open but it was little more than a clinic. His health over the years began to slowly deteriorate and his day-to-day involvement with the school became less and less. John Martin Littlejohn died at Badger Hall on 8 December 1947.

The British osteopathic schools and colleges

The British School of Osteopathy (BSO)

Founded in 1917 by John Martin Littlejohn and Francis Joseph Horn, it could be said that it began in various locations, in Thundersley and Enfield, but officially it was in consultancy rooms at 48 Dover Street, W1. With more students a bigger site was needed; this was found in Vincent Square and here the first graduates qualified in 1925. In 1927 the school moved to Abbey House, Victoria Street, Westminster. In 1930 the school moved again, this time to 16 Buckingham Gate, SW1, where the school stayed until 1980 when it moved to Suffolk Street SW1. The school's final move in the twentieth century was in July 1997 to Borough High Street, London, south of the river Thames.

The British College of Naturopathy and Osteopathy (BCNO)

The college was originally the British College of Naturopathy (BCN) and was founded by the British Naturopathic Association. In 1961 the BCN became the BCNO founded by Stanley Lief. In the past the BSO was against graduates of the BCNO being allowed on the General Council and Register of Osteopaths. As a consequence the BCNO formed their own register but they were accepted by the General Council in 1987.

The European School of Osteopathy (ESO)

The ESO and the John Wernham College of Classical Osteopathy began with the Institute of Applied Technique and Maidstone Osteopathic Clinic founded by John Wernham and T. Edward Hall in 1951. At the same time, in Paris, there was the École Française d'Osteopathie (EFO) where Tom Dummer (a BCNO graduate) joined the École Française in 1957. The school was forced to close because it was illegal for anyone except a medical practitioner to treat by means of manipulation of the spine and the then principal, Paul Geny, was sent to prison.

After his release Geny and 16 students were allowed to use the BCNO for a while with Tom Dummer in 1965. They stayed until 1968 when they moved to Maidstone, Kent as the Maidstone Osteopathic Clinic. As the EFO the school began to accept British students and run a four-year full time course; this eventually became the European School of Osteopathy. In 1979 the ESO moved to new premises, again in Maidstone and in 1983 graduates were allowed to apply for membership of the GCRO. In 1996 the school was named the John Wernham College of Classical Osteopathy and affiliated with the North East Surrey College of Technology awarding a BSc (Hons) in Osteopathic Medicine.

The London College of Osteopathic Medicine (LCOM)

The original BOA wanted a school based on the later American model of osteopathy. A clinic was opened in Vincent Square in 1927 and George Bernard

Shaw performed the official opening. In 1931 the school moved to Andrew Still House, 24–5 Dorset Square, NW1. After a number of years the realisation dawned that trying to pursue an American osteopathic curriculum in the UK was not possible. Eventually the course became an avenue for qualified British physicians to supplement their medical training with an osteopathic education.

George Bernard Shaw's support for osteopathy

The following is from the *Osteopathic Magazine*, 1927, at the opening of the London College of Osteopathic Medicine, by George Bernard Shaw.

'Feeling versus Cutting
You are going to form an Osteopathic Association. Well, there should be no such necessity. Your General Medical Council has no right to register any man as qualified, unless he has mastered the osteopathic technique; no practitioner should be hallmarked as competent unless he knows it. Some of them pretend to know it, and to know it in a proper scientific way, not like those American amateurs. They call themselves orthopedic surgeons. One of them was courteous enough to explain his position to me. He said in effect, "Suppose you have a diseased knee joint, what is the scientific way of dealing with it? Not feeling about with your fingers to find out what is wrong, like Barker and the osteopaths; the proper thing to do is to cut into the knee and see what is wrong with it." Now from the point of view of the gentleman who cuts into the knee there is no doubt a great deal to be said for this; but I, were I the possessor of that unfortunate knee, should regard cutting into it as the very last resort of helpless ignorance. I should certainly first consult a man who had learned to use his fingers a little, and whose motto was not "Seeing is believing" but "Feeling is believing". I am unscientific enough not to want my knee cut into if I can help it; and therefore I begin by consulting an osteopath. Supposing I try half-a-dozen osteopaths, and they cannot tell me what is wrong with my knee by feeling it, my knee is no worse; but if I go to a gentleman who breaks my knee open to see what is inside it, I shall be lame for months, and possibly for life. Besides, it hurts too much.'

The British Register of Osteopaths

The two chief functions of the Register of Osteopaths were:

- To regulate the standard of qualification and professional conduct, and
- To protect the public by supplying them with the names of those who are so qualified both from a technical and professional point of view.

These have also been summed up rather neatly by Miller (1949) who, differentiating between the Register of Osteopaths and the Osteopathic Association of Great Britain stated 'the purpose of the Register is to protect the public from the osteopath; the purpose of the Association is to protect the osteopath from the public.'

Nazi Germany

The following is an extract from the *Journal of Osteopathy*, September 1936, titled 'Official Report of the First Olympic Osteopathic Committee'.

'Under the auspices of the International Congress of Medical Advisors for Athletics, supported by the German Government and the University of Berlin, with Dr Emil Ketterer, leader of the guild of German sports doctors, and Dr Mallwitz, president of the organisation committee, the demonstrations of the Olympic Osteopathic Committee took place as scheduled on the morning of July 31, 1936, at the Institute of Sport therapy at Eichkamp.

Here the German trainers were treated and then our [Dr W. J. Douglas, Chairman of the Osteopathic Committee, Paris and Dr Clarence L. Johnson, Liverpool, one of the physicians in charge of the British Olympic Teams] services were enlisted for the contestants with much success. Several men beat their former records and attributed this to osteopathic treatment. The article following hereafter appeared in the German press. This is particularly interesting because the trend of physical medicine in Germany today is increasing due to some extent to the interest of Rudolf Hess, Minister of State, to create more cooperation between physical therapeutics and general medicine.

Berliner Tageblatt 1, August 1936: Friday morning there was a visit by the Olympic Osteopathic Committee, a group of American and English osteopaths, to the Sports Therapy Institute at Eichkamp in which through medical manipulative therapy and orthopaedic measures it was proven that sports lesions can be healed.

Morgenpost, 1 August 1936: Osteopathy aims to keep health in an ill body which is still NOT ill, and help to move those forces which work against illness. The osteopaths want to show with their method that every illness simultaneously requires some sort of change to the spine. If you correct the spine of the chest region you can help asthma and heart illness and stomach and bowel disease.'

A similar article on the same day appeared in the *Frankfurter Zeitung*.

The Osteopathic oath

'I do hereby affirm my loyalty to the profession I am about to enter. I will be mindful always of my great responsibility to preserve the health and the life of my patients, to retain their confidence and respect both as a physician and a friend who will guard their secrets with scrupulous honour and fidelity, to perform faithfully my professional duties, to employ only those recognised methods of treatment consistent with good judgement and with my skill and ability, keeping in mind always nature's laws and the body's inherent capacity for recovery.

I will be ever vigilant in aiding in the general welfare of the community, sustaining its laws and institutions, not engaging in those practices which will in any way bring shame or discredit upon myself or my profession. I will give no drugs for deadly purposes to any person, though it be asked of me.

I will endeavour to work in accord with my colleagues in a spirit of progressive cooperation, and never by word or by act cast imputations upon them or their rightful practices.

I will look with respect and esteem upon all those who have taught me my art. To my college I will be loyal and strive always for its best interests and for the interests of the students who will come after me. I will be ever alert to further the application of basic biologic truths to the healing arts and to develop the principles of osteopathy which were first enunciated by Andrew Taylor Still.'

Last but by no means least

'Disciples of Hoffman, Boerhaave, Stahl, Cullen, and Brown, succeed each other like the shifting figures of the magic lantern; and their fancies, like the dresses of the annual doll-babies from Paris, becoming, from their novelty, the vogue of the day and yielding to the next novelty their ephemeral favours.

I believe we can safely affirm that the inexperienced and presumptuous herd of medical tyros let loose upon the world destroys more lives than all the Robin Hoods, Cartouches, and Macheaths do in a century.

I hope and believe that it is from this side of the Atlantic that Europe, which has taught us so many useful things, will be led into sound principles in this branch of science [osteopathy], the most important of all, to which we commit the care of health and disease.'

Thomas Jefferson, author of the *American Declaration of Independence*.

References

Adams, W.P. (1999) The German Americans: An Ethnic Experience. *German American Corner: German-Americans: An Ethnic Experience,*
http://www.germanheritage.com/Publications/adams/index.html

Banta, D.H. (1971) Medical education. Abraham Flexner – a reappraisal. *Society Science and Medicine,* 5, 655–61.

Booth, E.R. (1924) *History of Osteopathy and Twentieth-Century Medical Practice*. Caxton Press, Cincinnati, Ohio.

Brashear, M.M. (1973) Dr Still and Mark Twain. Special article. *The Journal of the American Osteopathic Association*, September 73, 67–71.

Chila, A.G. (1990) Andrew Taylor Still Memorial Address: The Beginning of Osteopathic Medicine, *The DO*, October 68–79.

Kamphoefner, W.D. (1987) *The Westfalians: From Germany to Missouri*. Princeton University Press, Princeton, NJ.

Miller, R.F. (1949) The functions of the register. *The Osteopathic Quarterly*, January 2 No. 1.

Sartin, J.S. (1993) Infectious Diseases During the Civil War: The Triumph of the 'Third Army'. *Clinical Infectious Disease*, 16, 580–4.

Siehl, D. (1984) Andrew Taylor Still Memorial Lecture: The osteopathic difference – is it only manipulation? *Journal of the American Osteopathic Association*, 83(5) 47–51.

Still, C.E. Jr. (1991) *Frontier Doctor Medical Pioneer. The Life and Times of A.T. Still and his Family*. Thomas Jefferson University Press, Northeast Missouri State University, Kirksville, MI.

Further reading

Desmond, A. (1992) *The Politics of Evolution*. The University of Chicago Press, Chicago and London.

Gay, P. (1992) *Weimar Culture: The Outsider as Insider*. Penguin Books, London.

Hampson, N. (1990) *The Enlightenment: An Evaluation of its Assumptions, Attitudes and Values*. Penguin Books, London.

Marwick, A. (1989) *The Nature of History*. Macmillan, London.

Vico, G. (1999) *New Science*. Penguin Classics, London.

Williams, J.R. (1998) *The Life of Goethe*. Blackwell Publications, Oxford.

CHAPTER 2

Philosophy

'The osteopath finds here the field in which he can dwell forever. His duties as a philosopher admonish him, that life and matter can be united, and that union cannot continue with any hindrance to the free and absolute motion.'

A.T. Still

'Osteopathy is a philosophy.'

A. T. Still

Osteopathic medicine lies firmly within its philosophy or mode of consciousness. Modern physicists from Planck to Bortoft are indirectly proving that the osteopathic scientific paradigm is as sound as the analytical modern scientific paradigm. The two paradigms complement each other but they have to be recognised in their greater modes as distinct and not as different models within the same paradigm. Only when the osteopathic scientific paradigm is recognised can the original works of Still and his co-workers come to life in the form of osteopathy. Any judgement of osteopathic medicine before understanding its philosophy will be seen as interference, non-sense and poor science. Osteopathic medicine has been viewed as poor science because physiologists, anatomists and medical practitioners have used a mechanistic and cogwheel manner for their interpretation; this is still the case today. Life processes operate in patterns not abstractions (Hanson, 1958). Still spoke again and again of osteopathy being a combination of the three Ms, *mind, matter* and *motion*. He was nearly 150 years ahead of his time. Recently the late David Bohm proposed the concept that what we do is a combination of these three Ms in his works *Wholeness and the Implicate Order* and *Thought as a System* (1994). In addition osteopathy does not remove the practitioner from the phenomenon of the three Ms, adhering to Kuhn's (1996) approach in *The Structure of Scientific Revolutions* and Hacking's *Scientific Revolutions* (1981) in being extra-scientific and ultimately seemingly unstructured in its application. Historically the philosophy and psychology of America was introduced from Europe, particularly Germany, by Emerson and Coleridge (Littlejohn, 1899). The greatest input to American culture and society originated from the men and women of the 1848 emigration from Germany. The '48ers' were the heirs of the liberal tradition of Kant, Fichte, Schiller and others, who provided the German contribution to culture in America (Tolzmann, 1997). Friederich von Schiller in particular was the intellectual partner and good friend of Johann Wolfgang von Goethe. This German–American cultural dominance could be considered one of the main reasons why American medicine sought German know-how in developing a scientific system of health care and treatment at the end of the nineteenth century. It should be remembered that Still wanted to reform the practice of medicine, there was no indication of an alternative to the then system of practice.

Still tells us to 'find it, fix it and leave it alone' affirming his understanding of the body as an internally organising system. This organisational approach forms the essence of osteopathic philosophy. Any other approach breaks up the total mind set. Osteopathy directs natural proceedings trying not to 'do it' for the body. Bertrand Russell (cited in McConnell, 1938) reminds us that 'physical organisation is the physiological activeness, of function. A physical system expresses its energy in terms of function; for "energy is a certain function of the system, but it is not *a thing* [my italics] or substance persisting throughout the changes of the system".' And, as we shall see, of even greater significance is the beginning of the philosophy of *'oneness'* in Still's autobiography. McConnell (1938) writes that,

'in the light of the "oneness", the "organisation", of all parts of the body, wherein anatomy is inclusive of chemism, symptomatology, and pathology, as Dr. Still so emphatically states, and in the light of the facts that the organism is *in* nature, and the "specifiable things *as* links functionally significant in a process" show the intimate "interdependence of all organic structures and processes with one another," it is highly important to apply a structurally specific technique.'

Osteopathy is a science that is primarily concerned with the *Lebenswelt*, life-world.

The paradigm shift

'Galileo Galilei discovered the rotation of the Earth about the Sun, to the great agitation of the scientific and religious worlds. The Pope threatened the discoverer with excommunication. Bishops and other high dignitaries of Church laid heavy charges against him, and arraigned him before the courts. Finally he was made to retract and forswear by his colleagues. "Whatever you say, it still rotates!" were supposed to have been his last words before he died.'

Viktor Schauberger

Korr (1997) called for a paradigm shift to save osteopathic medicine. He went on as follows.

'Conventional clinical research protocols for the assessment of efficacy of most chemical and physical therapeutic agents are ill-suited for the assessment of osteopathic medical care, of manipulative treatment in particular. It is emphasised that osteopathic medical care must be evaluated as it is practised and not as a contrived, unreal version; and that it must be tested as a derivative of, and in the context of, that philosophy by criteria consonant with that philosophy.'

A paradigm is a belief structure that allows you to live with a view of your world, a *Weltanschauung*.. Any paradigm develops over time and becomes extremely comfortable, especially in our thoughts. This develops into a system of belief and at worst becomes a conviction. Our analytical paradigm has been practised but it is only one way of seeing, and it causes feelings of discomfort within individuals and societies if a new paradigm, let alone a new model, is experienced. Both Bohm (1994) and Still in his autobiography emphasised the difference between thoughts and thinking. Thoughts are the conditioning within us and thinking is the active process of awareness and relation to external objects and desires. Thinking can only take place on the basis of our conditioning or thought. Therefore we have no freethinking process. Any thinking that requires us to go against the grain of our thoughts makes us extremely uncomfortable.

William Kingdon Clifford, in *The Ethics of Belief* (1886), highlighted some of the following aspects on belief.

- Held beliefs cumulate and form an aggregate of beliefs forming a link between sensations (feelings) and action in every moment of our lives.
- Our cumulations of beliefs are so organised and compacted together that no part can be isolated from the rest.
- Every new belief is a new addition to held beliefs and modifies the structure of the whole.
- Any belief, no matter how small should never be taken as a minor issue, it sets us up to receive more like it, confirming those we already have and weakening others.
- Our words, our phrases, our forms and processes and modes of thought, are common property, designed by time, from generation to generation, to be handed on to the next generation, never changed but enlarged and purified.

Models and Paradigms (see Table 2.1)

Table 2.1 A comparison of models and paradigms.

Models	Paradigms
Designed to be tested (scientifically), or cannot be tested/disproved (metaphysical)	Assumed but not tested. (May become testable if the context is enlarged, or may be metaphysical.)
Models are constructed for usefulness, and many alternatives may be used by the same person for different applications.	Models are constructed within a paradigm's 'landscape' and use a similar symbol structure.
Although a model may become commonly used, it can easily be replaced with 'improvements'.	When a paradigm becomes 'subconscious' it begins to define the 'reality' of personal experience.
We are often very pleased to see new innovations, and celebrate the prospects of new model improvements with pleasure.	Without a paradigm, it becomes very difficult to interpret 'reality'. In fact, we may become blind to many of our observations when they do not fit our expectations.
If we *cannot* make a change to an entirely new and improved model, we are resentful and protest loudly and in extreme cases violently.	If we must change a paradigm that has defined our personal 'reality' it is very difficult, and causes high anxiety, confusion, and depression.
A certain model may become a strongly cherished symbol, and may be retained with nostalgia, but will not be confused with oneself.	One may fight for a paradigm, even give one's life for it if the interpretation of reality is dear, and defines one's self and self-value.
Use of models creates a jargon, which is intended to have clear definitions that can be used to explain and compare the terms.	A language may be built upon a certain paradigm (worldview), and make it difficult to communicate when the worldview is changed.
A model may reflect a skill, but not an awareness.	A paradigm may be associated with a 'consciousness' level.
Models may change, but they remain within the same paradigm.	Paradigms may become models, but a redefinition of the scale, scope, universe usually is required.
Difficult problems highlight the needed changes in the models. Businesses function within a common paradigm. New models are 'marketable'.	Many 'insoluble problems' have no solution until the paradigm is changed. It has been said, 'few real problems can be solved from which they arose'. The discussion of 'sustainability' has no solution within our prevailing paradigm.

Adapted from Guba (1990)

Hansonian interpretation

'We are prone to see what lies behind our eyes, rather than what appears before them.'

Thomas Huxley

In his work *Patterns of Discovery* (1958), Hanson demonstrated how 'the theory, hypothesis, or background knowledge held by an observer can influence in a major way what is observed' and that 'there is more to seeing than meets the eyeball'. This is a major problem with our interpretation when reading early texts on osteopathic medicine. Hanson experimented by making slides of playing cards from a normal deck. He then projected them onto a screen, for short periods, in front of an audience. Obviously the observers correctly recorded a number of the cards, the exception was a card that had the colour of its suit changed. This demonstrated a process of interaction between what is brought to the eyeball by light and what is actually interpreted by the observer. All senses behave in the same way. This meaning placed into what we see or experience (McNamara and Miller, 1989) is best seen in the present scientific model. We are led to believe that this is the only paradigm or way of 'seeing.' Max Planck (1949), the quantum physicist, reminded us that

> 'the best start toward a correct understanding of the scientific world picture will be to investigate the most primitive picture, the naïve world picture of the child. The more the child matures, and the more complete his world picture becomes, the less frequently he finds to wonder. And when he has grown up, and his world picture has solidified and taken on a certain form, he accepts this picture as a matter of course and ceases to wonder. Is this because the adult has fully fathomed the correlations and the necessity of the structure of his world? Nothing could be more erroneous than this idea. No! The reason why the adult no longer wonders is not because he has solved the riddle of life, but because he has grown accustomed to the laws governing his world picture.'

Science

'Old-time progressive politics rested on a long-term faith that science is the proven road to human health and welfare, and this faith shaped the techno-logical agenda for half-a-dozen World Fairs. This dream still carries conviction for many people today: what underlies their continued trust in science and industry is their commitment to the conception of 'rationality' that was established among European natural philosophers in the seventeenth century, and promised intellectual certainty and harmony. The widely scientific bles-sings of our age (above all, those in medicine) were not widely available before the late nineteenth century, but these blessings were happy outcomes of scientific inquiries that have made continuous progress ever since Galileo and Descartes, and so were the long-term products of the seventeenth century revolutions undertaken in physics by Galileo, Kepler, and Newton, and in philosophy by Descartes, Locke, and Leibniz.'

Stephen Toulmin, *Cosmopolis: The Hidden Agenda of Modernity*

The exposition of science is always an instruction for testing the totality of laws as they stand at that moment. It could therefore be put on a tape that would direct a testing machine. This is because the exposition displays the state of science at that moment as a complete and closed system, wholly contained in (that is, deducible from) its axioms and laws. The man who has to act now on present scientific knowledge has to accept that as an instruction, as a machine does. This is the nature of science as a mode of knowledge. It must be testable in action; so that, however it was discovered and however it will be corrected, at any moment it must be formally fixed as a system of instructions. But the thinker and experimenter does not have to accept the present state as closed, and its exposition as complete. He is free to work in the thinking language, and to explore its ambiguities to his mind's content (Bronowski, 1965). This standpoint is represented in extreme form by the modern theory of science, which strives to separate theory from fact. What remains unclear is the extent to which the so-called facts already harbour theories. This severing of theory from fact results in its losing the ground of reality beneath its feet: any assertion can be a theory, so long as it is interpreted in retrospect by means of experimental data (Hensel, 1998). Modern science binds the hands of osteopathic medicine. It externalises and abstracts what is essentially an experience, distorting, but not destroying, the possibilities by disempowerment of both osteopathic practitioner and patient. Experiments have to be verified and experience is not important: experiment and experience have their origins from the Latin *experiens*, meaning to try thoroughly. It is significant that the verb to experiment is now intransitive: one must experiment on something, thus distancing oneself from it, whereas the word 'experience' is direct; one experiences something at first hand. The stem *experiri* (Latin: to try) is related to the word peril, or trial to be passed through at some personal risk. Both experiment and experience may be dangerous (Lorimer, 1997). We have not even tried to develop, or try thoroughly, our experiences. Bronowski (1965) states:

'their theories [philosophers] are still dominated by their belief that science is an accumulation of facts, and that a generalisation grows of itself from heaping of single instances in one narrow field. They think that a scientist is persuaded that light arrives at the eye in a shower of quanta because he does an experiment, does it again, and repeats it to be sure. The classical error is to regard a scientific law as only shorthand for its instance. If we think like this, then naturally we can argue only among instances: "I have seen the sun rise every morning of my life, so I expect it to rise as long as I live." This is a fair expectation by habit, but it is not an induction; I might as well conclude "So I expect to live as long as it rises." An induction is not a guess at the next instance, and the next, and the next, but at the law which rules and, more deeply, which explains their occurrence. An induction in science is a generalisation which tries to thread its way through our experience and to guess what law has governed that. We are no more certain of the law in the past than in the future, for no law that we discover is certain and final.'

Historically we do not like uncertainty and the habits of certainty hunting have conditioned us to accept little that is not 'solid', in all its forms, as real science.

Stephen Toulmin, in *Cosmopolis: The Hidden Agenda of Modernity* (cited in Bortoft, 1997), reminds us that

'our modern scientific style of thinking has its roots within the successful history of mathematics and physics moving towards the already mentioned Cartesian–Newtonian model. Mathematical physics filled a cultural vacuum during a period of extreme scepticism following the Thirty Years War; the fight between Protestantism and Catholicism. People no longer knew what to believe and had come to the conclusion that knowledge and certainty were impossible. Descartes and others thought that this vacuum could be filled by mathematics. They had no idea that a mathematical approach would enable them to reach certainty. That was the cultural mission of mathematical physics.'

The predominant philosophy of the sixteenth century was humanistic, practical, sceptical, oral, and open to dialogue. Humanists were content to live in an open way where differences in opinion were tolerated and debated. Tensions in seventeenth century Europe degenerated into what is known as the Thirty Years War (1618–48) after the assassination of Henri IV of France in 1610. Henri was keeping the Protestants and Catholics at arm's length from each other in a very delicate balance, brokered by Michel de Montaigne. Once Henri was dead the news flooded across Europe and the wheels of instability began to turn. How important and respected was Henri IV? Toulmin compares the affection shown to Henri as similar to that shown to John F. Kennedy. In fact the assassination showed striking similarities.

The Jesuits claimed Henri's heart for a ceremony in his honour. At that ceremony was a young intellectual by the name of René Descartes. Every year since 1610 a memorial service in Henri's honour has been held and poems and essays submitted. It was one of these essays that first indicated the writings and thoughts of Descartes. It was a strange essay that showed his interest in the work of Galileo. As this terrible war continued people realised that if it was to stop there had to be some certainty in their lives. As the years went by the philosophical works of Descartes presented a counter to the uncertainty of the humanists and the religious conflict. By his method of 'theory-centring' and dehumanising he led philosophy into a dead end search for rationalisation. Expanding on the work of his hero Galileo he produced a series of certainties in a 'natural philosophy'. The quest for certainty was to present commonalties of the heavens and the earth in mathematical or quasigeometric form as a code of nature, to be decoded. This he hoped would damp the religious disputes. This quest was for religious stabilisation and faith.

The quest for certainty became more appealing and the chaos of the war diminished.

'In closing the *Principles of Philosophy*, for instance, Descartes refuses to claim logical or metaphysical certainty for his account of nature. He cannot formally prove that his system of natural philosophy is the one and only theory free of contradiction or inconsistency. We are to think of it, rather, as one tentative way of deciphering natural phenomena, and, as such, it has only a *moral* certainty.'

(Toulmin, 1990)

Mathematics or geometry is a series of 'certainties'.

Rightly or wrongly we are still looking for certainty. In our scientific quest we have specialised, abstracted and externalised. By this process we make the error of mistaking our manipulation of matter as an understanding of nature (Bortoft, 1999). As we shall see, this is not the only way to understand our world scientifically.

Still's science of osteopathy aspires as an organic way of seeing health and disease. It is this generally organic scientific mode of consciousness that needs to be investigated complementing the unifying principle and analytical practice of osteopathy. This has to begin if we are to understand the potential of osteopathic medicine. In its 'organicness' osteopathy is primarily ecological whereas allopathic medicine based on the Cartesian–Newtonian linear causation model is primarily aetiological. Keesecker (1955) wrote

'it is simpler to characterise the aetiological approach to the problems of health and disease than to describe the ecological viewpoint. The aetiological orientation is fixed and may be stated in a relatively simple way: What does the patient have, and what shall I give him? The ecological orientation is one demanding a medical philosophy. Its view is comprehensive, moving from the general to the specific.'

Modes of consciousness

'Why has not man a microscopic eye? For this plain reason – *man is not a fly.*'
Alexander Pope (1688–1744)

It is generally agreed that there are two extreme modes of consciousness, organic/holistic and analytical. Everyday, from minute to minute, we move between the two states of complementary consciousness, nobody is the same. In the organic mode we *belong* together with our environment, in the analytical mode we place physical things we think belong *together* within the environment (Bortoft, 1996).

In our earliest days we begin to externalise, i.e. relate to solid bodies: I am here, it is there. By using this process of one then another, distinction and separation, we have developed a sense of linear causation and logical thinking. We have practised this analytical mode of consciousness to the point that we no longer comfortably think about any other way of 'seeing'. Naturally this is related to language and its structure; especially the noun as the object. As Bortoft (1996) and others have discovered, 'it is this analytical structure of language which has made it inadequate for describing the domains which have been discovered in modern physics'. This difficulty in finding a language for describing observations in modern physics has also been inadequate in the observation of the phenomena in nature. Metaphysical or mathematical, mechanical or moral language, in each case one comes up against the limitations intrinsic to a particular way of relating to Nature. Goethe emphasised the senses in the understanding of our world. This would develop our way of thinking in a more 'real' form. Subjective experience is seen as too 'soft' for scientific attention. Only that which can be objectively demonstrated, quantified, and replicated is admissible to its realm (Korr, 1997). Bohm (1994) is insistent.

'Thought has produced tremendous effects outwardly. Yet the general tacit assumption in thought is that it's just telling you the way things are and that is not doing anything – that "you" are inside there, deciding what to do with the information. But I want to say that you don't decide what to do with the information. The information takes over. It runs you. Thought runs you. Thought, however, gives the false information that you are running it, that you are the one who controls thought, whereas actually thought is the one which controls each one of us. Until thought is understood – yet better, more than understood, *perceived* [my italics] – it will actually control us; but it will create the impression that it is our servant, that it is just doing what we want it to do.'

Bohm brings to the forefront the Goethean concept that it is not just what we see, it is primarily the meaning we have already placed into the phenomenon we are witnessing. Goodwin (1994) introduces Goethe's style of science as follows.

'Goethe himself ranked his scientific work significantly above his literary achievements, which themselves have given him the status of a creative genius of the first rank. So what are we to make of his science, which currently tends to occupy the fringes of conventional research, its originality keeping it maginalised? This is because Goethe believed in a science of wholes: the whole plant organism, or the whole circle of colours in his theory of colour. But he also believed that these wholes are intrinsically dynamic, undergoing transformation but in accordance with these laws or principles, not arbitrarily. So he was an *organocentric* [my italics] biologist, and a dynamic one to boot! It is only now that we can begin to recognise his insights, which involve an aesthetic appreciation of form and quality quite as much as dynamic regularity.'

The true organic/holistic mode of consciousness is non-external and non-verbal allowing the observer to become part of the experience witnessed. Any intellectualisation or cerebral interaction loses the experience and becomes analytical. You have a total and absolute relationship to your surroundings where no elements can be considered. There are no snapshots of time, spatial awareness or static appreciation. So far we have looked at what holistic consciousness isn't; we shall now look at some of its elements.

Holistic consciousness

'The reason why the adult no longer wonders (as does a child) is not because he has solved the riddle of life, but because he has grown accustomed to the laws governing his world picture ... he who has reached the stage where he no longer wonders about anything, merely demonstrates that he has lost the art of reflective reasoning.'

Max Planck

Goethe was remembered for his poetry and plays, especially *Faust*. Unfortunately he was also credited as one of the founders of Romanticism; he said, 'Romanticism is a sickness'. Like Newton he was interested in alchemy; unlike Newton this was not most of his work (White, 1997). As Newton's physics is beginning to collapse, Goethean science is beginning to be recognised, particularly within the field of quantum physics. Goethe's *Theory of Colour* is only now beginning to aid quantum physicists with a way of 'seeing'. For us to 'see' nature Goethe demanded an inner flexibility without inhibition in one mode of consciousness. He was aware that there were different ways of seeing and insisted that we do not restrict our observations to one particular mode. All are valid, since we form the constructs of our own awareness, but no single way should dominate. The wider the range of observation the greater our potential for understanding. Importance rests on the realisation that there is no 'right' way to observe Nature. The following is an extract from Goethe, written in the 1790s, and published posthumously in the Weimar edition of his works (cited in Naydler, 1996):

'...no one asks a question of Nature that they cannot themselves answer, for the answer is inherent in the question, in the feeling that the point can be discussed and pondered. To be sure, the questions vary according to the different types of humans. To orient ourselves somewhat among these various types, let us divide them thus into four spheres: utilisers, fact-finders, contemplators, and comprehenders.

(1) The utilisers, advocates and seekers of things practical, are the first to plough the field of science, metaphorically speaking, and they aim at practical results. Self-confidence derived from experience gives them assurance; necessity gives them a certain breadth.

(2) Fact-finders, those who crave knowledge for its own sake, require a calm, disinterested gaze, and inquisitive unrest, a clear mind. They are in contrast with the first group, but work out the results from the scientific point of view exclusively.

(3) The contemplators are somewhat more original, for the mere increase of knowledge unwittingly fosters interpretation and crosses over into it.

Even the fact-finders, however much they may make the sign of the crucifix at the very thought of imagination, before they realise it are compelled to call upon this selfsame power of assistance.

(4)   The comprehenders – in a deeper sense they might be called creators – are original in the highest sense of the term. By proceeding from ideas, they simultaneously express the unity of the whole, and it is almost the obligation of Nature to conform to the ideas.'

Goethe understood that science and art were at opposite ends of the same intellectual spectrum (Gould, 1987). He recognised the non-trivial patterns of connection. He straightened out the vocabulary of the gross comparative anatomy of flowering plants. He realised that to describe a leaf as a 'flat green thing' or a 'stem' as a 'cylindrical thing' was not good enough. We have lost *totemism*, the sense of parallelism between man's organisation and that of the animals and plants (Bateson, 1985). Gould, in addition, shows his understanding and brilliance in the field of geology (Gould, 1983). Goethe's ideas had more true science in them, they were hard and empirical (Gleick, 1987).

Gould (1993) poses two questions.

'Did Goethe get any mileage for his unconventional "artist's" approach in science? Did it work? The answer, I think, is undoubtedly "yes." We might hold that Goethe's general brilliance allowed him to succeed whatever cockamamie method he happened to use – and that his artist's vision of integration and imagination didn't really help after all. But we might also take him at his word, admit the efficacy of his approach, and try to appreciate the message of pluralism and the artificiality of conventional boundaries among disciplines.'

Counterfeit holism

'An impression can never by itself be associated with another impression. Nor has it the power to arouse others. It does so only provided that it is already understood in the light of the past experience in which it co-existed with those which we are concerned to arouse.'

Maurice Merleau-Ponty

Within the field of health care there are numerous claims to treating patients holistically. Unfortunately, this forms the essence of counterfeit holism. Wholeness is a consciousness not an action. You cannot intervene holistically at once with an action; it is only possible to treat parts. Commonly a practitioner will treat the body, intervening in various ways be it with nutrition, drugs, surgery or manipulation: these are all actions. Those making claims to treat 'holistically' will still have the analytical mode of consciousness as an underlying factor and epitomise the summation of parts (or actions) to form a whole. The conscious piecing together of the patient's problems in a mechanistic manner is a poly-reductionist and polyanalytical externalising of the patient's problems. As mentioned above osteopathic medicine should be organic in its philosophy, unifying in its principle and analytical in its practice; you cannot understand or implement osteopathy by focusing on any one of these three in isolation.

The hologram principle

A hologram is an image projected onto a photographic plate by a laser. Unlike a purely light impressioned photographic image the holographic image is three-dimensional. If both the photographic plate and the holographic plates are shattered the photographic plate shows pieces of the original image whereas the holographic plate shows the whole image in the each of the pieces, even though the image weakens (Bortoft, 1996). All natural forms are reflections of the whole in the pieces. We can see the smallest pieces of a leaf and know it belongs to a plant. As the pieces of the analytical approach breaks down the leaf into smaller and smaller pieces the form disappears. With the holographic plate as the broken pieces become smaller the image of the whole becomes smaller. The form of the original animal or plant is broken up to such a degree that death and an ability to express nature is destroyed (Fig. 1). We shall see this in the work of J. Curtis-Lake with regards to health in embryological development.

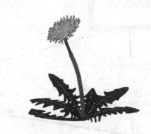

The whole plant

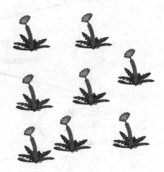

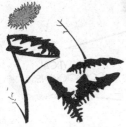

Photographic-analytical
consciousness

Holographic-organic
consciousness

Fig. 1 Modes of consciousness.

Unity and diversity

We have seen that the basic two modes of consciousness, organic and analytical, can be academically appreciated as two ends of the same phenomenon. A further analogy can be demonstrated in the understanding of unity and diversity. The organic approach sees wholeness initially and then considers the units without losing the holistic–universal paradigm at any point, *diversity in unity*. An analytical-general paradigm appreciates initially the sum of the parts into a sense of wholeness, *unity in diversity* (Fig. 2). A human being, is one organ, as is a flower. Goethe used the term *Urorgan* to demonstrate a oneness. There is only one, this is not a numerical one but a one with capital 'O' in the form of *Oneness* which expresses itself in multiple forms. This Oneness is expressed in all human form. Life expresses as a diversity not a unity or sameness.

Organic thought

'The world is ... the natural setting of, and field for, all my thoughts and explicit perceptions. Truth does not inhibit only the inner man, or accurately,

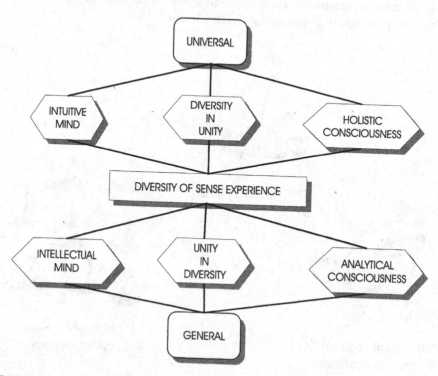

Fig. 2 Adapted from Bortoft (1996).

there is no inner man, man is in the world, and only in the world does he know himself.'

Maurice Merleau-Ponty

There is no balance in nature, only One. To understand this Goethe asked for an inner flexibility and openness. One of the first aspects is the habit of seeing nature as a solid object. We are only seeing the expression of nature in its physicality. But, we should not fall into the trap of perceiving nature as *nothing* when we should be regarding her as *no-thing*. Communication of this expression is through our language; this is why the poet and the scientist seem to be at opposite ends, rather than appreciating their methods of observation as having different modes of consciousness. These are two forms of observing the same thing. The main thrust of organic thinking is to appreciate that our sense of nature should not be totally substituted by symbols; mathematics being a good example. In the other we have developed a mathematical style of thinking. Goethe wrote (cited in Naydler, 1996) that

'Nature is no system; she has – she is – life and development from an unknown centre toward an unknowable periphery. Thus observation of Nature is limitless, whether we make distinctions among the least particles or pursue the whole by following the trail far and wide.'

We need to see with the eyes of a child (Planck, 1949).

'I've seen a child attempting to do some sort of puzzle, who tries without any sense of confusion or pain, just with interest – attempting again and again and again until maybe finally he succeeds.'

Bohm (1994)

Our major problem in the scientific approach is overshooting the mark in our eagerness to understand. We speculate well beyond the phenomenon that is happening in front of us. The way in which we see, or place meaning into what we see, has been practised. This organic view will be illustrated more fully in the section on form and function (page 62).

Scientist Rupert Sheldrake (1990) reminds us that William Wordsworth, the poet, inspired the title of the journal *Nature*. In the first issue, in 1869, it carried a collection of aphorisms expressing the thoughts of Goethe and Nature:

'Nature! We are surrounded and embraced by her; powerless to separate ourselves from her, and powerless to penetrate beyond her. ... We live in her midst and know her not. She is incessantly speaking to us, but betrays not her secret. ... She has always thought and always thinks; though not as a man, but as Nature. ... She loves herself, and her innumerable eyes and affections are fixed upon herself. She has divided herself that she may be her own delight. She causes an endless succession of new capacities for enjoyment to spring up, that her insatiable sympathy may be assuaged. ... The spectacle of Nature is always new, for she is always renewing the spectators. Life is her most exquisite invention; and death is her expert contrivance to get plenty of life.'

Phenomenology

'From things that have happened and from things as they exist and from all things that you know and all those things you cannot know, you make something through your invention that is not a representation but a whole new thing truer than anything true and alive, and you make it alive, and if you make it well enough, you give it immortality. That is why you write and for no other reason that you know of. But what about all the reasons that no one knows?'

Ernest Hemingway

In the early part of the twentieth century Edmund Husserl (1859–1938) developed a form of philosophy he termed 'phenomenology'. Husserl described this word as 'to the things themselves'. Literally, how would an object describe itself if it had the ability to speak (Spiegelberg, 1982), a consciousness of the first person? Martin Heidegger, Jean-Paul Sartre and in particular Maurice Merleau-Ponty further developed this philosophy. Phenomenology is the description, rather than an explanation, of the phenomenon you are witnessing where there is no beginning, end or a depth to that which we see. Husserl was concerned that science seemed to ignore the everyday experiences of everyday people. Science abstracts continuously.

'All my knowledge of the world, even my scientific knowledge, is gained from my own particular point of view, or from some experience of the world without which the symbols of science would be meaningless. The whole universe of science is built upon the world as directly experienced, and if we want to subject science itself to rigorous scrutiny and arrive at a precise assessment of its meaning and scope, we must begin by reawakening the basic experience of the world, of which science is the second-order expression ... To return to things themselves is to return to that world which precedes knowledge, of which knowledge always speaks, and in relation to which every scientific schematisation is an abstract and derivative sign-language, as is geography in relation to the countryside in which we have learnt beforehand what a forest, a prairie or a river is.'

Merleau-Ponty (1962)

Still and Goethe represented one way of a phenomenological approach towards man and the natural world, respectively. In his writings Still described what he saw: this has been interpreted as religious and poetic in style. Science did not and does not have the language to describe the phenomenon as it appears. Many have, and many still are, falling into the trap as seeing Still's style as a weakness or even daydreaming. It is this lack of perception that led to the criticism of Still, and Goethe, by those who suffered, and still are suffering, conceptual blindness. As with the Hanson interpretation it is the eyes that see but the mind that forms the meaning. Seeing the phenomenon takes practice and care must be taken not to place meaning into what we see and hear.

The poor descriptive language ability of science can be traced to the primary and secondary qualities of Galileo. Primary qualities were those that extended to the body by using quantitative symbols to desensitise the body appearing as objective (numbers, geometry and weights) whereas the secondary qualities, not to be trusted, were regarded as subjective and weak (sight, colour, taste and smell). Hersh (1998) in the preface to his work, *What is Mathematics, Really?*, wrote

'I show that from the viewpoint of philosophy mathematics must be under- stood as a human activity, a social phenomenon, part of human culture, his- torically evolved, and intelligible only in a social context. I call this viewpoint "humanist".'

Still and Goethe wanted us to bathe in the phenomenon and open our senses.

'[t]he observation of Nature requires a certain purity of spirit that cannot be disturbed or preoccupied by anything. The beetle on the flower does not escape the child; he has devoted all his senses to a single simple interest; and it never strikes him that at the same moment something remarkable may be going on in the formation of the clouds to distract his glances in that direction.'

Goethe (cited in Naydler, 1996)

For Husserl the solution to the phenomenological problem seemed to be the body, one's own as well as that of the other, as a singularly important structure within the phenomenal field. The body is that mysterious and multifaceted phenomenon that seems always to accompany one's awareness, and indeed to be the very location of one's awareness within the field of appearances (Abram, 1996).

Tucker (1919), the New York osteopathic physician, was well aware of the primary and secondary qualities and their place in metaphysics.

'We think of mathematics as existing in nature, since every quality of nature is definable ultimately in terms of mathematics. But nothing could be further from the truth. There is and can be no true mathematics in nature for the simple and perfect reason that there are no uniform units in nature. No leaf is just like any other leaf, no wave like any other wave, etc., *ad infinitum*. Now mathe- matics absolutely presupposes uniformity in that all ones are like other ones, or there could be no twos or any process built on them. There might be a pure mathematics of space and of time, except for the fact that space and time are not divided, either uniformly or otherwise. There can be no pure mathematics of force, for the quality of force partakes of that of the object in which it is expressed.

The metaphysical faculty of the human mind has, however, taken this general subject of the relations and proportions in nature, purified it of its accidents (that is of variable units) and deduced the pure science of mathematics toward which all natural phenomena of nature approximate to a degree that makes it the master science, next only to metaphysics itself, its parent.

So this faculty does to other groups of phenomena. It may be said to select and construct the living truth behind the inert phenomena of nature.

Nature in its upward struggle has perhaps been trying to purify its mathematical qualities and relations, as it has been trying to purify all of its subjects, and so to create broader and more perfect relationships and faculties. This and many other side lines of thought suggest themselves to us, but this is not the place to follow them.'

To understand the contaminating qualities of mathematics in relation to nature Tucker goes on to quote from the preface of Immanuel Kant's *Critique of Pure Reason*. Here we shall refer to an original 1910 publication and translation by J. M.D. Meiklejohn:

'In the earliest times of which history affords us any record, *mathematics* had already entered on the sure course of science, among the wonderful nation, the Greeks. Still it is not to be supposed that it was as easy for this science to strike into, or rather to construct for itself, that royal road, as it was for logic, in which reason has only to deal with itself. On the contrary, I believe that it must have remained long – chiefly among Egyptians – in the stage of blind groping after its true aims and destination, and that it was revolutionised by the happy idea of one man, who struck out and determined for all time the path which this science must follow, and which admits of an indefinite advancement. The history of this intellectual revolution – much more important in its results than the discovery of the passage round the celebrated Cape of Good Hope – and of its author, has not been preserved. But Diogenes Laertius, in naming the supposed discoverer of some of the simplest elements of geometrical demonstration – elements which, according to the ordinary opinion, do not even require to be proved – makes it apparent that the change introduced by the first indication of this new path, must have seemed of the utmost importance to the mathematicians of that age, and it has thus been secured against the chance of oblivion. A new light must have flashed on the mind of the first man (Thales, or whatever may have been his name) who demonstrated the properties of the isosceles triangle. For he found that it was not sufficient to meditate on the figure, as it lay before his eyes, or the conception of it, as it existed in his mind, and thus endeavour to get at the knowledge of its properties, but that it was necessary to produce these properties, as it were, by positive *a priori construction*; and that, in order to arrive with certainty at *a priori* cognition, he must not attribute to the object any other properties than those which neces-sarily followed from that which he had himself, in accordance with his con-ception, placed in the object.'

Maurice Nicoll wrote of Goethe's Faust in *Living Time and the Integration of the Life*, 1952:

'Goethe depicts Faust as having reached the place of *nothing* in his quest for truth. After investigating all branches of human knowledge, Faust finds no answers that satisfy him. He exclaims: "And here I am at last, a very fool, with useless learning curst, no wiser than at first..." There seems to be nothing. All his learning proves useless. Looking round him, he sees no way out. At this point he is faced with despair. His quest becomes meaningless. Meaningless is the worst thing that can assail us. Like the Medusa it turns us to stone. From what direction can Faust recapture meaning – new meaning? At first he sees no direction in which to go. "Fancy, too, has died away, the hope that in my day instruct and elevate mankind." Through the best, as we usually suppose, of the human aspirations – the "desire to help humanity" – he is nevertheless led to absolutely nothing.

In what direction does he turn? The movement of the soul is, of course, poetically treated. He opens an ancient book and catches sight of the sign of the *macrocosmos*, the great world that overshadows the visible fragment in the present moment. The hieroglyph is the seal of Solomon – the two triangles placed upside down, signifying the interpretation of lower and higher space, the passive and active mind. A change passes over him, and he exclaims: "Ha! What new life divine, intense, floods in a moment every sense. I feel the dawn of youth again... Was it a god who wrote these signs?"

Faust touches new energies. His despair turns to joy. He sees things *the other way round*. The active mind awakens. The invisible enters the visible on all sides. *Visibilia ex invisibilibus*. Faced by negation and so with petrifaction of soul, something is suddenly released in him and touches realities beyond sense. Has he not hit upon the divine science of Perseus, who escaped from being turned to stone by the Medusa (it would seem) through the art of seeing things the other way round? Perseus avoids death by looking at the Medusa in the mirror of Athena. Thereby he slays the Medusa and releases Pegasus who mounts to heaven. Is not this an allegory about man and his eternal nature?'

William Morton Wheeler (1865–1937), fortunately for osteopathy, gave a splendid comparison between osteopathy and medicine, in *The Naturalist versus the Biologist*. Here he compares the naturalist of the character of Andrew Taylor Still with the constructive biologist:

'On reviewing my students and the mature investigators I have known during the past half-century, I find that most of them belong to two extreme types, while the remainder are intermediate or ambiguous composites. These extremes correspond with the romanticist and classicist types respectively, which Ostwald distinguished among physicists and chemists, and also agree very closely with the two general psychological types which Jung calls extroverts and introverts. The more numerous romanticists or extroverts are the naturalists; the classicists or introverts are the biologists in the strict sense. The differences between these two types, which are very probably constitutional or dispositional, will be clear from the following very brief behaviouristic diagnosis:

The naturalist is mentally oriented toward and controlled by objective, concrete reality, and probably because his senses, especially those of sight and touch, are highly developed, is powerfully affected by the aesthetic appeal of natural objects. He is little interested in and may even be quite blind to abstract or theoretical considerations, and therefore inclined to say with Goethe:

> Grau, theurer Freun, is alle Theorie,
> Und grün des Lebens goldener Baum.

> Grey, my dear friend, is all theory,
> And green is the life of a golden tree.

He is primarily an observer and fond of outdoor life, a collector, a classifier, a describer, deeply impressed by the overwhelming intricacy of natural phenomena and revelling in their very complexity. He is, therefore, more or less irrational, intuitive, receptive, and passive in his attitude toward natural objects, synthesising rather than analysing, a poor mathematician, an amateur in the proper sense of the word. When philosophically inclined, he is apt to be a tough-minded Aristotelian. In his output he is clearly of the romanticist type, publishing copiously and easily, but often without much sense of literary form or proportion.

The biologist *sensu stricto* on the other hand, is oriented toward and dominated by ideas, and rather terrified or oppressed by the intricate hurly-burly of concrete, sensuous reality and its multiform and multicoloured individual manifestations. He often belongs to the motor rather than to the visual types and obtains his aesthetic satisfaction from all kinds of analytical procedures and the cold desiccated beauty of logical and mathematical demonstration. His will to power takes the form of experimentation and the controlling of phenomena by capturing them in a net of abstract formulas and laws. He is a denizen of the laboratory. His besetting sin is oversimplification and the tendency to undue isolation of the organisms he studies from their natural environment. As a philosopher he is apt to be a tender-minded Platonist. In his output he is a true classicist. The total volume of his writing is apt to be small, but high quality.

The naturalist seems to represent the more youthful, the biologist the more mature type. For this reason a naturalist may develop into something of a biologist, but a biologist never becomes a naturalist. The naturalist never feels really at home in a university environment, probably because university facilities include such a large number of introverts and because he is apt to be a mediocre student in many of the required, standardised subjects of instruction.

Now it is the holistic attitude that has always characterised the naturalist. Even that extremely practical but much-abused science, taxonomy, which would seem to contradict this statement, really supports it for classification is necessarily always a synthesis as well as an analysis. The naturalist and nature-lover will, therefore, always be with us. No matter how far the naturalist may specialise in his study of single groups of organisms or of the faunas and floras of particular regions or geological ages, he is always keenly aware both of the limitations of his speciality and of its relations to the whole realm of living things. Such modesty is not always apparent in the biologist in the strict sense, because he is not engaged in sympathetically exploring the contours of nature, but in determining the extent to which phenomena conform with his experimental, metrical, and therefore highly rational procedure.'

Goethe professed, 'the senses do not deceive; the judgement deceives' and that 'the Greeks spoke of neither cause nor effect in their descriptions and stories – instead, they represented the phenomenon as it was. In their science, too, they did not perform experiments, but relied on experiences as they occurred.' He saw the human being as the most exact instrument – as did Still. Modern science has been spending its time creating instruments of greater and greater complexity without being aware that it is still the human that has to interpret the meaning. It essentially doubles and distorts our encounter with solid objects. Osteopathic medicine only works in the present and it comes into being by its doing not by its intellectualising.

And finally Goethe wrote

'we get by in life with our everyday language, for we describe only superficial relationships. The instant we speak of deeper relationships, another language springs up: poetic language.'

'The eye, which is called the window of the soul, is the chief means whereby the understanding may most fully and abundantly appreciate the infinite works of Nature; and the ear is the second, inasmuch as it acquires its importance from the fact that it hears the things which the eye has seen. If historians, or poets, or mathematicians had never seen things with your eyes, you would be ill able to describe them in your writings.'

Leonardo da Vinci (1452–1519)

References

Abram, D. (1996) *The Spell of the Sensuous.* Vintage Books, New York.

Bateson, G. (1985) *Mind and Nature: A Necessary Unity.* Fontana, London.

Bohm, D. (1994) *Thought as a System.* Routledge, London.

Bortoft, H. (1996) *The Wholeness of Nature: Goethe's Way of Science.* Floris Books, Edinburgh.

Bortoft, H. (1997) Goethe's organic vision. *Network.* December 65, 3–7.

Bortoft, H. (1999) Personal communication.

Bronowski, J. (1965) *The Identity of Man.* Pelican Books, London.

Gleick, J. (1987) *Chaos: Making a New Science.* Cardinal, London.

Goodwin, B. (1994) *How the Leopard Changed its Spots: The Evolution of Complexity.* Phoenix, London.

Gould, S.J. (1983) *Hen's Teeth and Horse's Toes.* Penguin Books, London.

Gould, S.J. (1987) *Time's Arrow, Time's Cycle: Myth and Metaphor in the Discovery of Geological Time.* Harvard University Press, London.

Gould, S.J. (1993) *Eight Little Piggies: Reflections in Natural History.* Penguin Books, London.

Guba, E.G. (Ed) (1990) *The Paradigm Dialog.* Sage, London.

Hacking, I. (Ed.) (1981) *Scientific Revolutions.* Oxford University Press, Oxford.

Hanson, N. (1958) *Patterns of Discovery.* Cambridge University Press, Cambridge.

Hensel, H. (1998) Goethe, science, and sensory experience. In *Goethe's Way of Science: A Phenomenology of Nature.* Eds D. Seamon and A. Zajonc, Chapter 4, pp. 71–82. State University of New York Press, New York.

Hersh, R. (1998) *What is Mathematics, Really?* Vintage, London.

Keesecker, R.P. (1955) The nature of osteopathic medicine. *The Journal of the American Osteopathic Association.* November 55(3) 189–91.

Korr, I.M. (1997) Osteopathic Research: The needed paradigm shift. In *The Collected Papers of Irvin M. Korr,* Vol. 2. American Academy of Osteopathy, Indianapolis.

Kuhn, T. S. (1996) *The Structure of Scientific Revolutions.* Third edition. University of Chicago Press, Chicago.

Littlejohn, J.M. (1899) *Lectures on Psycho-physiology.* E.G. Kinney, Kirksville, MI.

Lorimer, D. (1997) Experiment and experience. Editorial, *Network,* December. 65.

McConnell, C. (1938) The osteopathic approach. *The Journal of the American Osteopathic Association,* 10 37 447–50.

McNamara, T.P. and Miller, D.L. (1989) Attributes of theories of meaning. *Psychological Bulletin* 106 (3) 355–76.

Merleau-Ponty, M. (1962) *Phenomenology of Perception.* Routledge and Kegan Paul, London.

Naydler, J. (1996) *Goethe on Science: An Anthology of Goethe's Scientific Writings.* Floris Books, Edinburgh.

Nicoll, M. (1952) *Living Time and the Integration of the Life.* Vincent Stuart, London.

Planck, M. (1949) The meaning and limits of science. *Science,* September 30 110 319–27.

Sheldrake, R. (1990) *The Rebirth of Nature.* Rider, London.

Spiegelberg, H. (1982) *The Phenomenological Movement: An Historical Introduction.* Third edition. Martinus Nijhoff, The Hague.

Tolzmann, D.H. (1997) *The German-American Forty-Eighters: 1848–1998.* Max Kade German-American Centre, Winter. http//www.serve.com/shea/germusa/tolz1848.htm

Toulmin, S. (1990) *Cosmopolis: The Hidden Agenda of Modernity.* The University of Chicago Press, Chicago.

Tucker, E.E. (1919) Dr Still, the metaphysician. *The Journal of the American Osteopathic Association,* 19(9) 486–94.

White, M. (1997) *Newton: The Last Sorcerer.* Fourth Estate, London.

Further reading

Adams, P. (1998) *House Calls*. Robert D. Reed Publishers, San Francisco.

Armstrong, K. (1994) *A History of God*. Mandarin, London.

Bostridge, I. (1997) *Witchcraft and Its Transformations: c. 1655 – c. 1750*. Clarendon Press, Oxford.

Brillat-Savarin, J-A. (1970) *The Physiology of Taste*. Penguin Classics, London.

Burke, E. (1998) *A Philosophical Enquiry into the Sublime and Beautiful and Other Pre-Revolutionary Writings*. Penguin Classics, London.

Clark, A. (1997) *Being There: Putting Brain, Body, and World Together Again*. MIT Press, London.

Clark, C.J.S. (1996) *Reality through the Looking-Glass*. Floris Books, Edinburgh.

Corfield, P.J. (1995) *The Power and the Professions in Britain 1700–1850*. Routledge, London.

Cytowic, R.E. (1997) *The Man Who Tasted Shapes*. Abacus, London.

Devlin, K. (1997) *Goodbye, Descartes: The End of Logic and the search for a New Cosmology of the Mind*. John Wiley & Sons, Inc., New York.

Englander, D., Norman, D., O'Day, R. and Owens, W.R. (Eds) (1994) *Culture and Belief in Europe 1450–1600: An Anthology of Sources*. The Open University and Blackwell Publishers, Oxford.

Gillott, J. and Kumar, M. (1995) *Science and the Retreat from Reason*. The Merlin Press Ltd, London.

Gjertsen, D. (1992) *Science and Philosophy: Past and Present*. Penguin, London.

Goethe, Johann Wolfgang von., (1840) *Theory of Colours*. Introduced by Deane B. Judd (1970). The MIT Press, London.

Good, B.J. (1994) *Medicine, Rationality and Experience: An Anthropological Perspective*. Lewis Henry Morgan Lectures. Cambridge University Press, Cambridge.

Hurd, D.L. and Kipling, J.J. (1964) *The Origins and Growth of Physical Science*. Volume 1. Pelican Books, London.

Illich, I. (1985) *Limits to Medicine*. Pelican Books, London.

Maull, N. (1978) Cartesian optics and the geometrization of nature. *Review of Metaphysics*, 32, 253–73.

Merchant, C. (1980) *The Death of Nature: Women, Ecology and the Scientific Revolution*. Harper and Row Publishers, San Francisco.

Merleau-Ponty, M. (1998) *Signs*. Northwestern University Press.

Miller, D. (Ed.) (1988) *Goethe: Scientific Studies*. Suhrkamp Publishers, New York.

Newton-Smith, W.H. (1996) *The Rationality of Science*. Routledge, London.

Novack, G. (1993) *The Origins of Materialism – The Evolution of a Scientific View of the World*. Pathfinder, New York.

Popper, K.R. (1992) *Objective Knowledge: An Evolutionary Approach*. Clarendon Press, Oxford.

Snow, C.P. (1993) *The Two Cultures*. Canto Edition. Cambridge University Press, Cambridge.

Tarnas, R. (1998) *The Passion of the Western Mind*. Pimlico, London.

Williams, B. (1978) *Descartes: The Project of Pure Enquiry*. Pelican Books, Harmondsworth.

Wilson, M.D. (Ed.) (1969) *The Essential Descartes*. A Mentor Book, New York.

CHAPTER 3

Dr Still, the Metaphysician

Ernest E. Tucker
DO, New York

[The following paper by Ernest E. Tucker, DO highlights the osteopathy of Andrew Taylor Still. Here it is published in full, as anything shorter would be an abstraction weakening the understanding of Still's mind as understood by Tucker. This work represents Husserl's phenomenology and Goethe's subjectivity both leading to the importance of developing intuition.]

Andrew Taylor Still, founder of the science of osteopathy, was a great metaphysical mind.

We knew him best through his creation, the science of osteopathy, that most practical, direct and effective of healing sciences. But always the faculty is greater than the fact it creates, the machine that can make matches is more important than the matches it makes – for they are an end; but it can go on creating more matches forever. To understand the faculty that produced osteopathy is to rediscover it at its original sources, and to open the way to endless further discoveries of the same kind. That faculty was a great metaphysical faculty, and osteopathy is a great triumph of metaphysics.

What is metaphysics, and wherein is osteopathy a great metaphysical triumph? Let us not get actual crystals mixed up with crystallography, the study thereof. Let us not get the metaphysical faculty, which Dr Still had, mixed up with metaphysics the study thereof, of which he was as innocent as a babe is of logarithms. The study of physiology is one thing, and the living animal so studied is another. We cannot create new animals by a study of physiology; but we can liberate them from disease and bring them to a maximum of efficiency. We can not create a metaphysical faculty by the study of metaphysics, but we can develop the one ourselves by studying in Dr. Still, and use it to great advantage in the criticism of his science and in the creation of new sciences.

Definition of metaphysics

What then is metaphysics, the study? Just a few words will be sufficient to get a viewpoint. Immanuel Kant is its great exemplar, to whom the reader is referred. Metaphysics is the study of the faculty of knowledge, of the scientific faculty, is the science of sciences. It distils, filters and refines all concepts into terms, as chemistry reduces all matter to elements. It eliminates all derived, secondary, acquired qualities, all probabilities and deals with things that are inherently necessary.

For instance, it discovers that in all of our mental concepts there are three elements never lacking, the concepts of time, of space, and of causality. It purifies these concepts of all accidents, and tries to give them ultimate definition – to find, that is, the final rock on which human knowledge and understanding rest. (Perhaps the underlying motive for this work was the attempt to discover Deity; and perhaps it has succeeded, though in a way strange enough by comparison with its original hope – but that is not part of this present story.) The irreducible elements of ideas it calls innate ideas, *a priori* concepts, intuitions; they represent the ultimate reality of thought, the ultimate foundation of science.

What then is metaphysics, the faculty? It is in effect the same process applied not consciously to thought itself, but unconsciously to nature. It is the faculty by which the mind thinks scientifically. For instance, take the matter of mathematics. Mathematics is a pure product of the metaphysical faculty. We think of mathematics as existing in nature, since every quality of nature is definable ultimately in terms of mathematics (see the table of periodicity of the elements, etc.). But nothing could be further from the truth. There is and can be no true mathematics in nature for the simple and perfect reason that there are no uniform units in nature. No leaf is just like any other, no wave like any other, etc., *ad infinitum*. Now mathematics absolutely presupposes uniformity in that all ones are like all other ones, or there could be no twos or any process built on them. There might be a pure mathematics of space and of time, except for the quality of force partakes of that of the object in which it is expressed.

The metaphysical faculty of the human mind has, however, taken this general subject of the relations and proportions in nature, purified it of its accidents (that is of its variable units) and deduced the pure science of mathematics toward which all natural phenomena approximate. This science gives it mastery over all phenomena of nature to a degree that makes it the master science, next only to metaphysics itself, its parent.

So this faculty does to other groups of phenomena. It may be said to select and construct the living truth behind the inert phenomena of nature.

Nature in its upward struggle has perhaps been trying to purify its mathematical qualities and relations, as it has been trying to purify all of its subjects, and so to create broader and more perfect relations and faculties. This and many other side lines of thought suggest themselves to us, but this is not the place to follow them.

Let us quote from Kant to further understand the value and importance of this faculty and this process. In his preface to the second edition of his epoch-making work, the *Critique of Pure Reason*, he shows how the sciences of mathematics and physics were lifted up and set on the high road of pure sciences.

'In the earliest times of which history has any record mathematics had already entered on the sure course of science, among that wonderful nation, the Greeks.... I believe that it must have remained long chiefly among the Egyptians, in a stage of blind groping after its true aims and destination, and that it was revolutionised by the happy thought of one man, who struck out and determined for all time the path which this science must follow, and which admits of an indefinite advancement. The history of this intellectual revolution (much more important in its results than the discovery of the celebrated passage around the Cape of Good Hope) and of its author has not been preserved. But Diogenes Laertius in naming the supposed discoverer of some of the simplest elements of geometrical demonstration – elements which according to the ordinary opinion do not have to be proved – makes it apparent that the change introduced by the first introduction of this new path must have seemed of the utmost importance to the mathematicians of that age, and it has been secured against the chance of oblivion.

A new light must have flashed on the mind of the first man (Thales, or whatever may have been his name) who demonstrated the properties of the isosceles triangle. For he found that it was not sufficient to meditate on the figure, as it lay before his eyes, or on the conception of it, as it existed in his mind, and thus attempt to get at a knowledge of its properties, but that it was necessary to produce *a priori construction*; and that in order to arrive with any certainty at *a priori* cognition, he must not attribute to the object any other properties than those which he had himself, in accordance with his conception, placed in the object.'

Let us try and paraphrase the part of this that is important to us in our study of disease and of Dr Still's faculty for observation of disease. In order to be certain of his conclusions, he must not attribute to the object any qualities which do not follow by necessity from the subject as he has defined it. He must not attribute even objective qualities unless they are inherent in the subject. We must purify the subject, and stay within the strict and necessary attributes of it as a subject. Let A, B, C be any isosceles triangle; what properties necessarily belong to any isosceles triangle? Let X be any animal organism in a state of disease; what things are necessarily true of it? What things are inherently necessary in it from the very fact it is an animal organism and that it is in a state of disease? It is not sufficient to meditate on the subject before us, as it lies before our eyes, nor on the conception of it as it is formed in our minds, i.e., the symptom-picture but it is necessary to see the qualities that we attribute to it as necessarily true, *a priori*, in the very fact as we define it; such that leaving out the necessary conclusions, the original fact or definition can no longer obtain.

This question we can answer to some extent right now, in advance of our study of Dr. Still's mind; and for an illustration of what is meant by this method of study, shall attempt to do so.

Living organism cannot manufacture alien processes

First it must be evident that the forces at play in the diseased state must be the same as those which are normally present and functioning in the organism in a state of health. These may differ in degree and in other respects dependent on that difference of degree; but they must be the same forces. Nature cannot manufacture properties only to exist as disease. A bell must react as a bell at all times and under all circumstances; it cannot manufacture qualities by which it reacts as other than a bell. This is a true metaphysical proposition, inherently necessary because a thing cannot both be and not be. So a living organism must react as what it is, if it reacts at all; it cannot manufacture processes that are alien to it. Disease cannot, therefore, be a process or a product of forces alien to the normal body.

The body may be put into an unnatural state by extraneous forces, as a bell may be broken by a cannon ball; but its reaction is true to its state. If it reacts at all it must react to qualities that are inherent in it – as we might say, *a priori*.

Simple as this statement is, axiomatic, necessary, it yet has to do battle with a vast mass of lore that has accumulated around the subject of disease; and it has not, unless very recently, played any part at all in the general study of disease.

It follows, however, that the state or condition of disease must necessarily be composed of two elements – the abnormal state into which the organism has been forced by some extraneous condition, and the reaction of that state; the former is the mechanical or chemical or nervous cause of the disease, the latter is the disease process itself. Of the two the former only is a strictly abnormal state itself. This metaphysical principle, perhaps unconsciously to him, certainly not defined by him, appears to have been a large part of the background of Dr Still's conscious thought. Certainly it is to his glory that he first applied it with consistency and courage to the problems of disease, with profit to the world scarcely second to that conferred by 'Thales or what ever may have been his name', or by the discoverer of the passage around the Cape of Good Hope. Possibly the science of healing may be rescued from the blind groping and set on the highroad of pure science by this method.

Let us make no mistake on one point. Dr Still was pre-eminently a practical man. He reasoned on the basis of things that worked. 'The God I worship demonstrates all His works.' It seems to me however, that it was the metaphysical background to his mind that lifted it to an apotheosis, a place with the gods; that made him to pick out and stick to the particular practical things that had eternal and elemental truth behind them; that emboldened him to bring all other 'practical' things to the same tribunal; whence the rejection of the vast superstition of curative drugs, and the genesis of the true science of osteopathy.

Approaching the study of metaphysics as a physician, particularly an osteopathic physician, having in mind at the same time both metaphysics and physiology and that inspiration for tracing things to their sources which is the inherent spirit of osteopathy, the two were seen in perspective of each other; and the source of the metaphysical principles, the innate ideas and intuitions, was seen in physiology.

For instance: the eye and hand and the physical body generally are moved through space. They are so moved by the nervous system. The nervous system to successfully move them had to learn, automatically and mechanically, the laws of space. These never of themselves presented themselves as laws, as principles, but were present in the mechanical side of the nervous system, as nerve coordinations that correspond with the laws of space. The mind, without necessarily recognising them as laws, yet used them nevertheless and moved in obedience to them; thought in accordance with them; and at last discovered them (by a process of awakening its own subject side – but that, too, is not part of our story). When, however, we school children studied geometry, we found that we knew much of it already, intuitively; and that a great part of it lay just beneath the surface in what we call our subconscious mind. It had merely to be realised and to be given strength by exercise.

Things taught to subconscious mind

Many other things are taught to the subconscious surface, so to speak, of our conscious minds in the same way and by the same action – by its operation of our bodies. Thus it learned the laws of nature as expressed in the body; by the operation of its own faculties it learned the laws and conditions of thought.

The things so taught are tremendous or transcendent value to us, and could we wholly define them in conscious thought, would be a body of arteries and propositions that would make our progress in science immeasurably more rapid. For they represent two factors – the things that were selected, developed and proved successful in the long school of evolution, and the master principles deduced therefrom.

Let us for the moment consider the institutions, time and space, and see wherein they are due to the mechanism of the mind. The concept of time arises necessarily from a comparison of a past state with a changed present state. The only thing capable of performing that feat of memory; one might almost say the human memory. It alone is capable of retaining a past state, and in the same place (the memory) of progressing to a present state, and by comparing then to generate the concept of time.

The same thing is true of space – the memory is the only thing capable of remaining in one place and at the same time progressing to another place and in comparing them to generate the concept of space. Or of comparing impressions received by different parts of the sensorium in one together so as to generate the concept of space. Thus, seeing problems of metaphysics and the facts of physiology at the same time, we correlate them and find the source of the metaphysical institutions in the physiologic functions.

It may be said that all the laws that exist or operate in the human body have probably to some extent taught themselves to this subconscious side of our minds. It may be said, further, that all laws that are in the universe exist or operate in the living body. These reveal themselves in the consciousness as intuitions. The summation of these intuitions corresponds, doubtless, with what we call God. The practical operation of them, of course, constitutes the consciousness itself. The analytical study of them and the purifying of them as subjects constitute metaphysics. The unconscious application of them to problems of nature is the metaphysical faculty and has been the genesis of science. What authority rests in them, and how does that authority compare with present experimental science?

Whatever authority the mind has rests in them. Our power to reason on the phenomena of nature rests solely in them. That authority, however, is the authority of things that work, that have worked so successfully that they have enabled us to reach our present state of development. They are themselves part of nature, that part which showed itself capable of being organised into such perfect coordination as we see in the living body and the consciously operating mind. Their authority we say is absolute, as far as it goes. They represent them as far as it does. They represent the thing that the Creator Himself laid down – the things that God did and the methods whereby He did them. We say that their authority is absolute as far as it goes – and that I think means that our concern should be not how far they may be trusted, but how far they can be carried; how far developed; for they are all that we have. They constitute the scientific imagination without which experimental science would be but a repetition of inert data that would lead nowhere.

Let us repeat that they represent that aspect of nature which has reached the highest evolution and development of coordination and function; the part by which, whether for good or ill, we are limited in our efforts to think and to understand; that part of nature by means of which we observe and interpret nature again. Our observation and our reason are just as excellent as is our individual development and use of this, the constitution and background of them; and no more.

Dr Still's application of principles

That these principles are the unconscious background of the thinking process of all of us is of course obvious in their very definition, as given here. But that they were more clearly felt, more courageously applied, more rigidly held to by Dr Still than is usual – that is my theme; and that in my opinion is what most lifted him above the level of his time, and incidentally is what enabled him to become the founder of the science of osteopathy.

Being innocent of all criticism of innate ideas, *a priori* cognitions, and the like, he couches his ideas in the language and the figure of his times, those of the Bible and ascribes the intuitions all to Deity. Nor, one might add, was he far wrong, since they represent the methods of the Creator. But his writings are as one might say riddled with God; in vast emotional passages, and in intellectual deductions. It takes courage to think always in terms of God; to carry ideas to their ultimate conclusion; to complete them as subjects, escaping from the 'tyranny of facts'; to see in their universal aspect; but he had the courage. He had the courage and the mental energy. He had the courage both to cast away the false, to walk forth into the blank spaces of nothingness and absence of all idea, with only these intentions for guide, and also to trust and follow wherever they led in the perception of truth; given by this process of thinking.

Again, first quoting Kant (Preface):

'A cursory view of this present work will lead to the supposition that its use is merely negative. That is in fact its primary use. But this assumes at once a positive value when we observe that it removes an obstacle which impedes and even threatens to destroy the use of practical reason.'

Still, *Autobiography*, we read.

'In sickness has not God left man in a world of guessing? Guess what is the matter? Guess what to give, and guess the result? And when dead, guess where he goes. I decided that God was not a guessing God but a God of truth. . . .

'All His works, spiritual and material, are harmonious. His law of animal life is absolute. So wise a God has certainly placed the remedy within the material house in which the spirit of life dwells. . . .

'Solemnity takes possession of the mind, a smile of love runs over the face, the ebbs and tides of the great ocean of reason, whose depths have never been fathomed, swell to your surging brain. You eat and drink; and as you stand in silent amazement, suns appear where you never saw a star, brilliant with rays of God's wisdom, as displayed in man, and with the laws of life, eternal in days, and true as the mind of God Himself. . . .'

'Having proved to my mind that God into the minutiae of all his works. . . .'

'Every step that drops even one grain of drugs sees more Deity and less drugs....'

'I took as my foundation to build on that the whole universe with its worlds, men, beasts, with all forms and principles of life, were formulated by the mind of an unerring God.'

Anyone at all familiar with his words will recognise the degree to which the intention of God, the sum of all intentions, lay at the back of them.

Observe that it is in the study of metaphysics that the subjects are consciously purified. In the intuitive mind, which uses therein, they are not so purified. It is more natural, indeed, to have a blending of reason and emotion and other qualities, as we have here. But these quotations, and many others, some of them of an equally intense poetic power serve to illustrate the intuition of order; on which alone the faculty of reason can be built, and – applying the intuition to the world again – on which alone creation could have progressed; one which, incidentally, any study of a living body must be based. 'If we have disorder and yet no disease, what is the use of order?' he asks in another work; and we must not forget also that these statements were designed not so much as an expression of accurate concepts, nor intended to stand as scientific dicta, but as the efforts of a teacher to arouse students' minds to a perception of the same intuitions.

Bodily order and disorder

These quotations all illustrate the negative side of intentions, attempting to clear away habits of thought that have lain across the path of our progress.

To those not familiar with the therapeutic world into which these statements were launched, it will be necessary to suggest a corollary to this intuition, and phrase it thus – that disorder added to order makes disorder. Applied to the body, it means that experimenting and guessing injected into the perfect order of the body make disorder. And even when a body is already disordered, then the injecting of further disorder, other disorder, different disorder, still makes nothing but further disorder. This corollary to the intuition of order is seen implied in for instance the following quotations.

'Soon I met a case of flux, and being a physician and familiar with the remedies recommended for such a disease, such questions as these arose: "What was God's remedy? Has God a drug store? Does he use sedatives for flux? Does He use sweating powders, such as Dover's and so forth? Does he use astringents?"...'

'As we are not willing to attribute to Deity anything but perfection, ... we must see and know that His work of animal life is partly a failure before we are justified in our conclusion to assist Him to subdue even a fever by the use of a drug of any kind. ....'

'Could you add or subtract a single bone, nerve, vein or artery that you know would be an improvement on the original? If not could you *add* and get beneficial results? Could you put machinery in there that would make better blood?'

These statements are what we would call ordinary reasonings, withal excellent ones. As Kant says, all reasonings go back to intuitions for their basis. Incidental processes of reasoning refer back to the machinery of reasoning power for their testing. The laws and the conditions of life are the vastest generalisations that have yet been made on our earth, the vastest and the surest that are accessible to the mind of man. If they have taught anything at all to the conscious mind, it is the intuition of order – condition of the workings of the body and of mind itself as well. All of us in our reasoning processes go back to this ultimate foundation, and read our conclusions of incidental things in the light of them. The difference is only that in Dr Still's case he applied so much more clearly and faithfully and uncompromisingly these intuitions that they led him to larger results.

In any case we see that his rejection of drugs as remedial agents was not on practical grounds merely, but on *a priori* cognitions, or the basis of the things that his own life and body had taught to his mind.

Dr Still relied on correction of disorder

In place of drug medication, Dr. Still placed entire reliance on correction of disorders. For many reasons: first, because they worked; second, because he knew of nothing else that did work. But there seemed to be more than this, for he positively and often more violently opposed any other reliance. 'Find it, fix it, and leave it alone,' said he in tones as of the decalogue. Looking, on account of this vigour, for something more than a mere practical reason, I again see an intuition. If this intuition were purified it might be called the intuition of the spontaneous. Life is spontaneous, as are all of its forces and processes. The force by which each part acts and reacts lies within it, and is wholly spontaneous, never compelled. Nothing in the body is compelled, except mechanically. The brain does not compel the body, nor yet does the body compel the brain; but both serve spontaneously a higher thing, the unity of the two. Nor is any organ or function of the body compelled; the energy of each lies within it, and its action is spontaneous, is a matter of coordinating – rather a matter of emulation and rivalry in service than of compulsion.

That this is certainly an intuition of the mind, taught to it by this deep principle of nature, is seen clearly enough at least in love and in the higher ethics. But its teaching is offset by the lessons taught the conscious mind on its other side – its outside – by the events of nature and its contact with them. I need not review the meaning and the lessons of force in nature. Between these two concepts, that of force and that of the spontaneous, there is war, and has been perpetual war since first the intuitions of man began to sway his conduct. And the matter has been tried out on the vastest scale of war that the world has seen. It is intuition versus experience.

Let us first clearly see it as a principle of nature, then as an intuition of the mind, and then indicate its meaning and value in therapeutics. Once we are caught in the grip of this intuition, we are likely to be led into all fields of human thought and endeavour, where its effect is seen to be tremendous, with a very great missionary zeal. As it begins to purify itself, we see a vast perspective of meaning. But though we may come to the border of these matters, and hint at them for the verification they give to our thesis, we may not here enter that territory.

First to see it as a principle of nature. Let us begin with the simple and the familiar – 'you bring a horse to water, but you cannot make him drink'. Extraneous forces can compel two objects to come together, but extraneous forces cannot compel them to react, much less to blend harmoniously, can indeed compel them to react, but only destructively, unless the forces that are involved in the reaction come from within, i.e. are spontaneous in the two. Only spontaneous forces can be constructive, can make a unity. It may be objected that the horse even when he drinks, forces the water to enter the system. That is true, but that is not constructive. The water does not become constructive until it enters the animal's vital processes and then it does so only through spontaneous affinities existing in it and also in the tissues themselves.

It is inconceivable that a unity should be created otherwise than by mutual spontaneous affinities. This is metaphysical proposition, inherently necessary; for otherwise we should have it built of qualities indifferent or negative, and in that case and to that degree it is certainly not a unity that would result.

(It may be necessary to redefine the word unity as intended here; to differentiate mechanical unity from vital, artificial from natural. It would seem, however, that merely to call attention to the difference would be enough.)

Creation of unity

Let us use a more convincing illustration. Two and two it is said make four. But two and two may lie side by side on the table or the paper through eternity, and will never become four, lacking an internal spontaneous affinity for doing so. They will forever remain two books and two books, or other object – or for that matter, one book, one book, one book, and one book – no two exactly alike. Only in the mind do they become four divorced from any special objective content. Nothing in the mind compels them to become four; the mind only observes the result of the action that has taken place between its ideas, taken place spontaneously in obedience to that action of all vital things that makes unity within itself. The only effort that the mind makes is to associate with this spontaneous result certain arbitrary shapes of figures, indicative of the two and the two, and of the resulting four.

Throughout the whole of nature this is true, though it would take us out of the preview of our thesis to review various aspects of nature and show its truth.

Fascinating it would be to compare the concept of Deity as taught to the outside of the mind by the huge and overwhelming forces of nature, and that taught to the inside by the intuition of the spontaneous; and to show that the former, as we more and more define our concepts, reveals itself as corresponding to the early concepts of the devil, the latter emerging as the true concept of God. Interesting it would be to compare with this concept of God the one taught by Christ: 'The kingdom of Heaven is within you'; 'God is Love', etc., i.e., spontaneous – no less than to compare with it the God-motive and what we may perhaps call the God-faculty evidenced in His healing. Suffice it for the present to compare with it Dr Still's own motive for healing, born perhaps of this same faculty in however less a degree.

As an intuition of the mind it is taught to it first by this condition of all vital processes – this spontaneous blending, and by the morbid state that results when compulsion or force upsets the perfect balance of the spontaneous forces of life; but as an intuition it is taught also by the mechanisms of the mind itself. The will is of course an element of force, of compulsion; but its office is to change and wrap the internal perfect harmony to adjust life to its environment – it again has reference to the vast external forces. Its value is temporary and for emergencies. After the will has thus acted, it is necessary for these spontaneous forces of life and of thought to build anew the harmony and balance, including the changes induced by the will. But it is the office of the reason to eliminate this warping element of will and to construct its processes on the basis of perfect harmony and blending; allowing the concepts to reveal their own innate and spontaneous affinities; first with the unity of life on the inside and then with each other, revealing the laws of nature on the outside. Out of this dual process are our facilities built and expanded.

To indicate the workings of this intuition in Dr Still's mind a few quotations will suffice; although we will find no violations of it – evidence of its footprints in intaglio everywhere.

'The human body is a machine run by the unseen forces of life, and that it may run harmoniously it is necessary that there be *liberty* of blood, nerves, arteries, from the generating point to destination. ...'

'God does not find it necessary to make these spots of beauty [in the peacock's tail] one at a time; He simply endows the corpuscles with mind, and in obedience to His law every one of these soldiers of life goes like a man in the army, with full instructions as to the duty he is to perform. ....'

'When we take up principles we get down to nature. It is ever willing and self-caring, self-feeding, and self-protecting. ....'

As to the meaning of this intuition in therapeutics, it may be briefly summed up in Dr Still's dictum, 'Find it, fix it, and leave it alone', which being explained means, find the disordered state that has been brought about by some abnormal force; correct it; and leave the rest to the spontaneous forces of nature. The rejection of medicines except as protective, as emergency, and as substitution measures, was also an expression of the same principle.

Whether the classic subject of metaphysics will bear the interpretation given to it here – that it is the things taught to the subconscious side of the mind by the machinery of the body and mind, I do not of course know. But certain it is that there are things so taught; and they correspond with the metaphysical cognitions. It appears natural that these things would be the best possible background for a study of the body and its diseases. It appears to be through them that osteopathy scored its great triumph. Further study of such intuitions and of their evidence in Still's mind, and of their bearing on therapeutics would be interesting and valuable, but cannot be included in this paper.

The Journal of the American Osteopathic Association.
June 1919, pp. 484–98.

CHAPTER 4

Form and Function

'He who neglects anatomy will wrong and kill his patients.'
Abu Al-Qasim Al-Zahravi (Albucasis)
936–1013 CE (Common Era or Christian Era)

Osteopathically it is important to see man from two major aspects: first in the phenomenological expression of form and function into the environment and second from the relationship of the autonomic nervous system. Form is the expression of the whole with an understanding of the space taken up by this whole. Autonomic nervous structure and function is paramount with regards to communication and coordination of internal organs and the myofascioskeletal system, known as *ergotrophism*. The sympathetic portion of the autonomic system controls and communicates with the circulatory system, hence its proper name of *vasomotor* system. As we shall see these two approaches eventually merge, developing the basis for both diagnosis and treatment from an understanding of the integration of expressive form and anatomical communication. Goethe was the earliest to remind us that when we are observing form or anatomical structure we are only dealing with matter. Louisa Burns, in an editorial in *The Journal of the American Osteopathic Association*, June, 1921, reviewed the address given to the profession in 1901 by Turner Hulett, entitled *The Biological Basis of Osteopathy*:

'Life is manifested through matter. Physicians have to do not with the nature of life itself, but with its material medium, a continuous stream of matter entering and becoming alive, at one point, then functioning as living substance, and lastly dying and passing out at another point. This metabolic cycle is the physiological unit. Nothing can enter it but food. It may be hastened or retarded, but cannot be changed qualitatively. Its interruption means death.

In living substance, as in the cell, the unit of organised life, this cycle may be conceived as being in progress at every point. Every change in environing conditions is responded to by adaptive change in the cell by change in the rate of the metabolic cycle, retarding here, accelerating there. This response will be manifested to the full limit of the responding power of the cell.

When the limit of the response is reached, death ensues. Below this limit we may have all degrees of response. When unimpeded it expresses normal vital activity, varied according to changing conditions of environment. When disturbed so as to impair the equilibrium of the vital activities, we call it disease.

This response is always such as tends to restore normal conditions. Disease is then the stimulus to its own cure. That cure shall result it is not necessary that stimuli shall be increased or multiplied. It is only necessary that physical conditions shall be made right, in order that existing stimuli may be effective.

These conditions are the elements of the environment, heat, light, moisture, circulation of fluids in and to the cell, condition of contractility in the cell substance, and free intercellular intercommunications.'

Seeing form

Developing the discipline of seeing the living form and structure Goethe termed *morphology*. Goethe coined this term as a way of seeing the wholeness of the organism, *Anschauung*. 'Seeing' physical form is seeing the way in which space is taken and filled three-dimensionally (Schad, 1977). Analytical science teaches us to think into the structure that appears in front of us. The study of form teaches us to change direction and think the structure out into the environment, developing the natural sense of *active absence* in the presence of the phenomenon we are witnessing.

There are two very different world views, the reductionists seem to be carrying out research to answer either/or questions, while those of the holistic school of thought use research designed to ask 'how?' (Reason, 1986). Goethe argued that *why* is not scientific at all. What we should be asking is *how*, 'how does the bull have horns?'. In the *Hologram Principle* we can begin to see that seeing form is not a summation of parts and *then* the whole; rather it is the whole, in nature, that is reflected through its parts.

Bortoft (1996) wrote

'the paradigm of modern scientific method is Kant's "appointed judge who compels the witnesses to answer questions which he has himself formulated". Science believes itself to be objective, but is in essence subjective because the witness is compelled to answer questions *which the scientist himself has formulated*. Scientists never notice the circularity in this because they believe they hear the voice of 'nature' speaking, not realising that it is the transposed echo of their own voice.'

Active absence

Babies express their consciousness into the environment as *egocentrism* (Cromer, 1995). At some point they will crawl towards something that attracts their attention via their senses. If a baby happens to be on a bed and what attracts him or her is on the other side of the room then he or she will try to get to the object irrespective of the impending end of the bed and the drop after that. Development leads to us see the world as a collection of objects. All mammals do this but man has progressed to seeing all things separately, one from another. We see ourselves as external to everything and have gone on to believe that we can be *objective* in the presence of any phenomenon. This is what we term awareness. Scientific experiments are a classic example; their objective approaches are in fact biased, as they are demonstrations of an already implemented analytical mode of consciousness. That thing is over there and we are over here.

We have always had trouble recognising the whole because our language has to recognise a 'thing'. It is impossible to recognise the whole as a thing. In recognising the whole as a thing we externalise it to other things and it becomes an object. Objects can be held in the hand, wholeness cannot. Many of my students have said 'then if it is not an object then it cannot exist because it would be nothing'. To maintain our sense of awareness we have to relate to *something*. Wholeness is not a *something* or a *nothing*; it is *no-thing*. It was the nineteenth century American writer Thoreau who wrote

'Man cannot afford to be a naturalist, to look at nature directly, but only with the side of his eye. He must look through her and beyond her. To look at her is as fatal as to look at the head of Medusa. It turns the man of science to stone.'

Nature is expressed through the physicalness of matter. This obsession with matter is hypnotising scientists. We are hod carriers of matter, mesmerised by symbolic quantitative measurements and generally insensitive to the qualitative expression of form.

To begin understanding no-thing we can use the concept of active absence. Active absence describes non-thing as essential for any thing to have meaning as a whole. It is the meaning we place into the phenomenon we witness, as the previously mentioned organic mode of consciousness, that allows us to become sensitive to the phenomena we see, hear, touch, taste and smell. An analogy of no-thing and a sense of meaning is a sentence. A word is not a sentence, a sentence is no-word. There has to be a sense of wholeness of the parts between reading the words and the sentence making 'sense'. There is definitely no-thing present to make sense of the sentence but this does not mean that there is nothing. This is the phenomenon of sensitivity known as *active absence*. Wholeness, and nature, is no-thing.

The previously mentioned egocentric mode of the baby is receptive to the environment, it is non-verbal, holistic, timeless, and non-linear, without discrimination. As we become older we become more active in the environment placing meaning into what we sense, resulting in a verbal, analytical, time framed, linear-causative, and logical mode of thought and thinking. It is as if we have literally changed direction i.e. from *receiving* the environment into our consciousness to acting into it and placing meaning *into* all phenomena. An explanation is our relationship with solid objects as the only reality. Bergson (1911) recognised this when he wrote

'that the human intellect feels at home among inanimate objects, more especially among solids, where our action finds its fulcrum and our industry its tools; that our concepts have been formed on the models of solids; that our logic is, pre-eminently, the logic of solids; that, consequently, our intellect triumphs in geometry, wherein is revealed the kinship of logical thought with unorganised matter, and where the intellect has only to follow its natural movement, after the lightest possible contact with experience, in order to go from discovery to discovery, sure that experience is following behind it and will justify it invariably.'

Form and function

'This separation between a pre-established structure and processes occurring in that structure does not apply to living organisms. For the organism is the expression of an everlasting orderly process. What is described in morphology as organic forms and structures, is in reality a momentary cross-section through a spatio-temporal pattern. What are called structures are slow patterns of long duration, functions are quick processes of short duration.'

Ludwig von Bertalanffy (1952)

In describing the phenomenology of form through the written word we immediately encounter the problem of abstraction. Words are abstractions and they force upon us a starting and finishing point that is unnatural in the expression of form. All starting and finishing points are artificial. Realisation of this disturbance is paramount if the reader is to let the human form 'speak' without placing too much of the individual's meaning into the phenomenon. As a starting point we can begin with the head and then an individual can see from as many different directions as there are people. Allen (1956) reminds us that A.T. Still understood this way of seeing.

'Still's centre of interest was man, whom he observed keenly and at first hand, without the bias or prejudice of preconceived ideas, nor was he influenced by what others thought they saw or believed. This is evident time and time again in what he has written. He saw man, too, as the perfect product of an Infinite Maker, and this has a direct and practical bearing upon his work, because it meant that he recognised that man's knowledge of man, however great, ends at the edge of the great unknown. This unknown beckoned his inquisitive mind onward and humbled him with a sense of littleness of what he knew. He knew that man, the whole, can never be only the sum of his measurable parts.'

This is consistent with Goethe's seeing the human being as the most exact scientific instrument. This contradicts what most contemporary scientists take for granted, and runs counter to the whole way in which science has been practised in modern times. Without the development of ever more refined and sophisticated non-human instruments, most of the advances in modern scientific knowledge simply would not have occurred. Why, then, should Goethe insist that the human being is the most exact instrument? As with Still, Goethe realised the phenomenon of Galileo's primary and secondary qualities. Only the human being can practise sensing the primary qualities and this takes instruction and time; he wanted to see the phenomenon as it was, not doubled and distorted with symbols and instruments. We have not mastered that which nature has endowed us.

The human form

Still, in his *Philosophy of Osteopathy* (1899), brought forward his concept of basic body division. This division separated the body into three:

'I have formulated a simple mental diagram that divides the body into three parts, chest, upper and lower limbs. The first division takes in head, neck, chest, abdomen and pelvis. The second division takes in head, neck, lower and upper arm and hand. The third division takes in foot, leg, thigh, pelvis and lumbar vertebra. I make this division for the purpose of holding the explorer to the limits of all supplies. In the ellipse of the chest is found all vital supplies; then from that centre of life we have two branches only, one of the arm, and one of the lower limb.'

Schad (1977) also described the human organism as *three-fold*. He pondered over questions about the physicalness of the human organism, asking whether it is an autonomous system, independent of the environment, or whether it is identical with environmental processes and laws. Our initial impression of the human is that we see a head, trunk and limbs, with the head at the highest point above the trunk and the base of the limbs attached to the trunk. We shall primarily consider the physical components; the other and complementary aspect is the function or physiology of the systems. As we shall see these aspects are one and the same.

A three-fold approach in its most basic form is the classification of the external expression into the environment of human form. These characteristics were originally grouped into four types:

- leptosome (slender type)
- athletic (competitive type)
- pyknic (corpulent)
- dysplastic (underdeveloped type).

Today we categorise the expression of man into W.H. Sheldon's three basic groups:

- *ectomorph*: generally tall, slim, delicate with a long neck, long fingers, narrow long feet and head dominant
- *mesomorph*: tends to be strong, athletic, proportioned and chest dominant
- *endomorph*: represents the old pyknic type; short in stature, with a short neck and abdomen dominant.

Littlejohn in his *Psycho-physiology* (1899) stated that Still's use of the word *machine* was not intended to be the same as a car or train. A Stillian approach is to understand that the human body and its expression should be considered as a mechanism because we are not dealing with nature directly but the interaction of matter. Matter is unified as an expression of nature and is presented in an environmentally interactive form. The human mechanism is the movement and relationship of that form from a micro- to a macro-level. Each part reflects the whole at all times, and all parts react to every other part at the same instant. The creations of man, while deadly and beneficial, are illusions created by the manipulation of matter, not nature. Hence they need maintenance and can also fall down, crash and explode.

Still continued from his *Philosophy of Osteopathy*:

'An organism and its environment are one, just as the parts and activities of the organism are one, in the sense that though we can distinguish them we cannot separate them unaltered, and consequently cannot understand or investigate one apart from the rest. It is literally true of life and no mere metaphor, that the whole is in each moment of the present. Organic wholeness covers both space and time, and in the light of biological fact absolute space and time, and self-existent matter and energy, are but abstractions from our partial aspects of reality.

Structure, composition and activity are inseparably blended together in life, and no phenomena in the organic world seem to us to be similar to the phenomenon of life. The fundamental facts with regard to life do not fit into the conceptions by means of which we at present interpret inorganic phenomena.

Life is something which the biologist as such must treat as a primary reality, and no mere artefact.'

Of major importance to Still is the Goethean middle (cavity) system of the body. This, you will see below, was demonstrated by Schad as the reciprocal action of the cardiorespiratory system. Breathing is central to the Stillian expression of health. The following quotation, cited in Frost (1918), is from Still's *Research and Practice* and demonstrates the importance he placed upon the lung as a functioning unit.

'The lung is one of the highest functionaries of the whole system. According to every method of reasoning the lung comes in as the Great I AM of living blood. As a philosopher who is able to reason you will see that the garden, the fountain of life, is the lung and that every atom of arterial blood is sent forth as ripe seed grown in the garden of life, the lungs.'

The similarities between Still's understanding and that of J.S. Haldane, the English physiologist, were very close if not the same; they could easily have been written by the same man. Still continues in his *Research and Practice*:

'All the organs of the system are subject to general laws of supply and action, and these laws extended to all parts of the system separately or combined; as much as so as earth is subject to sunlight and darkness. All organs and parts of the human body are the subjects of one general law of demand, supply, construction and renovation in order to keep up normal functionings.'

Seeing human form

We should be reminded that earlier we introduced the difficulty of an organised presentation of nature with the use of words. Again there is no particular starting or finishing point in nature, it is non-linear and outwith cause and effect.

In the mature human form we immediately see an upright and forward facing animal. Axially it comprises three main body cavities, the head, thorax and abdomen. We shall consider the pelvic contents as the lower part of the abdomen. The head is above the rest of the body representing its highest point in a case of which the bones have little relative movement to each other. The biology of form and the appreciation of three-foldness can begin with the comparative mammalian anatomy of the teeth. The most unspecialised teeth are those of man and it is from this point that all other teeth can be seen in a more specialised way. Unlike other mammals, man is not dominated by any particular dentition. Respiration and digestion begin in the head in relative immobility becoming more active as they descend into the thoracic and abdominal cavities. Food, for example, begins its digestion in the mouth in the form of a substance that is useless to the body and therefore has to be converted by the body into that which can be assimilated into body processes. Comparative anatomy is only the beginning of an appreciation of human anatomy. If human anatomy is considered on its own it has little relevance to any sense of holism. This dominance of the head keeps the organism's goal in sight and is the centre for the sense organs: sight, hearing, balance, smell and taste. It can be considered the centre of the *nerve–sense* system.

Moving downwards we see that the top of the neck is narrower than the base and gives way to the thorax. At once we are aware of the position of the clavicles at the base of the neck and the top of the thorax. These horizontal bones ossify before any other bone in condensed mesenchyme. They represent a legacy of the head in the upper thorax, as they are the only bones of membranous origin outside the head region. Moving centrally we see the stenoclavicular joints which are the only skeletal communication of the upper limbs to the axis of the body. In comparison to the head, the trunk and limbs display a far greater amount of physical and metabolic activity.

The upper ribs of the thorax are small, sturdy and close together. It can be said that they are ascending and closing to form the complete closed structure of the cranium. As we descend the thoracic cage the upper ribs become further apart, longer and thinner, initially attaching at their front individually to the sternum. They then attach to themselves at the front leaving the last two pairs of ribs holding back and floating. We can say that the thorax opens at its lower end to give way to the abdomen. Within the thorax are the heart and lungs. We can consider this region as the *respiratory–circulatory* system.

The abdomen has no bony protection. This is a dominantly soft tissue cavity, in fact any ossification in the abdomen tends to cause a functional disturbance. The abdominal cavity is intensely metabolic rather than 'physical', the cranium being the boniest, most secure and most physical of the cavities. Metabolism within the abdomen is closely related to limb function and activity. Korr (1991) reminds us that the myofascioskeletal system produces the most waste and uses more energy than any other system in the body involving all three cavities; particularly the abdomen. This, the last of the three cavities, can be considered the *metabolic– limb* system.

Being the largest of the three cavities, the abdomen takes in food, as foreign material, at one end and with intense metabolic activity converts it into 'human substance'. This resultant metabolic activity in relation to the demands of the myofascioskeletal system allows a human to maintain a high degree of independence within the environment. Mistakes are often made when the cavities are thought to be parallel or beside one another. They are within one another, sharing common systems while possessing their own dominant system. The thorax and abdomen can be seen as the most important cavities of the body in maintaining a greater degree of autonomy from the environment.

Therefore we have three cavities; the cranial cavity is completely surrounded by bone, the thoracic is partially surrounded while the abdominal is free of bone. Any hardening within these cavities is generally indicative of pathology, especially in the abdomen. All the cavities have limbs, i.e. parts that are able to manipulate objects in the outside world; flat bones and broad muscles accompany the attachments of these limbs to the cavities. Goethe considered the limb of the cranial cavity to be the lower jaw, with its flat temporal bone and the temporalis muscle. The thorax has the upper limbs, the flat shoulder blade and the rotator cuff and pectoral muscles; and the abdomen has the lower limbs with the flat bones of the iliac-pelvis and the gluteal muscles. Bones of the cavities are close to the surface of the skin seemingly containing and protecting the structures within. These bones ossify only when the internal soft tissues they contain have matured. Latey (1983) showed an osteopathic understanding of this relationship:

'Careful inspection of the side of a well preserved skull will usually reveal that the parieto-temporal suture is supplied with a set of powerful supporting and checking ligaments. These are arranged along the back half of the suture, getting larger, stronger and longer towards the posterior end. They do not cross the outer margin of the temporalis muscle, but, from their origins on the parietal bone, are inserted into the sutural edge of the temporal bone; with very few fibres crossing onto the surface of the temporal bone. It seems obvious that this is a joint, not a suture, permitting some sliding, swivelling, locking and swinging; transmitting very high musculoskeletal forces during muscular activity. The parieto-temporal, therefore, has several close and exact parallel functions with the sacro-iliac joint. One of these parallels is the difficulty in learning the palpatory "feel" of the joint in springing/torsion diagnostic manoeuvres.

'We are used to analysing the musculoskeletal stress patterns of the pelvic girdle and the shoulder girdle. The cranio-orofacial girdle is easily analysed in the same way thus:

Hip	Temporomandibular joint
Sacroiliac joint	Parietotemporal joint
Three gluteal muscles	Temporalis muscle
Quadriceps femoris	Masseter
Hamstrings	Pterygoids
(Toenails)	(Teeth)

'The longer groups of temporalis fibres cross the joint – just as the gluteus maximus crosses the sacroiliac. Temporalis acts within two extremely tough layers of fascia and is very sensitive to pressure: the gluteus medius and tensor fascia lata have many other similarities and will encourage more detailed investigations and analysis from other anatomists and osteopaths.'

Limbs are considered to be polaric to the body cavities. The limb's bones, for example, are deep within the soft tissues, becoming the internal structures of the limbs; in the cavity they are outside the structures. Limbs are highly metabolic, drawing from the abdomen and affecting all cavities in the process of waste removal especially during submaximal and maximal activity. Eventually the limbs continue into the environment 'breaking down' into an increasing number of smaller bones, muscles, nerves, and blood vessels as the human organism tapers into its environment (as opposed to the head, generally round in shape with flat bones, which does not taper). The head makes up for this by containing many differing tapering and therefore sensitive structures; tongue, nose, ears and even eyelashes.

One of the most important areas of anatomy for Goethe was the musculoskeletal system. In particular it led him to the discovery of the intermaxillary bone, which upset the long held belief that man was different from, and had no link with, other animals especially apes. This finding is consistent with Stillian philosophy where there is an underlying unity in animal forms. Goethe came to the conclusion that 'no individual human or mammal can be the pattern of the whole'. It was this *no-thing* that he termed the *archetype of forms*. This applies to plants and therefore expands to all material expressions of nature. Other holistic biologists such as Bölsche (1955) and Schad (1977) developed Goethe's idea, coming to the conclusion that no single skeletal system represents the whole; they are all expressions in the environment. Miller (1995) translated many of Goethe's works and found that he had developed an unparalleled understanding of comparative anatomy, especially of human osteology. Goethe wrote, 'the skeletal structure is the clear framework for all forms'. Holdrege (1998) shows clear direction when he says in the final part of his work

'The skeleton is my point of departure in considering the whole through its parts. The skeleton is the most definitely formed structure in an animal. It resists decomposition when the animal dies and can then be studied as a clearly formed memory of the whole. In penetrating this memory, the whole can come to life in us. I focus primarily on the limbs and skull – those parts of the body through which the animal, in movement and perception, relates most directly to its surroundings, thereby meeting and making its environment.'

Schad (1977) developed Goethe's method of understanding form when he wrote:

'In life, causes and effects take place simultaneously and complement one another. For this reason the organism always presents itself as a whole. Correlations, not causes and aims, determine the order of the life that forms a single whole, because life exists only as a continuing present.

The process of life, therefore, cannot be understood by either causal or teleological ways of thinking; they must be discovered as an active connection existing necessarily among phenomena in the present. It follows from this basic discovery that in trying to understand an animal, we must take form as the main thing the animal can tell us about itself. For form is simply the way any living being reveals to us its present order in space. ...We can keep a stone in a box and it will not change for centuries unless external factors act upon it. A living animal, however, cannot be preserved unchanged.'

Vibration, rhythm and motion

'Breathing is a form of motion, and it is the primary impetus that brings us into existence. Without a full, easy breath, no one can sustain a healthy life. More than an exchange of gases, breath has implications and consequences for the material, mental and spiritual planes of human existence.'

Robert Fulford, DO

Rhythmicity and motion occur within all the cavities and their relationship is reciprocal. The most rhythmic and the primary motion area of the cavities is the thoracic region. Rhythmicity and motion continues into the abdomen or meta-bolic–limb system and to a lesser degree into the head or nerve–sense system. A reciprocal rhythmicity occurs between the lungs and heart in the higher portion of the thorax, a 1:4 ratio respectively. This is still apparent and decreases as it ascends to the bonier skull resulting in a rhythm of between 6 to 12 cycles per minute. Descending the thorax the rib cage flares and opens, rapidly losing the rhythmicity. Abdominal motion is maintained through the enteric domain of the sympathetic nervous system, exhibiting a large degree of neurological indepen-dence from the brain and spinal cord. Additionally this gives way to the motion of the abdomen with the action of the diaphragm as a gross mover. Reducing rhythmicity and motion in man to a Newtonian–Cartesian construct, i.e. making similarities with, or substituting, mathematics and physics, in any way diminishes the ability to see form. Scientific and mathematical modes of consciousness are abstractions and can never reflect the whole in their parts.

Even though rhythmicity and motion are primarily observed in the thorax we can observe and palpate the effects all over the body. A less obvious rhythm and motion is that of the nervous system. As we have mentioned the nerve–sense centre is located within the head. In addition there is the *nerve–nutrition* system which is otherwise known as the *autonomic nervous* system. The autonomic nervous system is artificially split into the *sympathetic, parasympathetic* and *enteric nervous* systems. To understand rhythm and motion in particular, we have to pay some attention to the sympathetic and enteric nervous systems. Both these systems could be considered as divisions of the same system. They can be grouped as representing the sympathetic domain of the autonomic nervous system.

Robinson (1907) recognised this nerve-nutrition area of man and its role in rhythm within the entire organism. Robinson wrote:

'In mammals there exist two brains of almost equal importance to the indivi-duals and race. One is the cranial brain, the instrument of volitions of mental progress and physical protection. The other is the abdominal brain, the instrument of vascular and visceral function. It is automatic, vegetative, the subconscious brain of physical existence. In the cranial brain resides the consciousness of right and wrong. Here is the seat of all progress, mental and moral, and in it lies the instinct to protect life and the fear of death. However, in the abdomen there exists a brain of wonderful power maintaining eternal, restless viligance over its viscera. It presides over organic life. It dominates the rhythmical function of viscera. It is an autonomic nerve centre, a physiological and an anatomic brain. Being located at the origin of the coeliac, superior mesenteric, and renal arteries – the major abdominal visceral arteries – it is a primary vascular brain of the abdomen and a secondary brain of the visceral rhythm.'

As we shall see in the anatomy section, the ganglia, as the major driving force of the autonomic nervous system, orchestrate the role of reciprocal rhythm within the cavities into and from the limbs. Motor and sensory nerves run parallel with or traverse structures in the body. Sympathetic domain nerves form plexuses around structures, in particular the arterial vessels and gut. The vasoconstriction and vasodilatation of vascular structures is reciprocal with sympathetic nerve function. Rhythm is inherent in all cells and systems.

Robinson continues

'The abdominal brain is a receiver, a reorganiser, an emitter of nerve forces. It has the powers of a brain. It is a reflex centre in health and disease. The sympathetic abdominal nerve alone possesses the power of rhythm. Every organ possesses rhythm.

'The abdominal brain is not a mere agent of the brain and cord; it receives and generates nerve forces itself; it presides over nutrition. It is the centre of life itself. The abdominal brain can live without the cranial brain, which is demonstrated by living children born without a cerebrospinal axis.'

Rhythm and motion within all cavities have a common denominator, that of the sympathetic vasomotor system. This is the nerve–vascular communication between all cavities and its reciprocal relationship is vital for health. No cavity or its contents, unlike other mammals, dominates man; so the reciprocity of cavity function within each other should always be considered in health. Disturbance of rhythm and therefore motion is reflected in the matter and motion of the human form. As we shall see the vasomotor system or sympathetic domain of the autonomic nervous system imparts motion into all systems and cavities, including the central nervous system i.e. brain, spinal cord and coverings.

Charlotte Weaver, DO (1938), combined an understanding of rhythm and three-foldness in the human form, consistent with Goethe and Schad. Weaver was without doubt one of the greatest osteopathic physicians in a true osteopathic context of wholeness and its understanding of human form. The following can only be reproduced in its complete form when she wrote

'Throughout my entire research into certain heretofore unexplored functions of the central nervous system, I have been impressed with a sense of rhythmicity in the recurrence of certain structural arrangements in those progressive transmutational processes through which the unicellular zygote evolves into the mature human organism.

'Out of this growing sense of rhymicity in recurrence of certain structural arrangements grew a constant question in my mind as to what this rhythmicity might be, and why. And gradually I became able to formulate into words the law that:

(1)   the basic structural patterning of the human organism in each transient phylogenic stage of its evolvement is a *triadic* [emphasis added] arrangement in space of its contained materials, that is, of its chemo-synthetic materials, its vibratosynthetic materials, and those materials which accrue within the organism as the result of its own autochthonous integration of these two types of evolving forms of energy;

(2)   the fact that this is true because the human organism is a dynamic mechanism specifically evolved for the reception of

(a)   those certain, definite, evolutionally prepared chemical energy forms which are the chemical components of sea water, the chemical components of air, and the biochemical components of neutral fats, monosaccharid carbohydrates, and nucleoproteids, and

(b)   of those certain, definite, evolutionally prepared vibratory energy forms which are known by some under the broader, more comprehensive meaning of the term "heat", by others under the broader, more comprehensive meaning of the term "light", by others as "ether waves", and by others variously, and which the following table clarifies by giving numbers of vibrations per second in an ascending scale which is "foot-ruled" into contiguous segments by the respective gamuts of the various specific vibratoceptors of the human organism; for the transformation of these received energy forms into certain, other, definite types of energy forms which are of a higher evolutional order than are the received forms; for the integration into definite potentials of the newly achieved types; and for the subsequent adequate release of the energies so received, so transformed, and so integrated;

(3)   the law that this transformation and integration and subsequent adequate expression of its received evolving energy forms is achieved in the human organism by means of arranging them into a structural pattern which is internal to the organism and which arrangement is always such as to

(a) insure spatial regulation of those energy forms which the organism has selectively received while they are undergoing their processes of transformation and integration within the organism, and

(b) to make certain the possibility of controllable release of the transmuted energies;

(4) the law that in each transient ontogenetic stage of the organism these integrated energies are released in two specific ways which are the same for all stages, i.e.,

(a) in behaviourism, including growth, of the organism as it exists in each transient metamorphosis, and

(b) in the evolvement of the next new phylogenetic transformation of the next new phylogenetic transmutation of the organism;

(5) the law that in each stage

(a) the autochthonously integrated materials lie between the chemosynthetic and the vibrosynthetic materials,

(b) the vibrosynthetic materials lie in that portion of the organism which in the average posture of the organism is farthest away from the centre of gravity of the earth, and

(c) the chemosynthetic materials lie in that portion which, of the *three* [emphasis added], is nearest to the centre of gravity of the earth, this because of their comparative specific gravities;

(6) the law that in each transient stage the next transmutational form arises between the vibratosynthetic area and the integrating area;

(7) the law that integration in the organism is achieved at the expense of its contained energy forms, is reciprocally integrated by the chemosynthetic and the vibrasynthetic energy forms, but progresses under the dominance of its received vibratosynthetic energy forms;

(8) the law that each new transient transformation of the organism is achieved by means of a new *triadic* [emphasis added] arrangement in space of the materials which the organism will in that particular stage further fabricate;

(9) the fact that there are at least five distinct transmutational human forms up to and including the current neonatal form, and probably quite a few more:

(10) the fact that the current human adult form adheres to the laws governing structure and function of all earlier transient transmutational stages in that its structure is the result of a *triadic* [emphasis added] arrangement in space of its contained materials, and that its final energy-potential is expressed in behaviourism including growth and the achievement of its next transmutational form;

(11) the suggestion that the nature of the currently newly evolving transmutational form is deducible;

(12) the law that throughout the entire progress of the evolving organism the

final perfection of each, next, newly evolving transmutational form is absolutely dependent upon the structural integrity of the then current form;

(13)   the fact that these five successfully evolved transient forms are the zygote, the *triconcentric* [emphasis added] membranous embryo, the bilayered "embryonal area" with its autochthonously generated third or middle layer, the longitudinalised embryo in its morphologically *triregionalised* [emphasis added] status, and the segmented embryo.

'Applying these deduced laws and ascertained facts to the current adult human organism, the following facts are brought out:

(1)   The derivatives of the gut tube are the representatives in the adult organism of the chemosynthetic layer of the "embryonal area" which is formed in the triconcentric membranous embryo:

(2)   the derivatives of the neural tube are representatives in the adult organism of the vibratosynthetic layer of the "embryonal area";

(3)   the total so-called connective tissue system of the adult human organism represents the integrating layer, i.e., the mesoblast, that middle layer which is generated autochthonously by the proliferating cells of the vibratosynthetic layer as they come to lie within the colloid which is generated by the cells of the chemosynthetic layer of the "embryonal area";

(4)   the next stage after the formation of the "embryonal area", that is, the stage of polarisation, divides the "embryonal area" transversely into *three* [emphasis added] longitudinal divisions which I have termed the *cephalic, precaudal* and *caudal* [emphasis added] morphological developmental regions of the longitudinalising organism. Of these three morphological polarisation regions the following facts are notable, that is, in the cephalic region the vibratosynthetic layer is dominant, in the precaudal region the integrating layer is dominant, the caudal region attenuates and displays a tendency to disappear phylogenetically.

'In applying these deduced laws still further: In the cephalic one of the *three* [emphasis added] morphological polarisation regions again this *triadicity* [emphasis added] is evinced in the evolvement of the *three* [emphasis added] cephalic segments. In the neural tube these segments are realised in the *prosencephalon*, the *mesencephalon* [emphasis added], and the *rhombencephalon* [emphasis added] respectively. In the cephalic mesodermal tissues they are evidenced in the *three* [emphasis added] cephalic vertebrae. And, also, here again in the cephalic, one of the morphological polarisation regions the laws of structure and function apply. The interrelationship of the prosencephalon and vibratosynthesis are integrated in the mesencephalon. The next metamorphosis of the human organism will transpire between superior border of the mesencephalon and the adjoining border of the prosencephalon. This will transpire under the dominance of the vibratosynthetic functions.'

The external relationship of humankind

An external consideration of man brings into play the myofascioskeletal system and its direct relationship to itself, and to its internal and external environments. Immediately we are struck by the symmetry of the myofascioskeletal system in its relationship to the environment. As we have mentioned, each cavity contains a set of limbs. This expresses the symmetry even further. Muscle around the cavities tends to be flat and broad and the bone can be palpated easily through this tissue. Limb muscle around the limbs becomes greater as we descend from the jaw to the lower extremities and it is also voluntary as opposed to internal muscle which is structurally different and involuntary. The fact that certain cultures can alter their gut motility shows that no system is entirely independent of the intention of the organism. Contrary to popular belief the majority of voluntary muscle is in communication and forms a structural blending and physiological dependence with fascia rather than primarily with bone. Joints provide pivot points around which the myofascioskeletal system can express flexibility. Structures that are moved by voluntary muscle are encased in this highly metabolic tissue and muscles do not move structures outside of themselves. This is consistent with internal muscle actions.

All the limbs and systems of man are underdeveloped, even considered imperfect, compared to other mammals when viewed in isolation. The teeth can be considered the nails of the mouth; finger and toe nails are flat, delicate and practically useless. The mouth, hands and feet are not used for any particular purpose; they cannot shovel, paddle or grip very well. The jaw of the infant and its supportive myofascial structure are the first to develop, followed by the upper limb and then the lower limb. Babies will place objects in their mouths as soon as the upper limbs can manipulate. This is comparable with the fully developed primates who will still use the mouth to manipulate the environment. As the mouth of man begins to be released from the need to manipulate the environment it makes its contribution to communication. In comparison to other primates our jaw bone is held back; not protruding too far beyond the face.

Returning to the clavicles; it has been noted that horses and cats do not have clavicles. Orthopaedically this absence in some mammals has been accredited to the flexion and extension actions of the forelimbs. No limb, at its cavity base, works entirely in flexion and extension. Comparing man with these other mammals, the base bone, in man the humerus, is the longest of the upper limb bones. In the cat and horse it is short in comparison to the entire limb. The human limb begins by expression into the environment and the mammal begins by holding back, later to express into the environment as one toe, in the case of the horse. This shortening at the beginning of expression is vital for speed of movement. In man the entire upper limb is held back and very much shorter than the lower limb; this expresses the upper limbs' independence from the environment.

Man's limbs grow out into the environment, therefore the base of all the limbs is attached to the flat bones and supportive musculature mentioned earlier. As the muscles extend into the environment they become longer initially, only to increase in number and become shorter in length. Mid-limb muscles increase in tendon length, terminating in the fingers accompanied by very short muscles. This seems to express a combination of power and delicacy. In addition to the muscles increasing in number there is a reciprocal increase in the number and size of the bones. Here the human form is 'breaking down' into the environment in its most fragile expression. The finest expression of this is, for example, in the hands of a pianist.

Similar principles apply to the lower limb. The major difference is the dominance of the lower limbs' function with locomotion under the influence with gravity. In man this dominance of the lower limb releases the upper limb to manipulate objects within the environment. In mammals the most adaptive difference is the part of the peripheral limb closest to the environment. Again comparative anatomy is the only way to emphasise the observation. The femur, tibia and fibula of the horse are short in relation to the total limb length. Where the feet and toes of man are held back, those of the horse are expressed into the environment as one toe, the hoof. Humans stand on the same bones that horses have half way up their limbs. It seems comparatively that the more bones we have in contact with the ground the more variations in limb manipulation with the environment and the greater the movement over various types of terrain.

The upright posture of man is very special. Even our closest 'relatives' have trouble standing for any length of time. What would have happened to man without this upright posture? This special relationship has allowed us to express ourselves into our environment. The upright posture has to be one of the greatest factors in our freedom as an animal allowing us to express ourselves between the sky and surface of the earth.

Seeing man as whole we realise that every part is a 'reflection' of all other parts, in a physico-functional manner. By this it is meant that the hands and fingers, for example, have a certain width and length, respectively. If the hands were more shovel like and the fingers were more tapered then the food we ate and the tools we could use would be different. The food we could eat would have a profound effect of the arrangement of our teeth and the size and tapering of our feet and toes, and this in turn would have a profound effect on the terrain we could cover to catch or gather that food. Teeth arrangements would change our oro-facial features with a relative difference in our jaw width and length altering the shape of our nose and the position of the eyes. This can change our limb lengths, chest depth, etc. The changes are infinite and reciprocal for the survival of any species.

The internal form of humankind

Initially the overall arrangement of the internal form is polar to that of the myofascioskeletal system, it is asymmetrical. The only symmetrical system is the nervous system which is primarily related to the myofascioskeletal system. Beginning in the face we see the start of the processes of breathing and digestion. Both travel and function into the head turning downwards into the thorax via the neck. The lungs fill the thorax and stop whereas the digestive tract passes through the thorax, without any sign of altering form until it enters the abdominal cavity. On continuing into the abdominal cavity the gut comes into its own, expanding and forming an orderly twisting. It gives the impression of stalling its journey towards the exit at the bottom of the cavity; it is as if it knows it needs to 'waste some time'.

In the thorax the lungs intertwine with the heart and its great vessels. From the heart the aorta ascends and quickly changes direction to enter the abdominal cavity giving off branches to the head and upper limbs on the way down. It is in the abdominal cavity that the largest blood vessels form. The heart itself is slightly on the left of centre complementing the two lung fields on the left as opposed to the three lung fields on the right. This demonstrates reciprocity of form of the respiratory-circulatory system, where the cardiovascular system takes over from the respiratory supplying and removing metabolic products from the organism.

References

Allen, P. van B. (1956) Man, challenge to osteopathy, yesterday, today and tomorrow. JAOA Oct, 103–7.

Bergson, H. (1911) *Creative Evolution.* Translated by Arthur Mitchell. Henry Holt & Co., New York and Macmillan, London.

Bölsche, W. (1955) *Das Liebesleben in der Natur.* Fackelträger-verlag, Hanover.

Bortoft, H. (1996) *The Wholeness of Nature: Goethe's Way of Science.* Floris Books, Edinburgh.

Cromer, A. (1995) *Uncommon Sense: The Heretical Nature of Science.* Oxford University Press, Oxford.

Frost, H.P. (1918) Biological philosophy. *The Journal of the American Osteopathic Association,* 18(2) 78–80.

Holdrege, C. (1998) Seeing the animal whole. In *Goethe's Way of Science: A Phenomenology of Nature.* Eds D. Seamon and A. Zajonc. Chapter 9, pp. 213–32. State University of New York Press, New York.

Korr, I.M. (1991) Osteopathic research: the needed paradigm shift. *The Journal of the American Osteopathic Association,* February 99, 156–71.

Latey, P. (1983) *Structural Technique and the Cranium.* British School of Osteopathy Library, London.

Littlejohn, J.M. (1899) *Lectures on Psycho-physiology* G.G. Kinney, Kirksville, MI.

Miller, D. (ed) (1995) *Goethe: The Collected Works, Scientific Studies Vol. 12.* Edited and translated by Douglas Miller. Princeton University Press, Princeton.

Reason, P. (1986) Innovative research techniques. *Complementary Medical Research.* 1(1) 23–9.

Robinson, B. (1907) *The Abdominal and Pelvic Brain: With Autonomic Visceral Ganglia.* Frank S. Betz, Hammond, IND.

Schad, W. (1977) *Man and Mammals: Toward a Biology of Form.* Translated by Carroll Scherer. Waldorf Press, New York.

Weaver, C. (1938) The three primary brain vesicles and the three cranial vertebrae: III. The prosencephalon and the mesencephalon. *The Journal of the American Osteopathic Association,* June 37(10) 454–9.

Further reading

Fulford, R.C. (1996) *Dr. Fulford's Touch of Life: The Healing Power of the Natural Life Force.* Pocket Books, New York.

Kranich, E-M. (1999) *Thinking Beyond Darwin: The Idea of the Type as a Key to Vertebrate Evolution.* Lindisfarne Books, New York.

Kuriyama, S. (1999*) The Expressiveness of the Body and the Divergence of Greek and Chinese Medicine.* Zone Books, New York.

Schad, W. (ed.) (1982) *Goetheanistische Naturwissenschaft: Allgemeine Biologie.* Book 1. Verlag Freies Geistesleben, Stuttgart.

Schad, W. (ed.) (1982) *Goetheanistische Naturwissenschaft: Botanik.* Book 2. Verlag Freies Geistesleben, Stuttgart.

Schad, W. (ed.) (1982) *Goetheanistische Naturwissenschaft: Zoologie.* Book 3. Verlag Freies Geistesleben, Stuttgart.

Schad, W. (ed.) (1982) *Goetheanistische Naturwissenschaft: Anthropologie.* Book 4. Verlag Freies Geistesleben, Stuttgart.

Thompson, D. (1997) *On Growth and Form.* Canto (Cambridge University Press), Cambridge.

Weaver, C. (1938) The three primary brain vesicles and the three cranial vertebrae: I. The three primary brain vesicles. *The Journal of the American Osteopathic Association,* April 37(8) 345–50.

Weaver, C. (1938) The three primary brain vesicles and the three cranial vertebrae: II. The rhombencephalon. *The Journal of the American Osteopathic Association,* May 37(9) 402–9.

Weaver, C. (1936) The cranial vertebrae. *The Journal of the American Osteopathic Association,* March 35(7) 328–36.

Weaver, C. (1936) The cranial vertebrae. Part II. *The Journal of the American Osteopathic Association,* April 35(8) 374–9.

CHAPTER 5

Principles

The *Oxford English Dictionary* defines a principle as the following 'A funda-mental source from which something proceeds; a primary element, force, or law which produces or determines particular results; the ultimate basis upon which the existence of something depends; cause, in the widest sense.'

Basic osteopathic principles

There are five basic principles on which osteopathic practice is based.

(1) The body is an integral unit, a whole. The structure of the body and its functions are inter-related, and rely one on the other, for optimal health. To restore a body to a balance called health, requires treatment of the whole body, not just one part, for each part has a relationship to the rest of the body. Proper balance among the parts means health, while improper bal-ance can mean susceptibility to disease and illness.

(2) The body's systems have built-in repair processes which are self-regulat-ing and self-healing in the face of disease. The most obvious example is how the body reacts, diagnoses, and treats a break in the skin. From the initial opening to the eventual sloughing off of the final scab, and even after, the body is treating itself. Though an over-simplistic example, the principle is appropriate both for small and large health problems. According to the principles of Hippocrates, the measures

which aid the natural processes are the appropriate ones, and Still does not demur from this in any way.

(3) The circulatory system or distributing channels of the body, along with the nervous system, provide the integrating functions for the rest of the body. This is included for the sake of historical accuracy, and is usually described in Still's often, perhaps too often quoted: 'The rule of the artery is supreme'.

(4) The contribution of the musculoskeletal system to a person's health is much more than merely providing framework and support and both its response and vulnerability to stress should always be prime considerations. Improper musculoskeletal functioning can have serious and far-reaching ramifications for the health of the individual.

(5) While disease may be manifested in specific parts of the body, other parts may contribute to a restoration or correction of the disease. When this is found, it is called *compensation* or *adaptation*, and if inefficient may lead to referred symptoms.

'Classical' osteopathic principles and practice

Let us now consider the original, or 'classical' principles of osteopathy, and place them in context.

(1) Classical osteopathic theory believes that within the body are found (except where genetic and congenital defects exist) all the necessary mechanisms for self-sufficiency i.e. that the inherent repetitive forces within the patient overcome disease and that the role of the osteopath/physician is to harness and direct those forces.

(2) In helping the patient adjust to the nature and condition of his environment (internal as well as external), the means employed to save life, relieve pain or palliate should be such as to minimally interrupt or superimpose upon these self-reparative, physiological mechanisms.

(3) The body's immune response is dependent upon an unimpeded transmission of blood, nerve and trophic impulses and a major and frequently overlooked factor contributing to their interruption is to be found in the aberrant function of some aspect of the musculoskeletal system. These somatic signs and symptoms may be detected in the dysfunction of body mechanics and are not only often manifestations of underlying disease but also important contributing and/or maintaining factors.

(4) In the presence of such dysfunction (*the osteopathic lesion*) the body's self-reparative mechanisms may be significantly retarded and disturbed. Our unique contribution to medicine is to be found, therefore, to be the degree to which we ameliorate or correct such dysfunction, in all conditions of ill health, including the psychological.

(5) The manual treatment we employ to correct such dysfunction takes account (other than in the acute condition) of the unity of the body in regard to its body framework no less than its internal physiology.

(6) Diagnosis is, therefore, so directed as to detect any possible tissue abnormality in terms of tone, tension, mobility, rhythm, elasticity, resistance, flexibility and extensibility. That treatment and 'correction' is not a physical process but a process of coordination. It is an attempt, often requiring the expenditure of much time, to co-relate the structural and functional activities of the body mechanism.

(7) Such treatment has nothing to do with pushing or thrusting bones from one place to another (as if dislocated), nor the rubbing or gouging of soft tissues and vertebral (or cranial) adjustment is not the priority. It is recognised that we are dealing with living tissue and that 'correction' is a change of functional activity requiring integration throughout the body if physical treatment is to be expected to be converted into a significant physiological response.

(8) Our techniques pay particular attention to the bones of the body because every mechanical operation in the articulations of the body has its terminal point in a bone. However, we are concerned to use methods whose leverage appeals to muscular and ligamentous activity as well as fascial conciliation as it moves on bone as one articular unit. Further, it is suggested, the long leverages employed by Still and his early disciples go furthest towards accomplishing this goal.

Naturally it has to be realised that time has moved on and the principles of osteopathy should always be interpreted in the light of the knowledge of the time, as the original principles were. This does not in any way mean that the above are wrong. Many practitioners and students may interpret the word principles in their own way. Therefore it is relatively easy to talk of the principles of osteopathy as, 'that which is practised by an osteopath'. The most consistent 'principles' stated by osteopaths are that

- the body is a unit
- there is a capacity towards self-healing or regulation, and
- the structure–function relationship.

Sprafka *et al.* (1981) remind us that,

'it might be contended that nothing is uniquely osteopathic about these ideas, which are fundamental biologic principles that have been understood and expanded for many years. In the purest sense, the assertion is undeniably true. It was not the intent of Andrew Taylor Still or his more scientific, less evangelistic followers to assert that osteopathy was in any way a violation or a reinterpretation of basic biologic and anatomic principles as they were understood at the time. What Still was trying to demonstrate was that osteopathic medicine had a clearer understanding of basic biological principles which he felt were not held by allopathic, homeopathic, naturopathic, or the eclectic schools of medicine. The intent was to shift the focus of medical care away from curing by various forms of intervention and toward an understanding and appreciation of mankind's natural ability to function in an environment'.

Still did not intend to create an alternative or complementary system but a reform of the system of medicine practised at the time.

The Principles of Andrew Taylor Still

'Our platform

It should be known where osteopathy stands and what it stands for. A political party has a platform that all may know its position in regard to matters of public importance, what it stands for and what principles it advocates. The osteopath should make his position just as clear to the public. He should let the public know, in his platform, what he advocates in his campaign against disease. Our position can be tersely stated in the following planks:

First: We believe in sanitation and hygiene.
Second: We are opposed to the use of serums in the treatment of disease. Nature furnishes its own serum if we know how to deliver them.
Third: We oppose vaccination.
Fourth: We realise that many cases require surgical treatment and therefore advocate it as a last resort. We believe many surgical operations are unnecessarily performed and that many operations can be avoided by osteopathic treatment.
Fifth: The osteopath does not depend on electricity, x-radiance, hydrotherapy or other adjuncts, but relies on osteopathic measures in the treatment of disease.
Sixth: We have a friendly feeling for other non-drug, natural methods of healing, but we do not incorporate any other methods into our system. We are all opposed to drugs; in that respect at least, all natural, unharmful methods occupy the same ground. The fundamental principles of osteopathy are different from those of any other system and the cause of disease is considered from one standpoint, viz: disease is the result of anatomical abnormalities followed by physiological discord. To cure disease the abnormal parts must be adjusted to the normal; therefore other methods that are entirely different in principles have no place in the osteopathic system.
Seventh: Osteopathy is an independent system and can be applied to all conditions of disease, including purely surgical cases, and in those cases surgery is but a branch of osteopathy.

Eighth: We believe that our therapeutic house is just large enough for osteopathy and that when other methods are brought in just that much osteopathy
must move out.'

Still (1910)

CHAPTER 6

The Nervous System

'A physical organism which would not self-limit its own intellectual progress must, perforce, be an organism which has evolved the possibility of a stable intrinsic long-distance control of prehension, adaptability, defence, aggression, and the like; in other words, an organism with a central nervous system.'

Charlotte Weaver, DO

The nervous system can be broadly considered as having two basic functions: impulse based and non-impulse based. These two basic functions and the further sectioning of the nervous system, as is shown below, are purely academic. Structurally and functionally the nervous system works as a whole at all times. Areas may show signs of adaptive change, structurally and functionally: this is known as *plasticity*. As a whole the nervous system shows symmetry in its overall form; this has been attributed to its relationship with the myofascioskeletal system.

A nerve or neurone (L. *nervus*: tendon, leader, rope like, sinew) was originally thought to be a pulley to make the muscle move in a mechanical fashion. Changes between the central and peripheral system are not sudden (Fraher and Bristol, 1990) as is the impression given by most textbooks. These structures vary in size and shape all over the body, forming webs, nets, and short and long cords of varying diameters.

IMPULSE BASED FUNCTION

The motor neurone pool

Healthy skeletal muscle is in constant communication with collections of nerves within the spinal cord and brain referred to as the motor neurone pool. As with all areas of nerve tissue there are no absolute boundaries to the beginning or end of these pools, rather they dissolve into other areas. Even within the same spinal cord segment, motor neurones connected with different muscle groups are mixed and it would be anatomically and physiologically incorrect to separate muscle groups clinically, especially when considering antagonistic and synergistic muscle groups (Lüscher and Claman, 1992).

The motor neurone pool can be divided into the upper motor neurone and the lower motor neurone. A simple classification is:

- the upper motor neurone (UMN) consists of the cerebral cortex and terminates at the spinal cord
- the lower motor neurone (LMN) receives information peripherally and centrally.

Peripheral information reaches the LMN via the cutaneous receptors (touch, pressure, pain, vibration and temperature) and the proprioceptors: muscle spindles (via Types Ia and II fibres), Golgi tendon organs (via Type Ib fibres) and joint proprioceptors. Proprioceptive information can be subdivided as below. Central input is from the descending tracts of the brain and includes the pyramidal tract (corticospinal) and the extrapyramidal tracts (reticuloendothelial, vestibulospinal, rubrospinal tectoaspinal and olivospinal).

Proprioceptive information from the periphery can be from *homonymous* muscles where the input is from the same muscle as that supplied by the motor neurones and with which they synapse directly, or *heteronymous* muscles which may be agonistic, synergistic or antagonistic.

The upper motor neurones

Upper motor neurones (UMNs) are those nerve cells of the motor system that originate from the fifth layer of the cortex. Fibres descend into the motor nuclei of the cranial nerves and the anterior horn cells of the spinal cord. Those fibres that continue to descend cross in the medulla oblongata passing to opposite sides of the spinal cord as the lateral corticospinal tracts. Not every descending fibre in the corticospinal tract crosses over; those that do not continue in the anterior corticospinal tract. The UMN system is otherwise collectively known as the *pyramidal system*. These descending fibres continue on to tell the lower motor neurones what to do. Damage of the pyramidal system leads to the general clinical features of weakness, *hemiparesis*, of the limbs on one side and weakness of both lower limbs, *paraparesis*.

The extrapyramidal tract

As the name suggests these are those structures outside of the pyramidal system, comprising the basal ganglia and the cerebellum. The extrapyramidal structures initiate and control motor activity. Damage to this system is classically seen in Parkinson's disease where there is slow or no movement combined with involuntary movements, tremors, and a rigidity of muscles.

The lower motor neurones

Lower motor neurones (LMNs) are present in the cranial nerve nuclei and the descending anterior horn cells of the spinal cord. The complete LMN unit comprises a single anterior horn cell, the alpha motor nerves which continue on to leave the spinal cord at the anterior root and then into the muscle fibres. The LMN unit is stimulated via the corticospinal tracts, the extrapyramidal system, and afferent fibres from the posterior region of the spinal cord.

Damage to the LMN or the anterior horn results in changes to those tissues supplied by the affected nerves. This leads to muscle weakness, trophic wasting, fasciculation, hypotonia, reflex disturbance related to nerves or spinal cord segment affected, contractures, fibrillation potentials and trophic changes in skin and nails.

Tracts and fibres of the motor and sensory systems

It must be understood that the naming of tracts and fibres of the nervous system generally depends on where the neurones start and finish. There is no breaking up of the nervous system. Confusion in both students and practitioners results when trying to understand the apparent movement of tracts and fibres as a named collection of separate areas. In general, textbooks are unintentionally misleading by giving the impression that one section of the nervous system is different from the next; the system is a whole.

Efferent (motor) output

Descending or corticospinal tracts represent the efferent or motor output system. Corticospinal tracts are a collective name for the fibres that descend from the cortex of both cerebral hemispheres and move down on either side of the spinal cord. Fibres leave the cortex and descend through the posterior crus of the internal capsule, cross the cerebral peduncle of the midbrain, the pons, the medulla oblongata and the form of the tract slows to represent a bundle of fibres in the pyramid. Form tells us that the bundle in the pyramid or hindbrain section means that the tissue is slowing down to perform a particular function. At this hindbrain–spinal junction at least 80% of the fibres move to the other side; this is known as the *pyramidal decussation*. After fibres of the left have crossed to the right and vice versa, they continue descending the cord as the *lateral corticospinal tract*. The remaining uncrossed fibres that continue to descend the spinal cord are known as the *anterior corticospinal tract*.

Returning to the upper end of the corticospinal tract, the name has become synonymous with pyramidal tracts. In this upper region certain fibres leave the pyramidal tracts earlier and go on to supply the motor nuclei of the cranial nerves, these are the *corticobulbar fibres*.

Tracts descend the spinal cord in a column or *funiculus*. Lateral corticospinal tract fibres travel in the *lateral funiculus* for most of the spinal cord reducing the number of fibres until they reach about the fourth sacral level. Anterior corticospinal tracts descend in the *anterior funiculus* and are smaller than their lateral relations. Some fibres from the anterior corticospinal tract cross to the other side of the spinal cord to spinal neurones in a region known as the *white commissure*. Generally corticospinal tracts end in spinal interneurons and connect directly with spinal cord motor neurones.

The efferent or motor system begins in the pyramidal and extrapyramidal areas of the brain. Pyramidal tracts, originating as part of the neocortex, descend uninterrupted towards the brain stem and then onto the spinal cord. The phylogenetically older extrapyramidal system has subcortical grey areas that, as a whole, are more complex than the pyramidal system. These systems meet as lower motor neurones in the motor nuclei of the cranial nerves and the spinal cord ventral grey horns.

The pyramidal motor system

Pyramidal motor fibres originate in the frontal and parietal lobes of the cortex. Called the *primary motor area*, it covers a region of the frontal lobe of the cerebral hemispheres known as the *precentral gyrus* and the anterior section of the *paracentral lobule* located on the lateral and medial surface of the hemispheres, respectively. In addition this area corresponds with area 4 in Brodmann's cytoarchitectural brain map, with less than half of the pyramidal motor fibres originating from this area. Stimulation of neurones in this area express their excitation in the muscles on the contralateral side.

Within the pyramidal system is the corticobulbar or corticonuclear tract. These tracts continue on to the midbrain giving off fibres to the oculomotor and trochlear nuclei. Corticobulbar fibres that give up fibres for the nuclei of cranial nerves that originate in the pons and medulla travel on the medial aspect of the corticospinal tract. The corticospinal tract as a whole continues on to the front of the pons and the pyramid of the medulla whereas the corticobulbar tract section, as mentioned, leaves at intervals supplying the motor nuclei of cranial nerves in the pons and medulla. These nuclei include the trigeminal, abducens, facial, glossopharyngeal, vagus, accessory and hypoglossal nerves. A large number of the corticobulbar fibres cross each other to the other side of the nervous system while enough fibres are present on the same side of hemispheric origin allowing for compensation in cases of paralysis.

Afferent (sensory) input

Afferent input begins in the receptors of the somatic structures of the skin, subcutaneous tissue, fasciae, muscles, tendons and joints. The unbroken route from the receptor along the axon of the sensory nerve is termed the first order neurone. These receptors in their particular tissues are generally unmyelinated free nerve endings.

Receptors include the following.

- Pacinian corpuscles are present in serous membranes, joints, tendons, periosteum, interosseous membrane, skin and subcutaneous tissue. Due to their deeper location they respond to pressure, vibration, and muscle-tendon-joint proprioception.
- Krause end bulbs and Ruffini terminals respond to skin stimulation, in particular the dermis rather than the epidermis..
- Merkel's corpuscles are disc shaped receptors present in the epidermis.
- Meissner's corpuscles are present in the dermal papillae of the palmar skin of fingers.

Neurones entering the spinal cord from their respective receptors ascend towards the brain. Those fibres that join the spinal cord at its lowest level are more centrally or medially situated on the posterior surface of the spinal cord. As the cord is ascended additional fibres move outwards laterally around the cord.

The most centrally situated in the posterior aspect of the cord is the *fasciculus gracilis*. As we move around the cord this gives way to the *fasciculus cuneatus*. Due to fasciculus gracilis being the most centrally and posteriorly located tract it is present at the lowest or earliest part of the ascending spinal cord sensory tracts. It contains fibres that originate from the coccygeal, sacral, lumbar and lower lumbar segments. As we ascend the cord the more lateral fasciculus cuneatus begins to appear at the level of the mid-thoracic spine. Fibres contributing to this fasciculus originate from the upper thoracic and cervical-thoracic levels.

Moving more laterally on the dorsal aspect of the spinal cord we encounter the posterior (dorsal) and anterior (ventral) spinocerebellar tracts. Both of these tracts are known to have first and second order neurone inputs. First order afferent neurones begin in the posterior or dorsal root ganglia from numerous end organs. Second order afferent neurons are post synapse first order neurons, the axons of which begin in the spinal cord and end in the palaeocerebellar cortex. First order neurones give way to second order neurones, generally inputting information from the trunk and limbs.

Posterior spinocerebellar fibres begin around the second to third lumbar segment. They receive input from muscle spindles, tendon organs and sensation receptors of pressure and touch. This posterior tract ascends on the same side as it enters the spinal cord as thick myelinated fibres in the posterior or dorsal white column. The tract moves towards the lateral white column as it ascends entering the inferior cerebellar peduncle which lies in the lateral aspect of the floor of the fourth ventricle. It continues on to the cerebellum terminating on the lateral cuneate nucleus of the medulla oblongata. The posterior spinocerebellar tract receives fibres only from the lower trunk and lower limb.

Like the posterior spinocerebellar tracts the anterior spinocerebellar tracts' first order neurones receive their inputs from the lower limb receptors of the Golgi tendon, skin and joints involved in flexor reflex responses. The second order neurones generally cross the cord and ascend in the lateral white column as the anterior spinocerebellar tract. It ascends to reach the upper pons and continues on to the superior cerebellar peduncle to enter the cerebellum. A large number of these fibres cross again to end in the cerebral cortex.

In a similar way as the spinocerebellar tracts input information from the trunk and limbs the trigeminocerebellar tract inputs information from the trigeminal region. This input ends in the palaeocerebellar cortex.

The majority of the input to the CNS from the myofascioskeletal system originates from every part of the body; this flow of information never stops. The input flow gives a continuous source of information that allows the entire body to make those second-by-second adjustments of which we are not conscious. The input routes are widespread while showing selectivity to certain areas of the nervous system; this includes both the central and peripheral nervous systems. With regard to the peripheral system, this includes the autonomic nervous system which makes adjustments to the circulation (vascular and lymphatic), metabolism and viscera, in response to the needs of the myofascioskeletal system.

Korr (1975) suggests that it is the afferent sensory input from the proprioceptors in soft tissues, particularly muscle spindles, that is the source of disturbances that lead to facilitation of the spinal cord. These aberrant (disturbing) impulses from all over the body are generally non-specific and subconscious. They have been termed sites of 'endogenous origin' that maintain the facilitated segments in their state. This we shall look at in further detail when considering the osteopathic lesion. The main source of the endogenous input would seem to be the muscle spindles, as they would be

- sensitive to myofascioskeletal stresses
- capable of continuing impulses even at rest
- specific to nerve, joint and muscle segmental units.

Lastly, nerves branch from descending trunks, also supplying muscles, periosteum and skin innervate joints; this is regularly forgotten in the clinical setting. These nerves comprise myelinated and unmyelinated sensory afferent fibres and unmyelinated efferent sympathetic postganglionic fibres (Gardner, 1944; Freeman and Wyke, 1967; Langford and Schmidt, 1983). Joint receptors from group II afferent nerves end in corpuscular endings known as Ruffini type endings and are present in an ordered fashion in the fibrous capsule. These give feedback about direction, position, motion and velocity of the limb.

The reflex arc

'My diagram treats the final common path as if it consisted of a single individual neurone. It is, of course, not so. The single neurone of the diagram stands for several thousands. It may be objected that in the various given actions these motorneurones are implicated in particular sets – one set in one action, one set in another. That view seems unlikely. In the scratch reflex, I think we can exclude it.'

Sir Charles Sherrington

In the 1996 Olympic summer games in Atlanta, USA, Linford Christie was disqualified after his second apparent false start. Between the sound of the gun and the pressure being released from the blocks a possible human reaction time of 0.1 to 0.2 seconds was allowed. State of the art sports and neural physiology had set this time spacing. It was not until the press article by Highfield (1999) that it was documented that the scientists were wrong. Christie's entire body had left the blocks in 0.08 seconds. His body had in fact acted as an entire reflex proving that he was the epitome of a unifying (not just cerebral) organism in possibly its most natural disinhibited state. Adding insult to injury and embarrassment the scientist's only explanation was that Christie wasn't thinking, rather than accrediting him at that point in time as not practising an analytical non-organic mode of consciousness. Christie was the gun. We still find it hard to consider body and mind as One, with a capital 'O'. The Cartesian view of seeing the body as working via a prime mover, God, is still rooted in our mode of consciousness.

Concepts of a reflex arc can be traced to Descartes in his work *De Homine* or *Treatise of Man*, published twelve years after his death, as part of the Cartesian dualistic model. In his work he proposed a mechanism for the observed automatic response to outside stimuli. External motions affected the peripheral ends of nerve fibrils displacing the central ends which themselves become displaced. Displacement continues and the pattern of interfibrillar space was rearranged allowing the animal spirits to be directed to the appropriate nerves. This was the early reflex arc.

Modern versions of the reflex arc which have been misinterpreted are attributed to Sir Charles Sherrington. We are taught that the impulse moves in an arc returning to the point of impulse initiation. In fact it is more akin to a shower of impulses alerting the entire nervous system. In the knee jerk the entire nervous system is alerted, as with all stimulation of nerve endings. An extensor response takes place due to the initiated pathway being of a lowered threshold, allowing the impulses to express through muscular contraction in the same region as the original tap. In the case of the abdominal reflex no tap is needed, just the stroke of a finger across the skin of the abdominal wall. Facilitation in any part of the central nervous system will heighten the response of the stimulated surface or deep tendon body part.

A reflex that is not present does not mean the arc is 'cut', although no apparent response to the incoming stimulation suggests impaired function to the nerves in question. The nervous system as a whole would damp the incoming stimulation possibly due to plasticity and conditioning of the individual. Afferent impulses would be slowed and absorbed into the entire system. Reinforcing the reflex potential by pulling on clasped hands, clenching the jaw or any kind of artificial afferent bombardment is an abstraction and falsely summates the entire system. In a way it is similar to making the reflex happen for the practitioner rather than letting the body tell you what is going on.

Denny-Brown (1939b) reminds us that, 'the amount of relaxation in a muscle depends on the relative intensities of the excitatory and inhibitory effects. Similar antagonism occurs in visceral reflexes. Inhibition therefore does not necessarily cause complete relaxation'. We must also remove the concept of the spinal cord as relay station. Pascual-Leone and workers (1992) concluded that

'the seat of inhibition is therefore the spinal cord in the reflex activities. Establishing a synergism is the objective of osteopathic care. The reduction of inhibition procedures, you are not born inhibited, may be applied to any anatomical area that is felt is contributing to the upset in overall synergistic function. Time causes plasticity in even the most conditioned reflexes. Even the cortical map of adult humans shows signs of plasticity'.

This also means

'it's never too late to change!'

The entire body is involved in the reflex action, if this were not the case the entire body could never act in a reflex manner. As long as we are aware of what is possibly happening then the execution of the reflex abstraction as part of a neurological examination is valuable.

Models of reflexes

Osteopathic medicine supports the concept that a 'reflex' system of visceral and somatic interrelationships may give rise to manifestations related to disease at sites which are remote from the viscera or soma subsequently affecting the posture (Nicholas *et al.*, 1985 and Denslow and Hassett, 1944). It is well established, both anatomically and physiologically, that reflexes are final pathways during the somatic changes that result from the development of visceral disease (Warwick and Williams, 1978 and Pottenger, 1984). The onset of these reflex stimuli tends to be the pathological changes that occur in the viscera, these include: compression, ischaemia, spasm (if the organ possess contractile filaments) chemical irritation, inflammation, infection, and distension. These occur due to visceral afferents from the organ following the sympathetic course along the sympathetic chain and entering the spinal cord through the dorsal aspect of the spinal cord on the same side as the organ. After the impulses reach the dorsal root of the spinal cord the reflex process is established in the following manner.

(1) The reflex is established at the same level as in the formation coming into the spinal cord.
(2) It can then spread to other 'segmental' levels of the spinal cord.
(3) Depending on the sensitivity of the nervous system the stimulus can ascend the spinothalamic tract.
(4) Depending on the sensitivity of the nervous system the stimulus can amplify if the stimuli is not strong enough to ascend the spinothalamic tract.

This has been established in both laboratory prepared animal models and human subjects in a surgical setting (Johnston *et al.*, 1987).

As many circuits of reflexes can be developed as there are nerve connections. For clinical purposes reflexes have been grouped into:

- somatosomatic
- somatovisceral
- viscerosomatic
- viscerovisceral
- vestibulo-ocularcollic system
- miscellaneous.

Somatosomatic reflex

Use of the term 'somatic' includes the head, trunk, and walls of the body cavities as well as their limbs. Both receptors and effectors are in somatic tissue. A somatosomatic onset of a reflex may begin in the skin as a temperature variation, mechanical stress, chemical irritation or environmental stress. When conditions are such that the stimulus elicits and abnormally prolongs a muscle contraction in an area, the tissues become a secondary source of irritation with the potential to disturb homeostatic balance (Fig. 3). If the individual's inherent resistance cannot compensate for the imbalance, chemically recognisable symptoms are the result. It is possible that this state of muscle shortening may be classified as a *physio-*

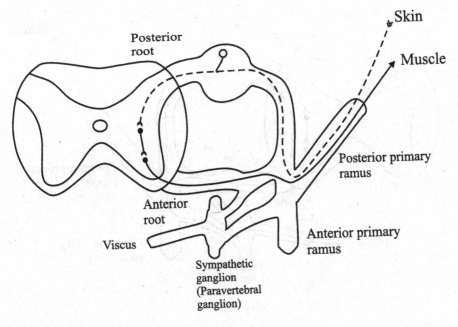

Fig. 3 Somatosomatic reflect pathways.

logical contracture. Physiological contracture is common in back pain patients where the muscle shortens via its parallel elastic component under passive tension; as the contracture continues the muscle loses its ability to hold the patient upright and he or she falls forward with a 'weak' and painful back.

Somatovisceral reflex

In this model the receptor is in the soma and the effector is in the viscera. An interneurone is present at the segmental spinal cord level. This interneurone or central synapse in the spinal cord is between the afferent neurone and the mediolateral cells of the grey matter of the spinal cord. Mediolateral cells are the cells of origin of the sympathetic paravertebral preganlionic outflow of the thoracic and lumbar regions. Parasympathetic reflexes act in the same manner at the cranial and sacral levels. Terminal fibres end in smooth muscle of the vascular system (i.e. this is the vasomotor system); stimulation of the nerves results in vasoconstriction (Fig. 4). Low thresholds of this reflex path result in vasodilatation and sweat gland activity as a local response in manipulative intervention. All stimuli originating from the soma will result within a degree of vasomotor response. This is a major factor in the concepts/principles of osteopathy – that a blood supply is essential for normal function, with a reduced blood supply disturbing the organism at both micro- and macro-cellular levels.

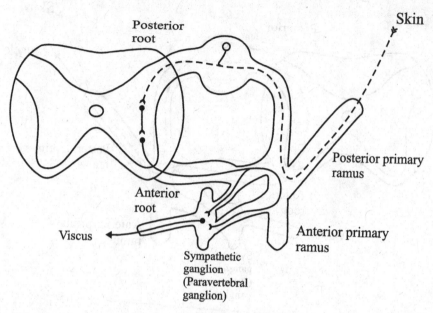

Fig. 4 Somatovisceral reflex pathways.

Viscerosomatic reflex

This is also known as the visceromotor, viscerotrophic or viscerosensory reflex; the variations in the name reflect the effector route ranges. Original visceral stimuli synapse in ganglia from an autonomic afferent neurone do *not* always result in a pure motor response of somatic structures (Fig. 5). Blood vessels in the skin, which are the recipients of aberrant visceral reflexes, lead to a disturbance in circulation resulting in characteristic trophic changes: thickening, flaking and redness. These afferent pathways from the viscera travel through the mixed sacral ganglia (parasympathetic and sympathetic) connecting with anterior horn cells or cranial nerve or both. Signs in the soma indicate that visceral nerve disturbance has summated to the point of somatic involvement.

Due to the paravertebral muscle rigidity associated with this reflex McConnell (1915) referred to this reflex as the 'secondary osteopathic lesion'. Pain and/or rigidity in the back is the most common symptom of visceral organic or functional disturbances. In addition this reflex would involve the dermatomes and myotomes generally at a subconscious level until the stimulus is strong enough to summate along the lateral spinothalamic tract, so becoming recognised as pain. In more chronic slow onset changes there is constant adjustment of thresholds with changes at a cellular level. This is commonly seen in the more viscerotrophic reflex presentation where neurotrophic supply is compromised leading to poor nutritional supply and, for example, eczema or skin breakdown.

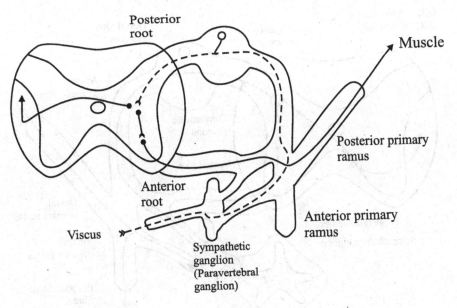

Fig. 5 Viscerosomatic reflex pathway.

Viscerovisceral reflexes

As we will realise with an understanding of the visceral or enteric nervous system, reflex impulses need *not* travel through the spinal cord or brain to complete a path. The gut, pancreas, gall-bladder and pelvic contents are viscera and organs that communicate between each other. Prevertebral ganglia in front of the spinal column and within these structures relay information back into the viscera causing adjustments to take place independently of the central nervous system (Fig. 6). So many neurones and ganglia are involved that the area of the abdomen has been called the second, little or abdominal and pelvic brain (Robinson, 1907; Gershon, 1998, and Jänig, 1995). Viscerovisceral reflex primary response is vasoconstriction of vessels and glands of one area in response to the changes in another. Kuntz (1953) documented the change in cardiac function with the ingestion of liquids into the stomach.

Vestibulo-ocularcollic system

This system has been attributed to the main role of head stabilisation and visual tracking. Stabilisation of the head movement involves a series or system of interacting reflexes involving information relating to the external environment and the internal environment of structures (Fig. 7). Head stabilisation involves the eye muscles and the balance centres of the ears in a vestibulo-ocular reflex

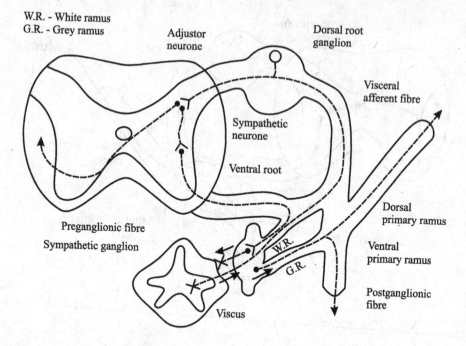

Fig. 6 The viscerovisceral reflex pathway.

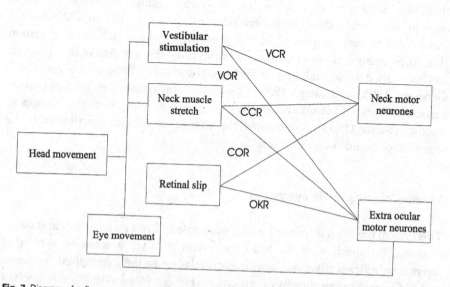

Fig. 7 Diagram of reflex systems in head movement. VCR, vestibulocollic reflex; VOR, vestibulo-ocular reflex; COR, cervico-ocular reflex; CCR, cervico-ocular reflex; OKR, opticokinetic reflex.

(VOR). This VOR is the principal mechanism that keeps visual images stable on the retina while the head is moving (Lisberger, 1988). Hair cells in the semicircular and otoliths of the inner ear are sensitive mechanoreceptors providing input to the central nervous system. Otolithic macular hair cells are sensitive to the position of the head in relation to the environment in both vertical and linear accelerations. All these reflexes are consistent with the nervous system in their expression of neural plasticity (Miles and Lisberger, 1981).

Movement of the head discharges semicircular canal afferents transmitting impulses to the second-order brain stem vestibular nuclei. Information is projected to the motor neurones, innervating the extra-ocular muscles, leading to short-latency reflexes, otherwise known as the 'three (tri)-neurone arc' mediating the VOR. If the eyes move, the visual images on the retina also move, giving rise to a 'retinal slip' signal. This visual stimulus evokes an optico-kinetic reflex (OKR). The OKR has a longer latency than the VOR, producing compensatory movements of the eyes and stabilising the retinal image. Head movements stimulate the VOR and the OKR in a synergistic fashion (Dutia, 1989). Fast, smooth and coordinated movements cannot take place by feedback alone because, in biological motor control systems, the delays associated with feedback loops are long and the gains are low. Therefore, internal predictive models of the motor structures (muscle and joints) are involved in these compensations. Internal models in the brain and body must be acquired through motor conditioning in order to accommodate the changes that occur with the growth of controlled objects such as hands, legs and torso, as well as with the unpredictable variability of the external world (Kawato and Gomi, 1992).

The cerebellum appears to be involved as a system whose main task is not to mediate the reflex *per se*, but to optimise its parameters. It is responsible for adjusting the directions, gains and time relations of these reflexes to optimise them for current conditions. Cerebellar function mediates both short- and long-term adjustments of reflexes to adapt to the particular needs of the movement. It is relatively difficult to discern much effect of the cerebellum on the 'normal' behaviour of any reflex (Stein and Glickstein, 1992).

Movement of the head is by the action of the neck musculature. Afferent information from muscle spindles of the neck accompanies that of the VOR and OKR in the form of the cervico-ocular reflex (COR). Neck integrity is important in mediating relative displacements between the head, the body and the environment. In addition a cervico-collic reflex (CCR) is where information from neck afferents is transmitted to neck motor neurones (Dutia, 1989).

The vestibulo-collic reflex (VCR) is the reflex acting on the muscles of the neck that arises from stimulation of the vestibular receptors in the labyrinth. Activating neck muscles, this reflex acts to counteract any head movement sensed by the vestibular apparatus; this activation helps maintain head stability in space (McKone, 1997).

Miscellaneous reflexes

Appenzeller and Oribe (1997) cite numerous additional reflexes which include: the gastroauricular reflex (Engel, 1922), the auricular phenomenon (Deutsch, 1919), the auriculogenital reflex (Bradford, 1937) in the cat, the auriculouterine reflex (Vasiliu, 1932), the oculocardiac reflex (Aschner, 1967), and the coughing reflex with heartburn (Berlin, 1959). A sacrogenital reflex occurs in two major ways: (1) when the skin over the sacral area is tickled it initiates a release of urine and, (2) if a patient has incurred minor impact trauma to the testes or ovary region, a sharp blow with the flat of the hand on the sacrum brings almost immediate relief.

The autonomic nervous system

'The science of osteopathy is not merely the punching in a certain segment or the cracking of the bones, but it is the keeping of a balance – by touch – between the sympathetic and the cerebrospinal system! That is real osteopathy!'

Edgar Cayce

Historically, the sympathetic division of the autonomic nervous system has been the most studied. Reasons for this are that the ganglia of the sympathetic division are macroscopic and easily seen in various species with the naked eye. It seems that Claudius Galen was the first to name this part of the ANS. He was born around 131 and died somewhere between 201 and 210 AD; he initially lived in Pergamos and finally in Rome. Due to his observations of the nerve trunks lying on the rib heads, either side of the vertebral column, he suggested there was 'sympathy' or consent' between body parts (quoted in *Opus de Usu Partium Corporis Humani*, (Paris edition of 1528)). He studied the sympathetic chain in animals, presumably not knowing that the nerves were a part of the cerebrospinal system. It appears that before his time the sympathetic ganglionic system of nerves was entirely unknown as regards their function. It is possible that Aristotle viewed them many times during his dissections without really knowing what the white cords and nodules were. There is also some evidence that the Arabians had some ideas concerning the sympathetic system. It was claimed that the Hippocratic school knew the sympathetic system. Hippocrates (460–370 BC) like Aristotle doubtless saw the cords and ganglia but may not have known their significance. Erasistratus (340–280 BC) believed that all nerves arose from the brain and spinal cord, presumably, again, not realising the significance of the sympathetic system.

Eustachius, an Italian anatomist who died in 1574, considered that the sympathetic nerves originated from the abducens or sixth cranial nerve. Some time later an English physician, by the name of Thomas Willis (1621–75), began to record his findings, and the realisation of the role of the sympathetic system began to develop. Willis realised the connection between the sympathetic system and the cerebro-spinal system. It was in 1660, while Sedleian professor of philosophy at Oxford, that he described the chief ganglia. René Descartes (1569–1650) was one of the first to describe the reflex movements of the ganglia. The ANS is additionally referred to today as the vegetative nervous system, but as we shall see it is neither totally automatic nor vegetative (L. *vegetus*; animated, lively or sprightly). (Today it means the opposite to the original meaning in that anything that vegetates is 'dead' or in a psychologically pathological state.)

The work of Gaskell (1899), Bayliss and Starling (1899), Robinson (1907), Langley and Anderson (Langley, 1921) and Strong (1940) created an early modern foundation for the understanding of the form, anatomy and physiology of the autonomic nervous system. Langley's divisions of the autonomic nervous system into the sympathetic, parasympathetic and enteric are still valid today. The development of modern neurotransmitter understanding is credited to the work of Elliott (1905), Loewi (1921), von Euler and Gaddum (1931), and in particular Dale (1935). We are now aware that the developing concept of the antagonistic mode of action of the ANS is a Cartesian construct and is wrong; parasympathetic cholinergic and sympathetic adregenic control of viscera and the cardiovascular system are complementary and reciprocal.

It was not until the 1960s that work began to shape our present understanding of the ANS. Workers found and developed the following points.

(1) Autonomic neuromuscular junction is not a synapse as in a fixed gap with pre- and post-junctional differences and specificity. It is now considered a varicosity of fibres with the distances from the receptor smooth muscle cells being of varying distances (Hillarp, 1959; Burnstock, 1986a).

(2) Nerves are non-adrenergic and non-cholinergic and they carry a range of neurotransmitters and trophic substances (Burnstock *et al.*, 1964; Burnstock, 1986b; 1993b; Burnstock and Milner, 1992; Rand, 1992; Snyder, 1992).

(3) Polytransmission occurs where nerves release more than one neurotransmitter actively. (Burnstock, 1976; Burnstock and Sneddon, 1985; Hökfelt, Fuxe and Pernow, 1986; Burnstock, 1990a).

(4) Sensory motor activity is an important factor in the normal regulation function in the gut, heart, lungs, ganglia and blood vessels (Maggi and Meli, 1988; Burnstock 1990a; 1993a).

(5) Large numbers of intrinsic ganglia in organs are capable of maintaining function independently of the brain and spinal cord (Kosterlitz, 1968 and Burnstock *et al.*, 1987).

(6) Plasticity of the autonomic nervous system not only occurs during development and ageing but also in the expression of neurotransmitters, receptors, trauma, surgery and disease (Burnstock, 1990b).

One of humankind's greatest assets is freedom to move within the environment. This high degree of independence has been attributed to the automatic adjustment of the internal environment to both internal and external needs. Adjustment and regulation of the human (and mammalian) internal environment is the task of the autonomic nervous system (ANS). As the cranial brain began to develop the ANS seems to function unnoticed as we go about our every day activities.

As we have read above, Langley divided the ANS into three divisions, with the enteric division as part of the sympathetic system. Debate still continues over the supply of autonomic fibres to striated muscle. Mitchell (1953) made a major contribution to the debate by adding, 'there has been much controversy about whether autonomic fibres do innervate striated muscles, or only their vessels, but after analysing the conflicting evidence Kuntz (1953) concludes that they do, and physiologists continue to argue about their possible effects on muscular function.' Many texts give the impression that the two major divisions are antagonistic, again this could not be further from the truth. While the divisions, in the main, have opposing functions the overall function is supportive and mutual for the good of the entire organism. One division speeds up a response, while the other slows it down. This harmony of function is expressed through the calibre of the peripheral arteries.

Sympathetic fibres are generally inhibitory, with the parasympathetic being generally excitatory. Communication between these two divisions will, for example, keep the heartbeat steady and cause glands to secrete and stop at the right time.

The ganglia

To regard ganglia as simple relay stations within the ANS is grossly to underestimate their functional capabilities. Within the autonomic nervous system they vary in structure from site to site. This variability is shown in the superior cervical ganglia with its mainly polymorphonuclear cells compared with the coeliac ganglia, which are composed mainly of large stellate cells. More importantly from an osteopathic view is that all ganglia seem to be surrounded by connective tissue capsule that is continuous with local structures. This capsule continues into the ganglia forming compartments or septa (Martin, 1937) supporting arterioles, venuoles (Spiegel and Adolf, 1920) and venous sinuses. Lymphatic vessels and glands surround the sympathetic ganglia and network draining into the local nodes. An example is the cervical sympathetic ganglia lymphatic system draining into the cervical lymphatic nodes (Rouvière, 1929).

ANS neurones are present at birth and by two years of age there are well developed inter-ganglionic nerve axons that continue to thicken with age. This indicates that the organisation of the sympathetic chain, landmarked by its ganglia, is anatomically mature at birth growing in size with the child. Development of size and distribution of the ganglia seems to be reciprocal with the demand of the organ they communicate with. With increasing age there is an increase in fibrous connective tissue replacing neural tissue and an increase in sclerotic changes. Obviously, fibrous changes affect the parasympathetic ganglia and Robinson (1907) noted that at post-mortem disease states were accompanied by advanced fibrous thickening noted around and within ganglia.

Norepinephrine released by sympathetic discharge, in the classic 'fight or flight' stress reaction, is the result of impulse activity. In addition it has been shown that the impulses have effects not just limited to their duration. Impulses crossing synapses (trans-synaptic) release norepinephrine and the impulses continue along the post-synaptic neurones causing slower and longer responses in metabolic tissue. Stimulation of metabolic (endocrine) tissue releases enzymes, e.g. trosine hydroxylase, as a response to perceived environmental stress. Trosine hydroxylase can continue to be released for up to four days after the instantaneous short-lived sympathetic impulse. This means we are still responding to the environment days after the original stimulation. Our behaviour will change in response to this enzyme release and its further stimulation within the four days, for example, reinforces adaptation and conditioning to environmental stimuli. It has been suggested that this anatomico-physiological relationship is the physico-emotional junction: one cannot work without the other. We can now see that the autonomic-endocrine system has something in common with the environment.

The sympathetic nervous system

'Vasomotion is the key to circulation of the blood; the balance wheel in the regulation of brain activity; coordinator between the pulmonic and systemic circulators; the normal regulator of many secretory processes in the body; the means of correcting inequalities in circulation through the spinal centres; to the determining of muscular activities; the correction of nerve impulses and the distribution of stimuli. It is the most powerful palliative treatment in osteopathy.'

J. Martin Littlejohn

'The sympathetic nerve presides over rhythm, circulation, sensation, absorption, secretion and respiration – nutrition.'

Fred Byron Robinson, MD

The sympathetic nervous system used to be known by a number of different names. These synonyms included the vasomotor nerve (nervus vasomotorius) named in 1840, by the German anatomist and surgeon Benedict Stilling

(1810–79). Other names for the sympathetic nervous system are systema nervorum sympathicum, the vegetative nervous system (systema nervorum vegetatorum), the ganglionic nervous system (systema nervorum ganglionicum), the nervous system of organic life, and the intercostal nerves (Thomas Willis 1621–1675).

The proper name for the sympathetic nerves is the nervus vasomotorius. This practically means the nerves belonging to arteries. Vasodilatation of arteries stretches the mesh of the vasomotor nerves contributing to the stimulation of their vasoconstrictive response. This reciprocal action is the main reason for the motion and rhythm of organs within the body cavities and the limbs.

An understanding of the general anatomy and physiology of the vasomotor system is essential for the theory and application of osteopathic medicine. It is through this understanding of the vasomotor system that the osteopath can construct a response to the needs of the patient. Through purely physical interventions a significant degree of influence over the circulation of the body can be achieved. An example is the maintained reflex cycle of joint restriction, myofascial shortening, ischaemia etc. which will compromise circulation.

The vasomotor anatomy is essentially that of the circulatory structural make-up of the autonomic nervous system. Presently, there is a dispute about the divisions of the autonomic nervous system (ANS). It has been traditionally divided into two parts: the *sympathetic* and the *parasympathetic*. More recently there has been an additional division of a self-sustained neural influence, that of the intestinal or enteric nervous system. This system affects immunomodulation (Metal'nikov and Chorine, (1926), Fecho, Maslonek *et al.*, (1993) and Jonakait (1993)), capillary permeability in the entire body (Engel, 1941) and has been indicted in the cause of disease (Fagius and Wallin, 1983, Shichijo, Ito *et al.*, 1993, and Speransky, 1944). As we shall see these divisions are anatomically artificial and both have communications, or at least connections, with each other. These systems must never be separated as they work together at all times for the benefit of the organism as a whole. They are in touch with each other. It is only when one begins to dominate (usually the sympathetic), that a problem may present itself.

Modern anatomical textbooks are in the main incomplete. With regard to the sympathetic nervous system their anatomy is highly selective. A good example of this is a lack of completion of the sympathetic chain into a type of anatomical cycle. The sympathetic chain communicates with and is completed in the cranium and the pelvis by the ganglion of Ribes (François Ribes, 1800–64, French professor of hygiene in Montpellier) and the ganglion of Impar (coccyx or coccygeal ganglion), respectively. The author has had to research back to find the origins of the full autonomic nervous anatomy and function. Modern texts are not so much concerned with the anatomical distribution but the chemical make-up (Fig. 8).

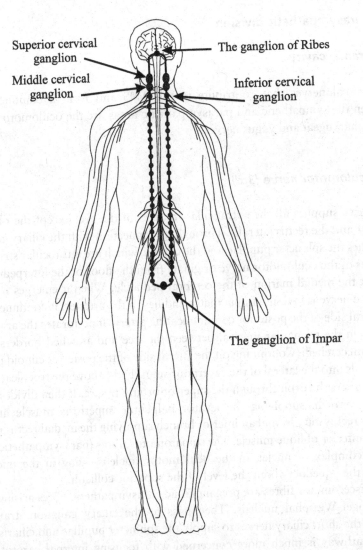

Superior cervical ganglion

Middle cervical ganglion

The ganglion of Ribes

Inferior cervical ganglion

The ganglion of Impar

Fig. 8 The Sympathetic Cyclic Chain.

Anatomy of the autonomic nervous system

'A brain (rather than the brain) is an apparatus capable of reception, reorganisation and emission of nerve forces. It may be composed of one or more nerve or ganglion cells.'

Fred Byron Robinson, MD

The autonomic nervous system can regarded as occupying the cranial, thoracic and abdomino-pelvic cavities.

The parasympathetic division

The cranial cavity

The cranial nerves that contribute to the ANS and form a communication between the sympathetic and parasympathetic areas are the oculomotor, facial, glossopharyngeal and vagus nerves.

The oculomotor nerve (3rd)

This nerve supplies all the extraocular muscles of the eye, except the oblequus superior and the rectus lateralis. Through its connection with the ciliary ganglion it supplies the sphincter pupillae and the ciliaris, which are intraocular structures.

Fibres of the oculomotor nerve originate from the floor of the interpeduncular fossa at the medial margin of the cerebral peduncle. When it emerges from the brain the nerve is invested in pia mater and lies in the arteries; it continues on to the lateral side of the posterior communicating artery. It perforates the arachnoid and lies in the triangular interval between the free and attached borders of the tentorium cerebelli. Continuing on the lateral side of the posterior clinoid process it descends into the lateral of the cavernous sinus, lying above the trochlear nerve. Here it enters the orbit through the superior orbital fissure. It then divides into a superior branch, supplying the levator palpebrae superioris muscle and the superior rectus muscle, and an inferior branch supplying the medial rectus muscle and the inferior oblique muscle. The somatomotor fibres (parasympathetic) arise from a complex of nuclei, in the oculomotor nucleus, lying in the midbrain beneath the aqueduct about the level of the superior colliculi.

The visceromotor fibres are preganglionic parasympathetic fibres arising from the Edinger-Westphal nucleus. They pass to the ciliary ganglion, travelling through the short ciliary nerves to supply the sphincter pupillae and ciliaris. This motor pathway is much more concerned with focusing internal carotid. This consists of postganglionic fibres from the superior cervical ganglion traversing the ciliary ganglion and emerging in the short ciliary nerves. They supply the vessels of the eyeball and may include fibres that supply the dilator pupillae. The sensory root is formed by a ramus communicans to the nasociliary nerve that contains sensory fibres from the eyeball. It reaches the ganglion in the short ciliary nerves passing through it without being interrupted.

The facial nerve (7th)

This nerve has both motor and sensory roots. The motor nerve travels to supply the face, scalp and auricle, the buccinator, platysma, strapedius, styloid and posterior belly of the digastric. The sensory nerve receives information from the corda tympani gustatory fibres from the presulcal area of the tongue and, from the palatine and greater petrosal nerves, taste fibres from the soft palate. In addition the sensory fibres carry the preganglionic parasympathetic (secreto-motor) innervation of the submandibular and sublingual salivary glands, lacrimal glands and glands of the nasal and palatine mucosae.

Therefore, the facial nerve can be thought of as having two nuclei, but this should only be from an anatomical rather than a functional viewpoint. These nuclei are the facial nucleus (motor fibres) and the superior salivatory nucleus (preganglionic secretory fibres); one motor and one saliva nucleus.

These roots give rise to the fibres that travel through the internal acoustic meatus, continuing onto the facial canal as a single trunk. At this point fibres leave the single trunk forming the superficial petrosal nerve, stapeius nerve and the corda tympani (these are the taste fibres to the anterior two thirds of the tongue and the preganglionic fibres to the mandibular and sublingual glands). The main body of fibres forms the ganiculate ganglion at the bend with the petrous bone; carrying onto the tympanic cavity, it turns downwards surfacing on the skull through the stylomastoid foramen, and then into the parotid gland. Around the parotid gland it forms the parotid plexus intertwining with the fascial muscles.

The source of the arterial supply to the facial nerve is intracranially from the anterior inferior cerebellar artery, itself from the superior branch of the middle meningeal artery and the posterior auricular or occipital arteries. Extracranially the source of the arterial supplies are the stylomastoid, posterior auricular, occipital, superficial temporal and transverse facial arteries. Venous drainage is via the venae comitanes of the superficial petrosal and stylomastoid arteries.

The glossopharyngeal nerve (9th)

This cranial nerve supplies sensory innervation to the middle ear, parts of the tongue and pharynx, parasympathetic secretomotor fibres to the parotid gland and motor fibres to the muscles of the pharynx. Due to this combination it contains motor, visceromotor and taste fibres.

The nerve originates as three or four rootlets from the medulla oblongata, forms a ganglion (the superior ganglion), passes out of the skull through the jugular foramen and forms another larger ganglion (the inferior ganglion). These ganglia are considered as two parts of the same ganglion. It then goes on to supply the taste and texture sensory fibres from the mucosa of the tongue (posterior third) and sensory fibres from the oropharynx, soft palate and fauces. The larger inferior ganglion has connections to the superior cervical sympathetic ganglion.

It continues on its course laterally to the internal carotid artery and the pharynx and the tongue. As it arches towards the tongue it divides into a number of terminal branches. These branches are the tympanic, carotid, pharyngeal, muscular, tonsillar and lingual.

The vagus nerve (10th)

The vasomotor importance of this nerve is its innervation of the heart, especially the smaller branches of the coronary arteries. The larger branches of the coronary arteries, as we will see, are innervated by the sympathetic system.

The vagus supplies the head, thorax and abdomen, where it divides into a plexus. This is the largest vegetative nerve of the parasympathetic division, which contains both motor and sensory fibres. It begins from eight to ten rootlets from the medulla oblongata then, as with the glossopharyngeal nerve, it forms two ganglia. A superior ganglion forms before the vagus nerve travels through the jugular foramen; it then forms an inferior ganglion. This superior ganglion is connected to the sympathetic chain via a filament from the superior cervical ganglion, its main concern being general somatic sensations mediated by the auricular branch of the vagus. The inferior ganglion of the vagus is also connected to the superior cervical sympathetic ganglion, the hypoglossal nerve, and a loop between the first and second cervical spinal nerves. The vagus nerve then continues to pass vertically down the neck in the carotid sheath between the internal jugular vein and the internal carotid artery. This course then differs from right to left.

On the right it descends behind the internal jugular vein into the superior mediastinum medial to the right pleura and the lung. It continues behind the root of the right lung joining with branches from the second, third and fourth thoracic sympathetic ganglia as the posterior pulmonary branches continuing on to form the right posterior pulmonary plexus. From this plexus two or three branches continue to descend to the dorsal part of the oesophagus where, forming a trunk with the left vagus, they form the posterior oesophageal plexus.

On the left the vagus begins with a similar course to the right. The left vagus enters the thorax between the left common carotid and left subclavian arteries, and behind the left brachiocephalic vein. As it continues to descend behind the root of the lung it divides into the posterior bronchial branches, joining with fibres from the second, third and fourth sympathetic ganglia forming the left posterior pulmonary plexus. Two branches from this plexus combine with a twig from the right posterior plexus on the front of the oesophagus to form the anterior oesophageal plexus. A trunk from this plexus, containing fibres from both vagus nerves, descends in front of the oesophagus entering the abdomen through the oesophageal opening of the diaphragm.

Within the abdomen the anterior vagal trunk supplies fibres to the cardiac antrum, dividing into the right and left branches. The left branch supplies the anteriosuperior surface of the stomach. The right branch has three main branches, the first supplies the pyloric canal, the pylorus, the superior and descending parts of the duodenum, and the head of the pancreas. The second part supplies the anteriosuperior surface of the stomach and the third branch follows the lesser curvature of the stomach as far as the angular notch.

The branches of the vagus nerve are as follows.

(1) In the jugular fossa:
 - meningeal
 - auricular.

(2) In the neck:
 - pharyngeal
 - branches to the carotid body
 - superior laryngeal
 - recurrent laryngeal (right)
 - cardiac.

(3) In the thorax:
 - cardiac
 - recurrent laryngeal (left)
 - pulmonary
 - oesophageal.

(4) In the abdomen:
 - gastric
 - coeliac
 - hepatic.

The accessory nerve (11th)

The accessory cranial nerve is formed from both cranial and spinal roots, known as the internal and external rami respectively. It is the cranial portion of the accessory nerve that can be considered as part of the vagus nerve due to the accessory distribution through the vagal branches. Its distributions are mainly in the pharyngeal and recurrent laryngeal portions of the vagus nerve.

The pelvic cavity

The pelvic cavity comprises the branches of the anterior rami of the second to fourth sacral spinal nerves forming the pelvic sacral plexus (pelvic splanchnic nerves). More importantly, they unite with branches of the sympathetic pelvic plexuses, forming mixed ganglia. These are small ganglia at the areas of unification and the walls of the viscera.

The sympathetic division

The thoracolumbar (sympathetic) outflow

The common misconception is that even though the sympathetic part of the autonomic nervous system originates from neurones in the thoracolumbar part of the spinal cord, ranging from the second dorsal to second lumbar segments, it is only parallel to this region that the immediate structure of the system extends. Confusion about its influence is restricted by the image of two chains of nerve tissue either side of the thoracic and lumbar spine. In reality the sympathetic portion of the autonomic nervous system forms a complete unbroken cyclic chain. At its highest point the chain completes in the head, anterior and superior to the anterior communicating artery, in the ganglion of Ribes, and in the pelvis as the ganglion of Impar. These are anatomically and therefore osteopathically significant as they complete the sympathetic nervous system, making it far more of a system than the parasympathetic.

The cranial section

On both sides of the neck the cranial part of the SNS begins with the preganglionic fibres at the first thoracic segment. It then continues as postganglionic fibres from the superior cervical ganglion (SCG) ascending as the internal carotid nerve. It continues posterior to the carotid artery; it enters the carotid canal in the temporal bone where it splits into a lateral and medial branch. These branches innervate the internal carotid artery and form the lateral and medial parts of the internal and carotid plexus respectively.

A vasomotor filament passes on to the ciliary ganglion entering the orbit of the eye through the superior orbital tissue. The fibres continue uninterrupted through the ciliary ganglion forming short ciliary nerves that supply the vessels of the eyeball.

The internal carotid plexus terminates around the anterior and middle cerebral arteries and the ophthalmic artery. As filaments converge from the left and right sides of the sympathetic nervous system, anterior and superior to the anterior communicating artery is the ganglion of Ribes. This completes the cranial end of the sympathetic cyclic chain.

The cervical section

In the main this is taken up with the superior cervical ganglion (SCG), the middle cervical ganglion (MCG) and the inferior cervical ganglion (ICG); this last ganglion is usually fused to the first thoracic sympathetic ganglion (the stellate or cervico-thoracic ganglion). The nerve cords between the ganglia originate from the white rami communicantes of the upper thoracic spinal nerves not the cervical spinal nerves. This area between the SCG and ICG does give back grey rami communicantes to the cervical spinal nerves as the chain continues up into the neck.

The superior cervical ganglion (SCG)

The SCG is the biggest of the three ganglia in the cervical part of the SNS. Their common site is anterior to the transverse processes of the second and third cervical vertebrae. It is believed that the SCG are the fusing of four ganglia originating from the upper four cervical nerves. Each SCG lies anterior to the longus capitis muscle and posterior to the sheath of the internal carotid artery. From out of the superior aspect of the SCG travels the internal carotid nerve and inferiorly it makes a connection with the middle cervical ganglion (MCG). This SCG has anterior, medial and lateral branches.

The anterior branches of the SCG
The anterior branches supply the common carotid artery and the external carotid artery and its tributaries. The plexus around the facial artery supplies a filament to the submandibular ganglion, the plexus around the middle meningeal artery goes on to supply the otic ganglion and the facial nerve ganglion.

The medial branches of the SCG
The medial branches supply cardiac accelerator fibres to the heart and the laryngopharyngeal branches in the form of the pharyngeal plexus receiving and forming connections with the glossopharyngeal and vagus nerves. On the right side this medial branch passes inferiorly along the common carotid artery to the posterior aspect of the aorta meeting and becoming part of the cardiac plexus. Its other connections include branches of the SNS, the external laryngeal nerve (a branch of the vagus), cardiac fibres of the vagus and the recurrent laryngeal nerve. On the left side this medial branch travels anterior to the left common carotid artery and continues past the left aspect of the aortic arch to the superficial aspect of the cardiac plexus. The communications of this left medial branch include the cardiac branches of the MCG, occasionally the vagus, forming a plexus on the ascending aorta.

The lateral branches of the SCG
The lateral branches supply grey rami communicantes to the four upper cervical, vagus, hypoglossal and glossopharyngeal nerves.

The middle cervical ganglion (MCG)

The MCG is the smallest of the three ganglia in the cervical part of the SNS. It is usually located anterior to the transverse process of the sixth cervical vertebra. It may be formed by the union of the fifth and sixth cervical nerves due to the supply of grey rami communicantes it gives to these two nerves. It has major thyroid and cardiac branches. Two cords from the MCG connect it to the cervico-thoracic ganglia with a posterior cord branching off to envelop the vertebral artery and an anterior cord supplying the subclavian artery called the ansa subclavia. This ansa subclavia connects with the phrenic and vagus nerves and is positioned anterior and posterior to the head of the first rib and clavicle.

The thyroid branches of the MCG travel along the thyroid artery to the thyroid gland. They connect with the superior cardiac, external laryngeal and recurrent laryngeal nerves with branches to the parathyroid gland. In the main these fibres are vasomotor and a minority of secretory fibres.

The cardiac branches of the MCG form the largest of the cardiac sympathetic supplies. Branches on the right travel inferiorly and posteriorly to the common carotid artery communicating with the superior cardiac and recurrent laryngeal nerves continuing on to the anterior aspect of the subclavian artery. It continues to travel inferiorly on the surface of the trachea joining the deep part of the cardiac plexus. Branches on the left enter the thorax between the left common carotid and subclavian arteries ending in the deep part of the cardiac plexus.

The inferior cervical ganglion (ICG)

As mentioned above, the inferior cervical ganglion is usually the combining of the inferior cervical ganglion and the first thoracic ganglion. Its other names are the stellate and cervico-thoracic ganglion. The ICG in its own right is probably formed from the fusion of the last two cervical ganglia and the first thoracic ganglion. The ICG in total is located at the base of the transverse process of the seventh cervical vertebrae and the neck of the first rib.

The ICG supplies grey rami communicantes to the sixth and seventh cervical and first thoracic nerves. There is a cardiac branch that supplies the deep cardiac plexus, the recurrent laryngeal nerve and the cardiac branch of the MCG. It communicates with the vagus and supplies local blood vessels.

Plexuses form around the blood vessels on the subclavian artery, which also communicates with the ansa subclavia, with plexuses continuing on to the axillary artery. Branches are given to the vertebral artery ascending to the basilar arteries and the posterior cerebral artery. When at the posterior cerebral artery the fibres communicate with the plexuses from the internal carotid artery. Additional branches go on to the internal thoracic artery.

There is communication of the ICG with the branches passing to the inferior thyroid artery and on to the thyroid gland. This communication of ICG branches continues with the recurrent and external laryngeal nerves, the cardiac branch of the SCG and the plexuses of the common carotid artery.

The upper limb communicates from the second to sixth thoracic spinal segments, forming a synapse with the ICG en route. After the ICG the postganglionic fibres continue on to the brachial plexus, mostly in the lower trunk. The majority of vasoconstrictor fibres of the arteries of the upper limb are supplied from the second and third segments of the ventral roots of the spinal cord. As the nerves travel past the axillary artery the blood vessels begin to receive their vasomotor supply from branches of the brachial plexus. An example would be the median nerve supplying the brachial artery and the palmar arches.

The thoracic section

Inferiorly, beyond the ICG the ganglia begin to align with every segment of the thoracic spine. Of clinical importance is the position of the thoracic ganglia. Each ganglion is anterior to the rib heads and posterior to the costal pleura. This is not the case with the last few ganglia as they align with the bodies of the vertebrae. The thoracic lateral chain of the sympathetic cycle continues on to become the lumbar lateral chain and passes through the medial arcuate ligament.

The medial branches from the upper five thoracic ganglia come together to form the thoracic aortic plexus with fibres from the greater splanchnic nerve. Fibres from the second to sixth thoracic ganglia form the pulmonary plexus and fibres from the second to the fifth ganglia communicate with the deep part of the cardiac plexus.

The medial branches from the lower seven thoracic ganglia supply the aorta and continue inferiorly to form the greater (from the sixth to tenth ganglia), the lesser (from the ninth to tenth ganglia) and the lowest (from the twelfth) splanchnic nerves. The greater and lesser splanchnic nerves travel through the crus of the diaphragm terminating in the coeliac plexus. Fibres from these nerves supply the aortico-renal ganglion and the suprarenal gland. The lesser splanchnic communicates with the aortico-renal ganglion and the lowest continues on to the renal plexus.

The splanchnic nerves and the vagus communicate in the coeliac plexus. The coeliac plexus continues with the arteries of the abdomen to supply the abdominal and pelvic organs.

The lumbar section of the sympathetic nervous system

There are four sympathetic ganglia in the lumbar spine. They lie anterior to the vertebral column usually along the medial margin of the psoas major muscle. The sympathetic chain continues inferiorly and posterior to the common iliac artery, becoming the pelvic chain as it enters the pelvis.

The first lumbar ganglion gives rise to the first lumbar splanchnic nerve joining the coeliac, renal and intermesenteric plexuses. The second lumbar ganglion gives rise to the second lumbar splanchnic nerve joining the lowest part of the intermesenteric plexus. The third lumbar ganglion gives rise to the third lumbar splanchnic nerve joining the superior hypogastric plexus (or nerve) with the fourth lumbar ganglion.

With regard to the vascular connections, all the lumbar ganglia communicate with the intermesenteric plexus. The lower lumbar splanchnic nerves communicate with the common iliac artery passing inferiorly to the external and internal iliac arteries and on to the femoral artery with its muscular, cutaneous and saphenous branches. Fibres from the lumbar plexus continue on to the obturator nerve and artery.

The pelvic section

The four to five ganglia of the sacral-pelvic section of the sympathetic chain are positioned anteriorly to the sacrum and medial to the anterior sacral foramina. The sympathetic chain travels inferiorly to where both sides meet anterior to the coccyx at the ganglion of Impar. There are no white rami communicantes of the remainder of the chain, similar to the cervical end, due to the anatomical position. The grey rami communicantes from these trunks give supply to the sacral and coccygeal nerves.

From the first ganglia fibres join the inferior hypogastric plexus (pelvic plexus) and a plexus on the medial sacral artery. The sacral plexus from the sympathetic chain supplies vascular branches to the popliteal artery and the continuing tributaries of this artery into the leg and foot. Remaining fibres of the sacral plexus communicate with the pudendal and superior and inferior nerves and their arteries.

Any preganglionic supply to the lower limb originates from the last three thoracic ganglia and two lumbar segments of the cords.

The plexuses

The plexuses are collections of ganglia and nerves in body cavities. Their anatomical courses tend to follow those of the large blood vessels with which they are functionally associated and so named. Here we shall take a closer look at the cardiac, pulmonary, coeliac, superior and inferior hypogastric plexuses.

Table 3 Sympathetic supplies and segmental roots.

Head and neck	T1–5
Upper limb	T2–5
Lower limb	T10–L2
Heart	T1–5
Bronchi and lung	T2–4
Oesophagus (caudal part)	T5–6
Stomach	T6–10
Small intestine	T9–10
Large intestine to splenic flexure	T11–L1
Splenic to rectum	L1–2
Liver and gall bladder	T7–9
Spleen	T6–10
Pancreas	T6–12
Kidney	T10–L11
Ureter	T11–L2
Suprarenal	T8–L1
Testis and ovary	T10–L2
Epididymis, dustus deferens and seminal vesicles	T11–12
Urinary bladder	T11–L2
Prostate and prostatic urethra	T11–L1
Uterus	T12–L1
Uterine tube	T10–L1

The cardiac plexuses

The cardiac plexuses are located at the base of the heart as the superficial and deep divisions. The superficial plexus is located inferior to the arch of the aorta, being formed from the cardiac branch of the SCG and the two cervical cardiac branches of the vagus. Branches from the superficial plexus travel to the deep plexus, the right coronary plexus and the left, anterior pulmonary plexus.

The deep plexus is located anterior to the bifurcation of the trachea posterior to the aortic arch. This deep plexus is the result of the cardiac nerves from the upper thoracic ganglia and the cardiac branches from the vagus and recurrent laryngeal nerves. Branches from this deep plexus communicate with the anterior pulmonary plexus, coronary plexus and the atria. The coronary and atrial plexuses send branches to the atria and ventricles.

The efferent preganglionic fibres from the upper four or five thoracic segments form a synapse in the thoracic and cervical ganglia. The postganglionic fibres are cardiac accelerators and coronary dilators and the efferent parasympathetic fibres from the vagus inhibit the heart and constrict the coronary arteries.

The pulmonary plexuses

The pulmonary plexuses are located on the anterior and posterior areas of the bronchial and vascular structures of the hila of the lungs. The origins of the plexuses are from branches of the vagus and the second to the fifth thoracic ganglia. Fibres from the pulmonary plexuses travel on to the lungs and mesh around the bronchi and pulmonary and bronchial vessels, continuing on to the visceral pleura.

The vagal fibres contract and the sympathetic dilate the bronchi. The sympathetic fibres provide motor impulses for the lungs while the vagus provides the regulator impulses. From a vasomotor aspect the vagal nerve dilates and the sympathetic fibres constrict.

The coeliac plexus

The area of this plexus begins around the twelfth thoracic and the first few lumbar vertebrae posterior to the stomach and anterior to the crura of the diaphragm, between the adrenal glands. The coeliac plexus wraps around and follows the coeliac artery and the root of the superior mesenteric artery, uniting the coeliac ganglia. These coeliac ganglia within the plexus receive the greater and lesser splanchnic, vagus and phrenic nerves. The plexus extends into a series of secondary plexuses wrapping around the arteries in the region.

The aortico-renal plexus, which forms the lower part of each ganglion, gives branches to the greater part of the renal plexus. The secondary plexuses are numerous and include the phrenic, splenic, hepatic, left gastric, intermesenteric, suprarenal, testicular or ovarian, superior mesenteric and inferior mesenteric. These secondary plexuses are consistent with other plexuses by wrapping around the arteries and following blood vessels to their respective organs.

The fibres of the renal plexus are primarily vasomotor and supply the vessels, glomeruli and tubules of the kidney. The efferent motor fibres from the tenth and eleventh thoracic levels supply the testes and ovaries. The parasympathetic supply is thought to have a vasodilator action and originates from the inferior hypogastric plexus. The vasoconstrictor fibres are supplied through the superior mesenteric plexus to the pancreas, small intestine and large intestine. The fibres of the inferior mesenteric plexus originate from the second and third lumbar splanchnic nerves and supply the transverse colon and rectum. The parasympathetic supply covering the area of the large intestine from the transverse colon to the rectum travels inferiorly from the vagus and superiorly from the pelvic splanchnic nerve.

The superior hypogastric plexus

The superior hypogastric pelvis is located anterior to the bifurcation of the abdominal aorta, the body of the last lumbar vertebra and the promontory of the sacrum. The plexus is the result of the unification of branches supplied from the aortic plexus and the third and fourth lumbar splanchnic nerves. As the plexus travels inferiorly it divides into the right and left hypogastric nerves becoming two separate inferior hypogastric plexuses. Areas supplied by the superior hypogastric plexus include the ureteric and testicular (ovarian) plexuses and the plexuses wrapping around the common iliac artery.

The inferior hypogastric plexus

The inferior hypogastric plexus is split laterally to the rectum and the posterior aspect of the urinary bladder, continuing on to the base of the broad ligament of the uterus in women. As it forms two bundles of plexuses, it is supplied by the hypogastric nerve which conveys most of the sympathetic fibres to these plexuses. The sympathetic fibres originate from the lower three thoracic and upper two lumbar levels. The parasympathetic fibres originate from the pelvic splanchnic nerves from the second, third and fourth sacral levels. This plexus provides branches to the pelvic viscera along the iliac artery or directly. Other branches' supply is directly to the rectum or along the middle rectal artery as the middle rectal plexus.

Motor fibres that include a vasomotor element supply the bladder wall. Sympathetic fibres, resulting in vasoconstriction and parasympathetic fibres resulting in vasodilatation supply the male genitalia. This action is the same in female genitalia with regard to the vagina, clitoris, vestibular glands and urethra.

Conclusion

The autonomic nervous system is a continuum that functions as a unit. Since it is our ANS, particularly the SNS that is linked to our stress response, then the vasomotor element is paramount in the day-to-day, year-by-year development of supply and drainage patterns of the body. Accessing the ANS can then be developed at many levels, including the narrative of psychology as well as osteopathic manipulative techniques. The key areas from a physically interactive perspective tend historically to indicate the sub-occipital and pelvic areas for the parasympathetic and the mid-thorax (ribs) for the sympathetic. These tend to effect a non-specific response that sets the stage for better adaptation by the patient.

The enteric nervous system

The enteric nervous system is thought to be the oldest part of the nervous system. Animal forms were originally a gut reciprocally supported by the nervous system. Research demonstrates the independence of the enteric system and its presence in all three body cavities. Nerves associated with the gut are the first to develop along its entire length. It is composed of ganglionated plexuses, the connections of these plexuses with each other, and nerve fibres which arise from them and supply the muscle blood vessels and mucosal lining of the gastrointestinal tract. The number of neurones in this part of the ANS is so large (approximately 10^8) that it rivals the number in the spinal cord (Appenzeller and Oribe, 1997 and Hoyle and Burnstock, 1989).

The enteric system has been called the 'second or original brain'. Its importance takes us back to a time when our primary concern was food and not being eaten by any other animal. If we wanted to catch food and avoid being eaten we had to be 'in sympathy' with our environment. As we saw under Robinson's description, the enteric system qualifies as a brain. This becomes even more apparent when we consider the anatomical and chemical origins and composition of the enteric system and its similarity with the cranial brain. Both originate from the neural crest in the embryonic stage and the neurotransmitters in the enteric system include the so-called cranial brain chemicals. Many of the cranial brain neurotransmitters are in greater quantity in the gut than in the head. As we shall see in the psychology section, Parkinson originally thought mental (as in cranial) nervous degeneration began in the gut and summated to express itself in the head.

The neurotransmitters

We can group the most common neurotransmitters in the nervous system into two main types. These are the *small-molecule neurotransmitters*: acetylcholine (Ach), dopamine (DA), norepinephrine (NE), serotonin (5-HT) and histamine, and the *amino acids*: Gamma-γ-aminobutyric acid (GABA), glycine, glutamate and aspirate. Of all these transmitters the most popular as we enter the twenty-first century is serotonin.

The localisation consciousness of the neurological world led us towards an understanding of the role of neurotransmitters in psychological expression. Serotonin (5-hydroxytryptamine, 5-HT), is present in animals and plants and is a product of tryptophan. Of particular interest is its action in the central and peripheral nervous system.

Serotonin was discovered in blood in 1948 and then at a later stage in the central nervous system. The chemical structure is simple and similar to norepinephrine and epinephrine. Serotonin is found in three main areas of the body: the intestinal wall (increasing gastric motility); in blood vessels (it acts to constrict large vessels); and in the central nervous system. In the peripheral nervous system it is involved in platelet homeostasis, increases capillary permeability where it is released in tissue injury and causes inflammation, increased gastric motility and carcinogenic tumours. In the central nervous system it is associated with mood, appetite, temperature function, endocrine function, behaviour, muscle contraction, and more commonly, as we shall see, depression. Serotonin is present in vast areas of the body even though the average person only has around 10 mg in their entire nervous system. The diversity of serotonin in the body is fairly unique and this is why it has such a powerful chemical and physiologically broad and non-specific effect on our function.

Serotonin works on two major areas of receptors: smooth muscle and nervous tissue. These two anatomical areas can be broken down into a group of labelled receptors. These are 5-HT1, 5-HT2, 5-HT3 and 5-HT4.

The 5-HT1 receptors

Overall these receptors are implicated in smooth muscle relaxation, cardiac and vascular smooth muscle contraction, junctional neurotransmitter release and the functional capability within the central nervous system.

- 5-HT1A receptors occur primarily in the central nervous system and are the main target in the therapy of depression.
- 5-HT1B receptors are found in rodents and seem to be absent in humans.
- 5-HT1C receptors seem to be similar to the 5-HT2 type and can also be named 5-HT2C. They are found in large numbers in the choroid plexus, implicating them in the regulation of cerebrospinal fluid production and cerebral circulation. This location increases the possibility of their involvement in cardiovascular regulation, analgesia and sleep.
- 5-HT1D receptors are mainly in the central nervous system, appearing to inhibit the release of neurotransmitters. The most common of the 5-HT1 receptors, they are also found in vascular smooth muscle regulating contraction.

The 5-HT2 receptors

These are found mainly in the vascular smooth muscle, lung, CNS, GI tract, lung and are associated with platelets. Their involvement seems to be with GI tract and vascular smooth muscle contraction, platelet aggregation, migraine, hypertension and nerve depolarisation.

The 5-HT3 receptors

The 5-HT3 receptors are found primarily in the central and peripheral neurons. They are implicated in the depolarisation of peripheral neurons, pain, and the emesis reflex.

The 5-HT4 receptors

These receptors are mainly in the GI tract, CNS and the heart. Activating these receptors increases cyclic adenosine monophosphate (AMP).

Serotonin and its functions are perhaps however at risk of being outshone by several new drugs that have entered into popular culture. One of the most important drug actions is the inhibition or serotonin uptake by selective serotonin re-uptake inhibitors (SSRIs). These selective 5-HT re-uptake inhibitors, also known as second generation antidepressants, include sertraline (Zoloft), paroxetine (Paxil) and the most popular, fluoxetine (Prozac). As with all drugs these do not go straight to the site of the brain receptor.

Vasoconstriction

Vasoconstriction of the blood vessels is by neurogenic, myogenic and chemical (metabolic) factors. The neurogenic component is largely sympathetic, there is a large myogenic influence. By myogenic it is meant that there are muscle fibres in the walls of the blood vessels that initiate vasoconstriction outside of the more general influence of the sympathetic system. A common example of myogenic influence would be in an emergency situation of vascular damage due to trauma. It is thought that the sympathetic influence on the resting tone of blood vessel walls in muscle, dermal and gastrointestinal tract tissue is between 15 and 20%. In the case of venous vessels the neurogenic component is the main influence on wall calibre. The only venous vessels where this is not the case and a myogenic component is a major influence are the portal and mesenteric veins.

A wave of myogenic activity along vessels which results in the relaxation, or decreased contraction, in walls distal to blood flow movement has been noted. This is again independent of overall neurogenic influence. As with the heart this is a sign of cell-to-cell propagation. The base resting tone of vessels before and after a capillary bed, pre- and postcapillary vessels respectively, show different base tones in different organs or tissues.

NON-IMPULSE BASED FUNCTIONS

'There is a mutual dependence of motor neurons and the muscles they innervate. The nerve determines the type of muscle and not vice versa. It has been suggested that the nervous system may have originated in the ancestral metazoans chiefly as a system of coordinating the regeneration and development of the body as a whole.

Gray's Anatomy (Warwick and Williams, 1978)

The 1936 Nobel prize for physiology and medicine was won by Otto Loewi (1873–1961) of the University of Graz, Austria and Sir Henry Dale (1875–1968), Director of the National Institute for Medical Research in Hampstead, London. Their research was one of the indirect contributions to osteopathic concepts, that of nerve nutrition to cells, organs and systems.

Loewi (1921) showed how the vagus nerve did not directly inhibit the action of heart muscle by impulses alone. He produced evidence that a chemical originating from the nerve cell body was the greater contributor to the inhibition of the heart muscle, known as *humoral transmission*. This chemical, christened Vagusstoff, was later to be similar to acetylcholine. Loewi went on to look at the accelerators of the heart from the sympathetic nervous system to investigate any similar humoral properties. Atropine, an alkaloid inhibits parasympathetic (vagal) function. This alkaloid does not paralyse the vagus nerve totally, but reduces, by humoral effect, the chemical action of the vagus on the heart.

Still, 1910, wrote in his *Osteopathy, Research and Practice*

'The osteopathic physician well knows that he must have two normally pure fluids, blood and nerve fluid. As a mechanical inspector he must ... hunt for such causes as would interfere with the production of pure arterial blood in quantities sufficient for all demands, or with the supply of nerve fluid to every organ.'

Trophism and axoplasmic flow

Neuroplasmic transportation is a general phenomenon of intracellular movement of material in all cells. In the case of nerves it is known as *axoplasmic transportation* (AXT) or flow. This is the other function of the nerve fibre and is no less important than the impulse based function in the healthy individual. This AXT can be disrupted as it is vulnerable to derangements, physical and chemical, and this may be the reason for certain tissue and neurological clinical presentations. The discovery of axoplasmic flow comes from the work of Speransky (1933).

This neuroplasmic material moves in a peristaltic manner along the axon supplying the necessary substances for normal nerve function that are not supplied by extracelluar fluids or blood. Turnover of this material may be several times a day with poor flow resulting in Wallerian degeneration (Korr, Wilkinson and Chornock, 1967). Disturbance of this flow can lead to degeneration of any tissue supplied by the affected nerves. These substances are moved in a trans-synaptic (across the synapses) manner and supply the tissue they innervate. Nerves vary in size and length and there are no natural barriers to movement of materials, only academic ones. Neuroplasmic flow is the flow of proteins, and can be slow or fast but is always bi-directional (Hirokawa, 1993). Most important is the understanding of the complete unity between the nerve, its neuroplasmic material and the tissue supplies.

Health of the nerve and the tissues it supplies is reliant on the unrestricted flow of neuroplasmic (cytoplasmic) material formed within the cell bodies. It is moved along the entire length of the nerve and all its branches in an active metabolically generated peristaltic manner by the axon. This neuroplasmic material may be replaced several times a day. Transported axoplasmic material includes enzymes, proteins, phospholipids, glycoproteins, and 5-hydroxytryptamine. Movement rates vary between substances and even between groups of entire nerves to and from the nerve cell bodies.

Nerves have been shown to instruct the tissue as to what kind of tissue it is supposed to be (Korr, 1979). The nerve determines the properties and type of tissue, chemically, structurally and functionally. Cytoplasm moves along the nerve supplying nutrients to the nerve and the target tissue at such a rate that the entire nerve cytoplasm can replace itself two to three times a day. Cytoplasmic movement along the entire length of the nerve shows that the organ and its cells receive nutrients from the nerve tissue and not only from lymph, plasma, or cerebrospinal fluid.

Trophism of peripheral nerves supplies tissues and organs with substances that are vital for normal maintenance and self-repair. This affects other functions such as hormones, metabolic clearance, nutritional integrity and the environment for microbes. Stressor factors have also been shown to affect the movement of materials leading to long-term detrimental response of tissues and organs through the development of osteopathic lesions. In turn trophic disturbance will affect the healing rate, pre- and postnatal development, and disturbed hormonal and lymphatic responses.

Morphogenesis

The trophic action of the nerves on the organ or tissues influences the form or morphology of the organ or tissue; this is known as *morphogenesis*. Korr (1972) gave the example used by Hix, a colleague, in that when the nerve supply to a kidney of a puppy was interrupted in the tenth or eleventh day of life the development of the kidney was retarded. After this time the kidney would continue to form. Experiments demonstrated that there is a critical point in the development of tissues related to the trophic growth factor functions of nerves particularly in embryonic development; including muscle. Muscle formation in the differentiation process of embryonic tissue has to have a nerve supply i.e. intact nerve-muscle junction, for the muscle to differentiate from the original embryonic tissue.

Regeneration

In lower animal forms, for example newts, amputation of entire limbs or the tail results in regeneration. After amputation or trauma the damaged tissue undergoes a form of differentiation in the form of a *blastema*. This process of regeneration seems to be related to the amount of neural tissue to total limb mass. The greater the amount of cross-sectional neural tissue and the lower the amount of limb mass, the greater the process of regeneration.

THE IMMUNE-NEUROENDOCRINE SOMATIC SYSTEM

In the treatment of disease, injury and ill health the osteopathic profession has always emphasised the reflex neurolymphatic response resulting in a lymphatic circulatory and immune disturbance. Undisturbed lymphatic circulation tends to be segmental in arrangement suggesting a reflection of the embryonic development patterns. Fine, paired, and unnamed arteries, particularly in the abdomino-lumbar region, originating from the aorta supplying the nodes (Sasaki, 1990) are paramount for the local and general homeostatic adjustment capabilities of the organism. Cells, organs and ultimately the entire organism rely on effective *metabolic clearance rates* (MCR). Clearance of by-products of metabolic activity varies; the metabolic activity itself advances from person to person and system-to-system and determines whether the demand is normal or excessive. Osteopathic medicine has emphasised the role played by emotion, the autonomic nervous and myofascioskeletal systems, and the diaphragms, particularly the thoracic diaphragm.

Osteopathic principles do not allow systems to be considered separately in clinical practice. Academically three main systems have been brought together in the discipline of psychoneuroimmunology, with the addition of a fourth, the myofascioskeletal system, being the most energetic. Eventually, with the addition of all systems, we should no longer consider people, social aspects, and the above systems abstractions. In this way we find ourselves back where we started, talking with and examining the patient. For years it has been demonstrated that there is a direct and reciprocal communication between the immune, nervous and endo-crine systems. Particular attention has been paid to the interrelatedness of the immune and nervous systems both in their anatomical connection and the common hormones and peptides. Thus the two systems actually represent a totally integrated system (Blalock, 1984).

Immune-neuroendocrine system

Direct communication of the autonomic nervous system with the lymphatic system has been recognised since the beginning of the twentieth century (Pot-tenger, 1984 and Robinson, 1907) and more recently by Bellinger *et al* (1994). Robinson (1907) highlighted the rhythm and motion of lymph as important mechanical factors in the continued maintenance of health. The presence of smooth muscle filaments and nerve fibres in the walls of the vessels was con-firmed by more sensitive investigation techniques (Rusznyák *et al.*, 1967). It has been shown that the lymphatic vessels contract and relax; in particular the thoracic duct contracts every 10 to 15˚seconds. Pulse waves of between 6 to 8 seconds with a mean pressure increasing from 15–20 mmHg that are asynchronous with respiration and limb movement suggest an intrinsic rhythm within the structures (Degenhardt and Kuchera, 1996).

The neurolymphatic system was demonstrated by Metal'nikov and Chorine (1926), who also emphasised the physiological conditioning and plasticity capabilities of the immune response. Nerve endings are directly in communication with the immune system and other tissues. Innervation includes bone marrow, thymus, spleen and lymph nodes (Blalock, 1984). Lymph glands are mainly innervated by large parenchymal sympathetic nerves with the cells of the immune system possessing β-adrenergic receptors (Appenzeller and Oribe, 1997). Blalock (1984) continues to present the biochemical reasons for the interrelation of the immune and neuroendocrine systems in the discipline of neuroimmunoendocrinology.

Peptide hormones and lymphokines (interferon) act through similar mechanisms in the nervous and lymphatic systems. Due to this common ground, Payan et al. (1984) agree with Blalock (1984), concluding that

'it is my opinion that one important aspect of this communicality of signals and receptors is that the immune system serves a sensory function. It has receptors and senses noncognitive stimuli (bacteria, viruses, antigens, etc.) that are not recognised by the central nervous system. This information is then relayed to the neuroendocrine system by lymphocyte-derived hormones and a physiologic change results. Contrariwise, central nervous system recognition of cognitive stimuli results in similar hormonal receptors on lymphocytes, and an immunologic change results.'

This communication is continuous by moving across synapses (Maycox et al., 1990) and shows plasticity in times of stress, infective, psychological and physical. Our nervous systems continually have to adjust to traumatic environmental demands; this has an effect on the immune cytokines, cell proliferation, degree of tissue survival, nerve outgrowth and neurotransmitter expression of cells of the nervous system. The opposite is also true: neurotransmitter and neurotrophic molecules originally defined by their function in the nervous system variously affect immune system function. This crosstalk between the nervous and immune systems using molecules common to both demonstrates regulatory interaction between the two systems (Jonakait, 1993). To present the neuroendocrine peptides and the immune system relationship simply we can initially involve the peptide neurotransmitters and associated hormones. Clinically the interrelation of the immune, nervous and endocrine systems is seen in the patient who presents with long-term effects of stress on his or her immunity and myofascial tissues; the patient looks as though he or she is being eaten 'from inside out'.

Investigators have placed paramount importance on the hypothalamic–pituitary–adrenal (HPA) axis. The HPA axis is a schematic representation of a 'linear' communication route between the hypothalamus, pituitary and adrenal glands in the stress response of immune–neuroendocrine interaction. As an expression of function the hypothalamus releases peptides known as *releasing factors* or hormones that affect pituitary hormones. The releasing factors are the following:

- corticotrophin-releasing hormone (CRH)
- growth-hormone-releasing hormone (GHRH)
- thyrotropin-releasing-hormone (TRH)
- luteinizing-hormone-releasing hormone (LHRH).

The pituitary gland, which sits in the sella tursica in the base of the skull, is connected to the hypothalamus by the pituitary or hypophyseal stalk. Pituitary gland structure reveals anterior and posterior compartments. The anterior compartment contains five different cell types releasing the following:

- adrenocorticotrophic hormone (ACTH, a corticotroph)
- growth hormone (GH, a somatotroph)
- thyroid-stimulating hormone (TSH, a thyrotroph)
- luteinizing hormone (LH, a gonadotroph) and follicle-stimulating hormone (FSH, a gonadotroph)
- prolactin (PRL, a lactotroph).

The releasing hormones from the hypothalamus and the hormones released from the pituitary are as follows:

- CRH – ACTH
- GHRH – GH
- TRH – TSH LHRH – LH/FSH
- prolactin release is held in check by dopamine.

Release of these hormones from the pituitary gland has an effect on certain organs. The level of response from those organs provides negative feedback to control the release from the pituitary gland and/or hypothalamus.

Central to the functioning of the HPA axis is the cell type known as the *corticotroph*, which produces, processes and stores a protein called *pro-opiomelanocortin* (POMC). Products of POMC include ACTH, corticotrophin and β-endorphin.

A stress response can be the higher centre cognitive recognition by an individual's central nervous system (CNS). CRH is immediately released from the hypothalamus to the pituitary gland via the portal circulation. CRH causes the release of ACTH into the blood circulation. ACTH acts on the adrenal gland causing the production of glucocorticoid hormone. Glucocorticoid hormone produces many of the signs of stress altering metabolic and immune function. It also has a negative feedback function inhibiting the further release of CRH and ACTH.

The above is naturally a simplification of the communication response of the metabolic and immune response. In addition the HPA axis involves the free cells of the immune system. These cells produce peptide hormones and neuro-transmitters that are also present in the central nervous, endocrine and myo-fascioskeletal system. All these systems communicate with each other and they are bi-directional. What can be definitely proven is that ACTH, endorphins and CRH are common in lymphocytes and macrophages even though they were earlier thought to be isolated in the neuroendocrine system.

These neuropeptides and hormones are not only present in the brain. A large number are in the gut in amounts that is comparable to the CNS. Due to the massive presence of small ganglia in the neural network of the gastrointestinal tract, pancreas and biliary systems, a range of transmitters is also present. The enteric nervous system is a far simpler neural system than the CNS, but this does not reduce its overall power on the entire organism. We have seen that the enteric reflex system is largely independent of the CNS: this principle applies to its peptides and other transmitter chemicals. Neuropeptides and their receptors thus join the brain, glands, and immune system in a network of communication between brain and body, probably representing the biochemical substrate of emotion (Pert *et al.*, 1985). Again, a large number of these chemicals are common to the other systems.

The following is a short list of neuropeptides, neurotransmitters and hormones involved in the communication between the myofascioskeletal, enteric, endo-crine, immune and central nervous systems.

- acetylecholine (ACh)
- ACTH
- corticosteroid hormones
- cytokines (Interleukins, IL)
- encephalins
- endorphins
- GH
- neuropeptide Y
- nitric oxide (NO)
- substance P
- substance K
- vasoactive intestinal peptide (VIP).

These chemicals are delivered via the circulation and/or direct neurotrophic communication. As we have mentioned above, the communication is bi-directional, and includes one of the most common chemicals known as *cytokines*. The cytokines are part of a group known as *endogenous pyogens* i.e. fever inducing chemicals, which include *interleukin 1* (IL-1), *interleukin 6* (IL-6) and the *interferons* (IFNs) having a widespread effect on all the systems (Fresno *et al.*,

1997). In combination these cytokines make you feel hot, sleepy and with diminished appetite, resulting in the characteristic myofascial aching associated with influenza symptoms. Crosstalk between systems and tissues is now apparent and in particular the cytokines are not only present in nerve tissue but are also manufactured in the CNS, being released by stress including changes in the environment. This is via the sympathetic nervous system (Kluger, 1991). Autonomic nervous function is indicative in a body's being preconditioned to express itself as fever or ill health. Under healthy conditions of running or physical activity cytokines are released but return to normal as soon as inactivity occurs. Under long-term low-level stress conditions individual heightened sympathetic tone affects muscle tone with poor clearance of metabolites. The CNS, specifically the spinal cord, induces the release of cytokines generally with poor metabolic clearance of tissues locally. As we shall see in the pathology section this is the classically described facilitated segment factor in the ill patient resulting in a local tissue acidic shift. Generally this provides the ideal environment for the multiplication of micro-organisms. Cells of the immune system are not only capable of responding to neuropeptides, but also of synthesising them (Fabry, Raine and Hart, 1994) indicating how open and barrierless systems are becoming understood. We would expect the functional integration of the body's cells through networks of neuropeptides and their receptors to be critical to the health of the organism as a whole (Pert et al., 1985).

The somatic-immune system

The role played by the myofascioskeletal system in immune stability of an organism is paramount in osteopathic principles. This somatic–immune connection is on a general and local level. The entire somatic component unspecifically expresses a reflex feedback of disturbance. Over time, considering intensity, the entire somatic component disturbance leads to what can only be described as a physiological breakdown in somatic–visceral communication. Reflexes become generally aberrant with an ANS, particularly vasomotor, disturbance. Locally muscle expresses immune functions at a cellular level. In reality both the global and local somatic–immune functions occur simultaneously.

General repeated low-grade vasomotor tone, vasodilatation and leakage of cells into surrounding tissue leads to fibrosis with myofascial and joint disturbance. This disturbance completes a cycle of aberrant afferent reflex dysfunction with the lymphatic system as one of the systems affected by this disturbance. Since the myofascioskeletal system is the biggest energy user and waste producer of the body the general MCR is disturbed leading to an acid shift in the acid–alkaline optimum of the body; micro-organisms prefer a more acid environment.

Somatic communication with the immune system is at both a motor and autonomic nervous system level. At a somatic spinal cord level the muscle spindle plays a key role in the feedback to CNS with regard to body tone and movement economy. High resting tone leads to a poor body economy with regards to posture and movement with accompanying fatigue and an increased need for metabolic clearance. Spinal motor neurones communicate with visceral motor neurones at academically segmental levels both on the same side and on the opposite side of the spinal cord. This is diagrammatically represented in Fig. 9 as a somatic-immune reflex pathway. This afferent CNS aberrant neural bombardment eventually leads to facilitation of spinal cord segments with direct and indirect sympathetic vasomotor outflow disturbance. This afferent flow can originate from the stimulation of nociceptive receptors in somatic structures via the sympathetic system. The thymus, spleen and other lymphoid tissues are innervated by autonomic postganglionic neurones that appear to modulate the T-independent B cell antibody response and circulation (Bullock and Moore, 1981; Miles *et al.*, 1981; Williams *et al.*, 1981; Bullock, 1985 and Stekel *et al.*, 1997). Burns (1933) cited Robuck, who in 1915 discussed the place of bony lesions in lowering immunity, and included with this discussion some phases of the pathology of the osteopathic lesion.

It should not be forgotten that the spinal cord comprises ascending and descending tracts. Disturbed somatic afferent impulses ascend to the medulla oblongata on its way to the reticular formation. Hind brain disturbance leads to aberrant parasympathetic outflow leading to an overall disturbance. Since lymphoid glands and vessels are heavily supplied by the vasomotor sympathetic system, fever and lymphoid gland enlargement have been shown to occur in small mammals and children by increased sympathetic activity where there is no infection, due to sudden environmental changes perceived as threatening (Kluger, 1991).

Muscle cell immunology is primarily concerned with the role played by *myoblasts* and *myotubes*. Disturbance of muscle cells and fibres as a result of injury, metabolic and/or physical, leads to the formation of myoblasts that go on to fuse forming primitive myotubes. Myoblasts and myotubes express antigens and interact with lymphocytes. Hohlfeld and Engel (1994) demonstrated that viruses can directly affect and infect muscle fibres in the expression of acute influenza and cocksackie virus myositis. They show that the muscle is the preferred site for the injection of vaccines as human myoblasts function as local antigen-presenting cells providing the signals necessary for triggering antigen-specific lysis and immune T-cell proliferation. This 'local' activity taken on a more general basis is experienced as the massive viral myositis felt by patients with the onset of 'flu' like symptoms.

Through extensive analysis of immunological concepts, Szentivanyi (1989) came to the following conclusions.

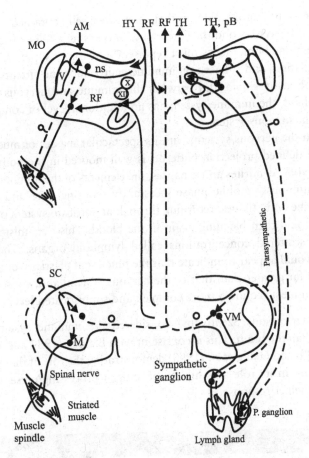

Fig. 9 Somatic-immune reflex pathways. V, nucleus of trigeminal nerve; X, nucleus of dorsalis nervi vagi; XII, nucleus of nervi hypoglossi; SC, spinal cord; ns, nucleus solitarius; M, spinal motor neurone; AM, amygdalar nuclei; a, nucleus ambiguus; RF, reticular formation; HY, hypothalamus; MO, medulla oblongata; TH, thymus; VM, viscero motor neurone; pB, nucleus parabrachials.

- The significance of the pharmacological mediators of immune responses in normal physiology is that they are the chemical organisers of central and peripheral autonomic action.
- This suggests an inseparability of the immune response system from the neuroendocrine system.
- Such inseparability indicates the *de facto* existence of immune/neuroendocrine circuits and the necessity for a bi-directional flow of information between the two systems.
- One must distinguish between the concept of autoregulation as one that primarily revolves around one effector molecule of immunity, the antibody, and satisfies the requirements of antibody diversity and specificity, in contrast to the more complex requirements of immune homeostasis.

- In contrast to autoregulation that is always self-contained, homeostatic control is always beyond the constraints of one single cell or tissue system.
- Thus, immune homeostasis must represent a far more sophisticated level of autoregulation, and is based on immune/neuroendocrine circuits.
- While the many similarities between the immune and nervous systems are fully realised, the immune system has an additional level of complexity over that of the nervous system.
- Although the nervous system, with its spectacular masses of much revealing and well defined projection patterns, is well moored in the body in a static web of axons, dendrites and synapses, the elements of the immune system are in a continuously mobile phase incessantly scouring over and percolating through the body tissues, returning through an intricate system of lymphatic channels, and then blending again in the blood. This dynamism is relieved only by scattered concentrations called lymphoid organs. These circumstances would appear to indicate that the functional plasticity of the immune system is far greater than that of the nervous system, and, consequently, its regulation must require a more complex and sophisticated level of control.

For the above reasons Szentivanyi considered the immune system as more 'intelligent' than the brain. This is consistent with Blalock (1984 and 1994), Van Buskirk (1990) and Heilig *et al.* (1993) demonstrating the role of the sympathetic nervous system in its role as inhibitor of antigen processing/presentation and, indirectly, T helper response.

THE MYOFASCIOSKELETAL SYSTEM

'Function of muscle – the all-important factor – cannot be satisfactorily taught in the dissecting room. It can only be taught on the living, and is largely a question of comparison – a comparison between the normal and the paralytic.'

Sir Colin Mackenzie

Golgi tendon organs are contraction-sensitive mechanoreceptors of mammalian skeletal muscles innervated by fast-conducting Ib afferent fibres. Control of posture and movement requires permanent monitoring of muscle length and tension, which is provided in mammalian muscles by two kinds of mechanoreceptors, spindles and tendon organs, which are sensitive to changes in muscles' length and tension, respectively (Jami, 1992). Anatomically, the spindles are arranged in parallel to the extrafusal fibres and are suited to sensing length changes in muscle. The tendon organs are located in series with the muscle fibres and detect force generated by the muscle fibres. Spindles are sensitive to very small changes in muscle length, producing a reflex activation, or shortening, of the stretching muscle. Tendon organs were thought to respond only to high levels of force and provide protection against the development of too much force by inhibiting the muscle (i.e. muscle of origin of the reflex) (Howell *et al.*, 1986).

Understanding the model of the gamma gain system is one of the central osteopathic concepts. This anatomic and physiologic motor-sensory feedback mechanism is an abstraction within the model of the motor neurone pool at the spinal cord level. The gamma gain system, at its simplest interpretation, involves the motor-sensory nerves, muscle, tendons, joints and investing fascial tissue. Simply, the gamma gain system alters the sensitivity of the nerve, muscle, tendon, joint and fascial relationship for the good of the organism. The muscle spindle – the word was coined by Kühne in 1863 (Sherrington, 1894; Rasch and Cole, 1960) – is the most active component of the system. Obviously taking one spinal cord level is an abstraction and so can not exist.

Muscle spindles are found in large numbers in most striated muscles of mammals. These sensory receptors signal information about muscle length to the CNS, information used in the control of muscle contraction and in body perception. They are sensitive to dynamic and static changes, being controlled by efferent neurons from the CNS. Sensory organs are located mostly at or near the equatorial region of the muscle, the largest axon to the spindle, the Ia (primary afferent) axon, has extensive annular terminations on all the intrafusal fibres of the spindle in their nucleated regions (the primary ending). Smaller group II axons terminate in 'flower spray' endings disposed principally on the nuclear chain and bag 2 (the secondary ending). Most spindles have only one sensory region (simple spindle); some have more than one sensory region (tandem spindles).

Primary endings arise from the large Ia sensory axon that divides repeatedly as it approaches the intrafusal muscle bundle. The main Ia axon has a diameter of 12–20 μm in its course from dorsal root to muscle. Of the two branches produced at its division on approaching the spindle, one often travels exclusively to terminals on the bag 1 fibre while the other innervates the bag 2 and chain fibres; occasionally a few on the bag 1 fibre. Although some of its terminations have an annular form, many do not encircle the intrafusal fibres to the extent seen in primary endings. The overall appearance is more patchy, as suggested by Ruffini's description of the secondary ending as flower spray. Whereas the primary ending is distributed over the nucleated region of the intrafusal fibres, the secondary terminals overlie regions of the fibres more completely occupied by sarcomeres, which are presumably more contractile (Hunt, 1990).

The term 'tension' (i.e. the constrained condition resulting from elongation of an elastic body) is used in physiological studies to designate the force that has to be opposed to a muscle to maintain it at a given length. When a non-contracting muscle is extended, it develops, by virtue of its elastic properties, a 'passive tension'. By analogy, the term 'active tension' is often used to designate the force developed by contraction. Both active and passive tensions are usually measured with transducers (strain gauges) and are expressed in 'gram' units rather than newtons, dynes or gram-force. As the muscle lengthens the spindle is stretched and stimulated to release impulses along the nerve fibres. Signal changes, i.e. the rate of impulse discharges, are proportional to the amount of lengthening the muscle performs (Rasch and Cole, 1960). These capsules containing the intrafusal fibres run the entire length of the muscle from tendon to tendon.

So-called mechanical properties of muscle tissue, length and tension are physically inseparable parameters, but while spindles monitor muscle length rather than tension, assessment of muscle tension rather than length is considered to be the task of tendon organs (also called musculotendinous end organ, Golgi organ or tendon spindle). However, tendon organs are not equally sensitive to passive and active tensions. In recent years the most important advance in our knowledge of tendon organs was the demonstration that contraction is their adequate stimulus and that an individual receptor can monitor the activity of a single unit.

Commonly accepted ideas that have to be revised represent the tendon organ as a stretch receptor with a high threshold and a low dynamic sensitivity. In fact, muscle stretch does not consistently or significantly activate tendon organs, whereas contraction does. Moreover, tendon organs display a very low threshold and an appreciable dynamic sensitivity when tested with their adequate stimulus: they can signal very small and rapid changes in contractile force. This is likely to have functional consequences that are not yet fully appreciated. As originally reported by Golgi, they are mostly found at points of attachment of muscle fibres to tendinous tissue, including deep intramuscular tendons or aponeuroses.

Recent studies have shown that there is no 'private' pathway for Ib input at the segmental level, since a variety of peripheral and central inputs converge on the interneurons mediating autogenic inhibition. Information from tendon organs is co-processed with information from other receptors and dispatched, as from a turntable, via different 'alternative pathways' selected by descending motor commands. The fact that inputs from tendon organs reach the cerebral cortex suggests that they contribute to conscious sensation, allowing assessment of the force developed in a voluntary contraction. It is difficult to disentangle the relative contributions of spindles, tendon organs and other muscle receptors, but this contribution to consciousness seems likely, as in the spinal cord, in light of centrally generated information derived from motor commands (Jami, 1992).

Contractions of muscle

Muscle contractions occur in one of three ways:

(1) shortening of the distance between fixed points and areas, i.e. bone and fascia (isotonic or passive tension)

(2) increasing tension within the muscles without shortening (isometric or active tension)

(3) a combination of the two.

Understanding this basic model is important in clinical presentations.

Fascia

It was not until the latter part of the nineteenth century that connective tissue began to be studied in any detail, when chemists and physicists became interested in its composition. Prior to this A.T. Still conceived his new method for the treatment of disease, with connective tissues playing a central role in the new concept. Connective tissue proper, derived from mesoderm, may be subdivided into three descriptive types: *loose* or *areolar*, in which the fibres form a loose network, the interspaces (areolar) of which are filled with semi-fluid, amorphous ground substance; *dense (fibrous) connective tissue*, which is characterised by a great many more closely packed fibres with correspondingly fewer matrices; and *special connective tissues*, which represent modifications of the loose variety and comprise the adipose pigment and haemopoietic tissues.

Connective tissue contributes to the representation of form, being the phenomenological soft tissue relation of body. In the Newtonian–Cartesian model it provides intervisceral support and binds every cell of the body. As a bed for all vessels and nerves, connective tissue serves a mechanical and physiological role, manufacturing intercellular substances, blood and lymph cells, heparin and antibodies. The significance of the reactivity of this tissue in the prevention and control of noxious forces in the body, antibody production and phagocytic cell activity, together with its role in the inflammatory reaction and in the prevention of spread of infection, cannot be overstated.

Osteopathic physicians have always appreciated the value of connective tissue in synchronising motion between muscles, viscera, vessels and nerves. As with the skeletal system constant adjustment and motion both physiologically and anatomically is recognised as a major factor in maintaining health. Contractility of this tissue continues throughout life; this quality supersedes all others, with elasticity decreasing with increasing age. Fascial attachments shorten after a period of great activity followed by a period of inactivity. With increasing age the ligamentous components become thicker and tighter.

That part of treatment in which fascia is important must take advantage of the properties and functions of fascia (Cathie, 1974). The properties of this connective tissue can be summarised as follows.

- It provides sensory nerve endings.
- It possesses properties of contractility and elasticity.
- It provides extensive attachments for muscles; more than bone.

- It regulates circulation especially that of the low pressure venous and lymphatic systems.
- It gives support, feedback and stabilisation for balance; suggestive of its involvement in motion.
- It assists in the initiation of motion, its control and interrelation of parts during motion.
- Fascial change will precede changes in cartilage and bone in the degenerative disease characteristic of ageing.
- Chronic passive congestion is predisposed by fascial contraction and thickening.
- Chronic passive congestion precedes the abnormal production of fibrous tissue, followed by an increase in the hydrogen ion concentration of articular and periarticular structures.
- Many fascial specialisations have postural function. In these, definite stress bands can be demonstrated.
- A burning type of pain will often accompany sudden stress on fascial membranes.
- Fascia (connective tissue) is an arena for inflammation, especially in viral infections.
- Infections and fluid often track along fascial planes.
- The dura mater is a connective tissue specialisation surrounding the central nervous system. In the skull it is attached to bone and to the nuchal ligament. Changes in tension and structure are important in the production of headache, and many disturbances of the brain.

The myofascioskeletal system is generally viewed as a complex system of levers, pulleys and joints functioning interdependently under the motive power of inertial forces and forces supplied by the contractile properties of muscle. This is an example of reverse anthropomorphism, arising from the early puppets created by jesters for entertainment. Some of the earliest Japanese puppets, a few thousand years ago, were the earliest to posses 'strings' attached to pieces of wood. They were human-like in their movements and as a system of levers and pulleys this attribute was turned back onto the body (Fig. 10). This is the origin of the link system approach to the human body. It permits us to characterise motion, and limits to motion, under normal and pathologic influence, and to understand the effects that local dysfunctions produce for the rest of the body. Frequently, we fall into the trap of assuming that muscle is the single motive force acting on the myofascioskeletal system. Indeed, it is a major factor, but a variety of inertial forces are also highly influential (Wells *et al.*, 1980); in health the body never stops moving.

Movement is again considered as a poly-reductionist interlink system in all animal forms. This oversimplification leads to the breakdown and rationalisation of abstracting parts from the whole. Observing normal motion is a phenomenon

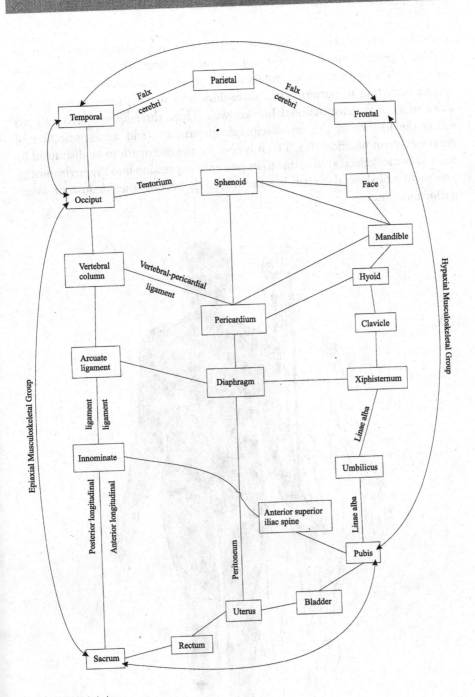

Fig. 10 Fascial chains.

of totality and constant adjustment. Osteopathic manipulative therapy is an analytical process but it is never applied on this interlink understanding but always with a holistic consciousness in the present. It considers lesions of the system occurring in patterns in a three-dimensional time-frame rather than a series of stepwise abstractional breakdowns. These three-dimensional patterns reflect the history of the myofascioskeletal structure and are a reflection of nervous system function (Fig. 11). It is easy for the osteopath to be distracted by the myofascioskeletal system due to its power of expression into the environment. The myofascioskeletal system has unfortunately become the Medusa of osteopathic medicine.

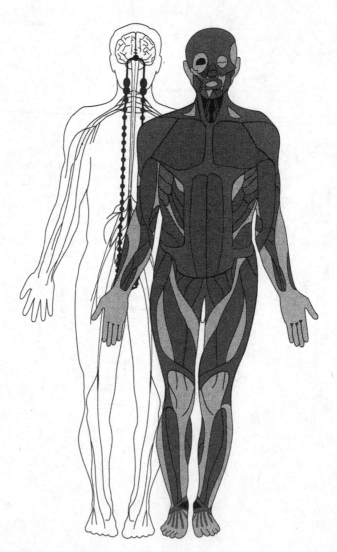

Fig. 11 Myofascial reflection of the nervous system.

THE CONCEPT OF BODY UNITY AND DIVERSITY

'The superior man in the medicine of the future will not be the great laboratory worker, or the man who is known for his studies in metabolism or the expert gastroenterology, or neurologist, or the surgeon or he who stands pre-eminently above his confrères in his knowledge of disease of the heart and arterial system or of the lungs, but the man who recognises the fact that the truths derived from all of these sources of study and investigation must be interpreted as belonging to the human patient as a whole – in other words, the internist who recognises both the psychical and the physical man and appreciates the unity of medicine. The distinguished specialist will be one who regards his field of study in its intimate relationships to the body as a whole.'

Francis Marion Pottenger

'There never was in the world two opinions alike, no more than two hairs or two grains; the most universal quality is diversity.'

Michel Eyguem de Montaigne

The concept of body unity and diversity (multiplicity) is not new; it can be traced back to the works of Hippocrates. The *unifying of bodies* and the *unifying of the body* are two different approaches. Unifying of bodies essentially does away with any individual qualities; it looks for commonalities between bodies. Unifying of the body includes diversity and tends to include non-common factors individual to the patient. Both work well, but both are limited. As we have seen in osteopathic philosophy, if we want to understand wholeness or an organic view we have to be aware of our choice of words in describing our thoughts. Andrew Taylor Still emphasised 'to find health should be the object of the doctor'. As we have read health is not only the absence of disease. The key word in our understanding has to be unity, the idea of interrelation derives from a consciousness of compartmentalisation. Beginning with pieces and showing how they relate is the analytical approach known as counterfeit holism. This philosophical point must be kept in the mind of every osteopath. Body unity of any kind is a human construct derived from abstractions of the body out of the environment; it is analytical in relation to real organic wholeness. Our dominant western philosophical mode of analytical consciousness makes it difficult to start with the organism-as-a-whole-in-its-environment.

This section will consider the body in its own right as an organism that, without a doubt, possesses a high degree of environmental independence from an anatomical/physiological aspect but *not* from a form/functional, or phenomenological, aspect. Anatomical/physiological and form/functional aspects must not be confused; one is a dominantly analytical symbolic construct, the other is a phenomenological expression. Unfortunately, it is nearly impossible to write about diversities between people: it would mean a section on every person that attended an osteopathic surgery. This demonstrates the totality of the osteopathic philosophy, principles and practice, i.e. it has to be done to the patient by the osteopath and not intellectually analysed. Osteopathy is a doing medicine, performed in the present with a timeliness. This was the humanistic philosophy before Descartes dragged it into a dead end (Toulmin, 1990).

Compartmentalisation of the disciplines within medicine has led to the further disempowerment and deconstruction of the patient. Specialists no longer talk the same language, so a cardiologist sees the entire body as a cardiovascular system, a urologist sees the entire body relating to the urinary system and the gastro-enterologist sees the patient as a gastrointestinal tract. While their contributions towards better health cannot be questioned, there are still too many investigations, too many medications and too many operations that would not be necessary if the concept of unity and diversity was applied. There could also be considerable economic savings. Still's philosophy urges us to see the human form as a unit, presenting as a whole. If we are to observe systems academically we must always try to do introduce an organic, intuitive consciousness. An example is the original meaning of the word evolution, before Darwin's use, which was the unfolding of the embryo as a whole, a phenomenology of the forming animal.

From the clinical standpoint what seems to be an isolated clinical entity is in fact the expression of the disturbed form, of the whole in a part *not* a part in the whole. This part-in-the-whole approach has led to the unity-out-of-diversity treatment of body systems. We see the cardiovascular, neurological, and gastrointestinal systems, each as a common unity, without diversity between patients. This is the mathematical Newtonian–Cartesian model applied to body systems. We unify between patients to form a commonality and certainty while ignoring the diversity of form and function which disturbs the modern scientific model. At best we see the individual in all the complexities of heredity, social and physical environment, past injuries, and experiences. This then becomes the key to pathogenesis, rather than the non-specific stress factor which happened to be most recently operating on him (MacBain, 1956).

In the last millennium there have been many concepts of unity and the maintenance of the inter-relationships between and within body systems; these included the 'milieu interne' of Claude Bernard, the general adaptation syndrome of Hans Selye, the homeostasis of Walter B. Cannon and the adjustments of A.T. Still. All express the organism-as-a-whole philosophy in their own way. The unifying body concept is built around the integrating function of the nervous system. In particular the medical profession is only just beginning to recognise that the nervous system acts as a whole all the time. Its unifying action is total, constant and spontaneous, varying in degrees. There is no such thing as the 'all-or-nothing law'. Organisms are never nothing or no-thing, in part or in total, at any point in time.

Andrew Taylor Still presented his system of disease prevention and treatment to the world in 1874. It is both unified and diverse in approach, with a consistent philosophy enacting in its principles and practice. He always stated that man was a unit, a machine (mechanism) made up of many parts contributing to the overall function, allowing a degree of independence and survival in the world. During the latter part of the nineteenth century, during Still's life, the versatile and broad physician was slowly disappearing. Society was demanding and rewarding the specialist. Only when Still's postulates of unification in both of its forms are understood and practised can they be used in diagnosis, the understanding of cause, and the treatment of disease and disability. In particular, only with this philosophy and principles can osteopathic manipulative treatment come to life.

Here we will develop *The Journal of the American Osteopathic Association's* January 1953 Symposium: *Osteopathic Contribution to the Concept of Body Unity*. This symposium called upon the expert contributions of A.A. Eggleston, J.S. Denslow, A. Levitt, G.W. Northup, C.A. Rohweder, and R.N. MacBain. We have looked earlier at the nervous system and its various reflexes that unite the body anatomically and physiologically. The above physicians went further and looked at the clinical inter-relatedness of the tissues that were supplied by these reflexes.

We shall briefly look at various components considered historically and clinically important in osteopathic medicine with a sense of inter-relatedness. These components are

- somatic
- visceral.

The somatic component

Osteopaths have regarded the integration of the somatic or myofascioskeletal system as a major component in the concept of body unity. Two reasons for this concept are first, that all organs and tissues have an anatomic and physiologic inter-relationship with somatic components through the various academic divisions of the nervous system. Second, observation, palpation and other investigatory methods have shown disturbances in somatic structures that seem to be remote from areas of pathological disturbance. Treatment of these distant somatic structures has an influence on the course of the pathological state.

For academic purposes the inter-relationship of organs and tissues has been neurologically reduced to an understanding in the form of segmentation. With this in mind we are then vulnerable to oversimplification and therefore construct doubt when we cannot put things together once we have academically pulled them apart. Applying the mathematical mode of consciousness to the myofascioskeletal system has led to the 'level and pulley' approach to understanding. The nervous system looks from inside out, we look from outside in. Fragmentation of the system into muscles is one problem; abstracting the whole system from the body is another.

Returning to the first point, if a tissue has a nerve supply then it is related to other nerves etc. Eventually there is a communication through the central nervous system within the 'motor neurone pool'. We can hard-wire the communication of tissues and organs to and from the somatic system in an anatomical manner. Unfortunately this does not reflect the physiologic function of the system or systems in relation to the soma. Injury, inflammation or degenerative change in one area is communicated to all other parts through pathways in an *oligodynamic* manner. Oligodynamic organismic responses involve a degree of excitation and inhibition determining the extent to which the impulses or trophic disturbance reach somatic structures. With varying amounts of excitation and inhibition particular to the individual we cannot have a clear cut situation of linear causality in response to a particular effect. This stands for disease as well as health. Somatic representation or reflection is never absolute and this should be remembered in examination, diagnosis and treatment. The biggest mistake made by medical professions is oversimplification.

Our second issue, continuing from the first, is that the relationship of the somatic system to the concept of body unity is seen in a clinical context. Clinically it is the bi-directional influence of the soma and other organs and systems that bring the osteopathic concept of unity and diversity into focus. It seems that other disciplines recognised this inter-relationship. As you will see in the psychology section even Freud recognised a somatic-psychic relationship. Speransky, while investigating the functions and behaviour of the nervous system in the origin and course of experimental lobar pneumonia, found that the course of the disease might be influenced favourably, and often dramatically, by the procainisation of the paravertebral muscles at the rhomboid area. Travell recognised myofascial trigger areas on the surface of the body caused a 'somatic blockade' of impulses to and from the spinal cord. In particular Travell demonstrated the relationship between these trigger points and cardiac disease.

With paravertebral muscles in particular it has been found that they reflect spinal cord function and health. Low resistance areas (LRA) present as inconsistent patterns in the paravertebral muscles and skin, that have to be 'read'. By inconsistent it is meant no two patients are the same. Palpation of these tissues has to be performed *intelligently*, as the origin of the word means 'to see through'. At a clinical level the practitioner must have an organic consciousness at the point of palpation. This is discussed in the clinical section.

The visceral component

As we have seen it is the relationship of the viscera to the myofascioskeletal system that has been called the 'metabolic limb system', by Schad. It is generally through the metabolic demand of the limbs and the energy supplied and waste removed by the viscera that this system works. Dr Still identified certain abnormal changes in the body whereby the viscera and organ systems may become disturbed in structure and function, leading to a general deterioration in health. This phenomenon of disturbed structural integrity with related disorders in the viscera and organ systems which make up the internal environment of the body, has become known as the *osteopathic lesion*. Broadly speaking, this is an abnormal body change that is frequently primary in time and relation to visceral disease, and as such it is capable of damaging its host, favouring poor metabolic clearance leading to an individual relative metabolic toxicity.

Speransky demonstrated his theory that disease was a reaction of the entire organism to whatever the irritation may be. According to Speransky the nervous system is the coordinating factor in the process and the pattern of response manifested in health or disease is determined by the pre-existing state of the individual's nervous system. This is particularly pertinent when we consider the gut as the 'second brain'. The only place an osteopath can experience body unity is in the presence of the patient. Only here will he or she be able to witness the phenomena of collective, reciprocal and interactive function.

The term 'visceral component' in the concept of body unity deals with the role which the body viscera, and the organ systems, have in the overall expression of health and disease. As we are aware, all cells are bathed in intercellular lymph through which the cells, and therefore collectively the organs and systems receive nutrients and deposit waste/metabolic by-products. Naturally the health of the cells depends on the movement and constitution of the intercellular fluid. This fluid can be influenced by physical, chemical and psychological factors which excite or depress metabolic function.

Viscera do not work as an independent collective. Function and communication are spontaneous varying in degree depending on the total economy needs and wishes of the organism-as-a-whole. Adjustment of the viscera to the needs of the myofascioskeletal system, via the nervous system, is the prime metabolic objective. MacBain (1951) wrote

'No system or organ has the entire load of adaptation – every function may enter into the response to environmental change when the necessity rises, and the more complex the organism, the greater the range of adjustment ... The mechanisms of the body are or become inadequate or over-respond or else the environmental change is overwhelming when disease becomes established. In any case, there is a complex and multiple failure involving total function, not merely one subdivision of the life process.'

It is in the abdomen that the aorta, great veins and lymphatics make their presence felt, anatomically and physiologically. Circulation is the fundamental essence of metabolism for the entire organism. Disturbance of the delicate abdomino-circulatory system will have consequences for the entire body. Low-grade dysfunction over long periods of time becomes a silent killer, especially to delicate central nervous system tissue. Parkinson recognised that the initiation and summation of enteric nervous disturbance led to brain damage and the disease which is named after him.

We have seen the role played by the enteric nervous section of the autonomic nervous system. Miller (1942), Kuntz (1953) and Robinson (1910) indicated patterns of clinical disease that were partially or wholly expressions of autonomic activity; they showed that the autonomic nervous system may react as fully and vigorously in the absence as in the presence of somatic damage. They also showed that through mechanisms of central autonomic regulation of visceral functions, widely divergent clinical phenomena may resemble each other and even defy clinical differentiation. Miller (1942) demonstrated that gallbladder disease stimulates coronary occlusion, pulmonary disorders, peptic ulcer, appendicitis, and other conditions.

The usual term of stress is an oversimplification of the course of visceral disturbance and its non-specific effects on the entire organism. Symptoms of disease occur because of reactions on the part of the viscera and other organ systems to injury, insult, infection and other short- or long-term stress factors. Response to these factors brings into action repair of injured tissue and other adjustments. In addition there is the continuing dynamic immunological adjustment to the internal and external environments.

The role of the posture completes a cycle of visceral–postural–visceral disturbed expression. Faulty body stance in its outward expression, (reduced in the Cartesian–Newtonian interpretation as mechanics) is always reciprocally related to the clinical observation of visceroptosis. These adjustments include fascial chain integrity disruption leading to disturbance of the reticuloendothelial system, which has the major role of providing the body with white blood cells and in detoxifying the organism. Considering the extent of the fascial system, especially when taking the abdomen and contents as a starting point, the circulation and therefore intercellular fluid disturbance can be appreciated over time. This is non-specific and leads to every disease presenting differently in every patient.

This leads to an appreciation of nutrition as part of the overall continuum with function and structure. Body and food are reciprocal; for food to be digested it must have something in common with the body. Proper digestion begins in the face and assimilation via circulation continues in the abdomen. Faulty structural relationships 'scramble' the signals leading to metabolic adjustments within the organism and therefore expression into the environment. Nutrition and structural integrity are interdependent. Poor nutrition in a poor or structurally compromised organism is the worst possible combination.

Among the long-term effects of visceral–autonomic (vasomotor) and trophic disturbances, possibly as a result of structural or form expression disturbance, can be included conditions of the thyroid, vagotonia, hypercholesterolaemia, hyperinsulinaemia, hypoglycaemia, and the degenerative diseases. Viscera of the human environment function in patterns in relation to the extremes of local enteric adjustment and myofascioskeletal, particularly limb, demands. Therefore disturbance of the viscera may be reflected in the soma and the soma will economically alter the demands and function of the viscera. Stressed or poorly adjusting functional activities of these viscera can lead to disorders in immunity via poor movement of metabolic by-products.

At the beginning of the twenty-first century we are seeing the slow demise of quantitative nutritional dominance. Qualitative whole food needs to be metabolised by an economically functioning myofascioskeletal system. Deposits of unmetabolised poor quality food are seen in many patients and, worse, in many children. Instead of using, working or exercising the system as a whole we limit the intake of natural products, i.e. sugar, salt, cholesterol, etc. The metabolic–limb system consciousness is now dominated by the fitness and health industries. These monopolising industries use the snapshot of simplistic compartmentalisation, symbolic of Newton and Descartes, to paper over individual bodily unifying humanistic needs in health and disease.

References

Appenzeller, O. and Oribe, E. (1997) *The Autonomic Nervous System. An Introduction to Basic and Clinical Concepts*. Fifth edition. Elsevier, London.

Aschner, J. (1967) *The Neurologic Examination* (ed. R.D. De Jong) p. 315. Hober Medical Division, New York, London.

Bayliss, W.B. and Starling, E.H. (1899) The movements and innervation of the small intestine. *Journal of Physiology* (London), 24, 99–143.

Bellinger, D.L., Madden, K.S., Felten, S.Y. and Felten, D.L. (1994) Neural and endocrine links between the brain and the immune system. In: *The Psychoimmunology of Cancer: Mind and Body in the Fight for Survival* (eds C.E. Lewis, C. O'Sullivan and J. Barraclough). Oxford Medical Publications, Oxford.

Berlin, R. (1959) The gastroauricular phenomenon. *The Lancet*, I, 734–5.

Blalock, J.E. (1984) The immune system as a sensory organ. *The Journal of Immunology*, March 132(3) 1067–70.

Blalock, J.E. (1994) The syntax of immune-neuroendocrine communication. *Immunology Today*, 15(11) 504–11.

Bradford, F.K. (1937) The auriculo-genital reflex in cats. *Journal of Experimental Physiology*, 27, 272–9.

Bullock, K. and Moore, R.Y. (1981) Innervation of the thymus gland by the brain and spinal cord in mouse and rat. *American Journal of Anatomy*, 162, 157–66.

Bullock, K. (1985) Neuroanatomy of lymphoid tissue: a review. *Neural Modulation of Immunity* (eds R. Guillemin, M. Cohn and T. Melnechuk). Raven Press, New York.

Burns, L. (1933) Principles of therapy dependent on the osteopathic pathology of sprains and strains. *The Journal of the American Osteopathic Association*, 33(11) 100–2.

Burnstock, G. (1976) Do some nerve cells release more than one transmitter? *Neuroscience*, 1 239–48.

Burnstock, G. (1986a) Autonomic neuromuscular junctions: current developments and future directions. *Journal of Anatomy*, 146, 1–30.

Burnstock, G. (1986b) The non-adrenergic non-cholinergic nervous system. *Archives of International Pharmacodynamic Therapy*, 280 (suppl.), 1–15.

Burnstock, G. (1990a) Co-transmission. The fifth Heymans lecture – Ghent, February 17, 1990. *Archives of International Pharmacodynamic Therapy*, 304, 7–33.

Burnstock, G. (1990b) Changes in expression of the autonomic nerves in ageing and disease. *Journal of the Autonomic Nervous System*, 30, 525–34.

Burnstock, G. (1993a) Introduction: changing face of autonomic and sensory nerves in the circulation. In *Vascular Innervation and Receptor Mechanics: New Perspectives* (eds L. Edvinsson and R. Uddman) pp. 1–22. Academic Press Inc., San Diego.

Burnstock, G. (1993b) Physiological and pathological roles of purine: an update. *Drug Development Research* 28, 195–206.

Burnstock, G. and Sneddon, P. (1985) Evidence for ATP and noradrenaline as cotransmitters in sympathetic nerves. *Clinical Science*, 689(suppl.10) 89s–92s.

Burnstock, G., Campbell, G., Bennett, M. and Holman, M.E. (1964) Innervation of the guinea-pig taenia coli: are there intrinsic nerves which are distinct from sympathetic nerves? *International Journal of Neuropharmacology*, 163–6.

Burnstock, G., Allen, T.G.J., Hassall, C.J.S. and Pittam, B.S. (1987) Properties of intramural neurones cultured from the heart and bladder. In *Histochemical and Cell Biology of Automatic Neurons and Paraganglia. Experimental Brain Research Series* 16 (ed. C. Heym) pp. 323. Springer Verlag: Heidelberg.

Burnstock, G. and Milner, P. (1992) Structural and chemical organisation of the autonomic nervous system and special reference to nonadrenergic, noncholinergic transmission. In *Autonomic Failure*, third edition (ed. R. Bannister) pp. 107–25. Oxford University Press, Oxford.

Cathie, A.G. (1974) The fascia of the body in relation to function and manipulative therapy. In *1974 Year Book*, pp. 81–84. American Academy of Osteopathy, Chicago.

Dale, H. (1935) Pharmacology and nerve endings. *Proceeds of the Royal Society of Medicine*. 28, 319–32.

Degenhardt, B.F. and Kuchera, M.L. (1996) Update on osteopathic medical concepts and the lymphatic system. *The Journal of the American Osteopathic Association*, February 96(2) 97–100.

Denny-Brown, D. (ed.) (1939a) *Selected Writings of Sir Charles Sherrington* p. 1. Hamish Hamilton Medical Books, London.

Denny-Brown, D. (ed.) (1939b): *Selected Writings of Sir Charles Sherrington* p. 265. Hamish Hamilton Medical Books, London.

Denslow, J.S. and Hassett, C.C. (1944) The central excitatory state associated with postural abnormalities. *Journal of Physiology*, 5, 393–402.

Descartes, René (1972) *Treatise of Man (De homine)*. Translated by Thomas Steele Hall. Harvard University Press, Cambridge, Massachusetts.

Deutsch, M. (1919) Ein Beitrag zur Symptomatologie der Beginnenden Lungentuberkulose. *Medizinisch Klin*, 43, 1090–1.

Dutia, M.B. (1989) Mechanisms of head stabilisation. *News in Physiological Sciences*, 4, 101–4.

Elliot, T.R. (1905) The action of adrenalin. *Journal of Physiology* (London), 32, 401–67.

Engel, D. (1922) Über das Reflektorische Ohrenjuncken bei Sodbrennen. *Med. Klin*. 47, 1495–7.

Engel, D. (1941) The influence of the sympathetic nervous system on capillary permeability. *Journal of Physiology*, 99, 161–81.

Fabry, Z., Raine, C.S. and Hart, M.N. (1994) Nervous tissue as an immune compartment: the dialect of the immune response in the CNS. *Immunology Today* 15(5) 218–24.

Fagius, J. and Wallin, B.G. (1983) Microneurographic evidence of excessive sympathetic outflow in the Guillain-Barré Syndrome. *Brain*. 106, 589–600.

Fecho, K., Maslonek, K.A., Dykstra, L.A. and Lysle, D.T. (1993) Alterations of immune status induced by the sympathetic nervous system: immunomodulatory effects of DMPP alone and in combination with morphine. *Brain, Behaviour, and Immunity*, 7, 253–70.

Fraher, J.P. and Bristol, D.C. (1990) High density of nodes of Ranvier in the CNS-PNS transitional zone. *Journal of Anatomy*, 170, 131–7.

Freeman, M.A.R. and Wyke, B. (1967) The innervation of the knee joint. An anatomical and histological study in the cat. *Journal of Anatomy*, 101, 505–32.

Fresno, M., Manfred, K. and Rivas, L. (1997) Cytokines and infectious diseases. *Immunology Today*, February **18**(2) 56–8.

Gardner, E. (1944) The distribution and termination of nerves in the knee joint of the cat. *Journal of Comparative Neurology*, 80, 11–32.

Gaskell, W.H. (1899) On the structure, distribution and function of the nerves which innervate the visceral and vascular systems. *Journal of Physiology (London)*, 7, 1–80.

Gershon, M.D. (1998) *The Second Brain*. Harper Collins, London.

Heilig, M., Irwin, M., Grewal, I. and Sercarz, E. (1993) Sympathetic regulation of T-helper cell function. *Brain, Behaviour and Immunity*, 7, 154–63.

Highfield, R. (1999) Study clears Linford Christie of false start in the Olympic final. *Daily Telegraph*, London. May 17, p. 7 and Editorial p. 21.

Hillarp, N.-Å. (1959) The Construction and Functional Organisation of the Autonomic Innervation Apparatus. *Acta Physiologica Scandnavica*, 46(suppl. 157) 1–38.

Hirokawa, N. (1993) Axonal transport and the cytoskeleton. *Current Opinion in Neurobiology*, 3, 724–31.

Hohlfeld, R. and Engel, A.G. (1994) The immunobiology of muscle. *Immunology Today*, 15(16) 269–274.

Hökfelt, T., Fuxe, K. and Pernow, B. (eds.) (1986) Coexistence of neuronal messengers: a new principle in chemical transmission. In *Progress in Brain Research*, Vol. 68. Elsevier, Amsterdam.

Howell, J.N., Binder, M.D., Nichols, T.R. and Loeb, G.E. (1986) Muscle spindles, Golgi tendon organs, and the neural control of skeletal muscle. *The Journal of the American Osteopathic Association*, 86(9) 599/119–602/118.

Hoyle, C.H.V. and Burnstock, G. (1989) Neuronal populations in the submucous plexus of the human colon. *Journal of Anatomy*, 166, 7–22.

Hunt, C.C. (1990) Mammalian muscle spindle: peripheral mechanisms. *Physiological Reviews*, 70(3) 643–63.

Jami, L. (1992) Golgi tendon organs in mammalian skeletal muscle: functional properties and central actions. *Physiological Reviews*, 72(3) 623–67.

Jänig, W.M. (1995) Ganglion Transmission *in vivo*. In *Autonomic Ganglia*, (ed. Elspeth M. McLachlan) Chapter 9. Harwood Academic, London.

Johnston, W.L. *et al.* (1987) Somatic manifestations in renal disease: a clinical research study. *The Journal of the American Osteopathic Association*, January, 87(1) 22–35.

Jonakait, G.M. (1993) Neural-immune interactions in sympathetic ganglia. *Trends in Neuroscience*, 16(10) 419–423.

Kawato, M. and Gomi, H. (1992) The cerebellum and VOR/OKR learning models. *Trends in Neuroscience*, 15(11) 445–53.

Kerr, H.E. (1936) The role of fascia in osteopathic problems. *The Journal of American Osteopathic Association*, May, 36(9) 418–20.

Kluger, M. (1991) Fever: role of pyrogens and cryogens. *Physiological Reviews*, January 71(1) 93–127.

Korr, I.M. (1979) The segmental nervous system as a mediator and organiser of disease processes. Originally published in *The Physiologic Basis of Osteopathic Medicine* The Collected Papers of Irvin Korr, 1979. American Academy of Osteopathy, Chicago.

Korr, I.M. (1975) Proprioceptors and somatic dysfunction. Originally published in *The Journal of the American Osteopathic Association*, 74, 638–50. *The Collected Papers of Irvin Korr*, 1979. American Academy of Osteopathy.

Korr, I.M., Wilkinson, P.N., and Chornock, F.W. (1967) Axonal delivery of neuroplasmic components to muscle cells. *Journal of the American Osteopathic Association*, 66(9) 1057–61.

Kosterlitz, H.W. (1968) The alimentary canal. In *Handbook of Physiology*, (ed. C.F. Code) vol IV, pp. 2147–72. American Physiological Society, Washington, DC.

Kuntz, A. (1953) *Autonomic Nervous System*. Lea & Febiger, Philadelphia.

Langford, L.A. and Schmidt, R.F. (1983) Afferent and efferent axons in the medial and posterior articular nerves of the cat. *Anat Rec*. 206, 71–8.

Langley, J.N. (1921) *The Autonomic Nervous System*, Part 1. W. Heffer, Cambridge.

Lisberger, S.G. (1988) The neural basis for the learning of simple motor skills. *Science*, 242(4) 728–35.

Loewi, O. (1921) Über Humorale Übertrangbarkeit der Herznervenwirkung. XI. Mitteilung. *Pflugers Arch. Gesamte Physiolo*. 189, 239–42.

Lüscher, H-R. and Claman, H.P. (1992) Relation between structure and function in information transfer in spinal monosynaptic reflex. *Physiological Reviews*, January No.1 72, 71–99.

MacBain, R.N. (1951) Body unity – in health and disease. *The Journal of the American Osteopathic Association*, 50(12) 605–10.

MacBain, R.N. (1956) The somatic components of disease. *The Journal of the American Osteopathic Association* 56(3) 159–165.

Maggi, C.A. and Meli, A. (1988) The sensory-efferent function of capsaicin-sensitive sensory nerves. *General Pharmacology*, 19, 1–43.

Martin, C. (1937) Relaciones anatomopatol – gicas entre la arterioesclerosis aortica y los ganglios simpáticos. *Bol. Soc. Biol Concepción* 11, 45–65.

Maycox, P.R., Hell, J.W. and Jahn, R. (1990) Amino acid neurotransmission: spotlight on synaptic vesicles. *Trends in Neuroscience*, 13(3) 83–7.

McConnell, C.P. (1915) Etiology of the osteopathic lesion. *The Journal of the American Osteopathic Association* 15, 173–80.

McKone, W.L. (1997) *Osteopathic Athletic Health Care: Principles and Practice*. Stanley Thornes, London.

Metal'nikov, S. and Chorine, V. (1926) Roles des réflexes conditionnels dans l'immunité. *Annales de L'institut Pasteur*, 11, 893–900.

Miles, F.A. and Lisberger, S.G. (1981) Plasticity in the vestibulo-ocular reflex: a new hypothesis. *Annual Review of Neuroscience*, 4 273–99.

Miles, K., Quintans, J., Chelmicka-Schorr, E. *et al.* (1981) The sympathetic nervous system modulates antibody response to thymus-independent antigens. *The Journal of Neuroimmunology* 1, 101–5.

Miller, H.R. (1942) *Central Autonomic Regulations in Health and Disease, with Special Reference to the Hypothalamus*. Grune and Stratton, New York.

Nicholas, A.S. *et al.* (1985) A somatic component to myocardial infarction. *British Medical Journal*, 291, 13–17 6 July.

Northup, T. (1976) The musculoskeletal system: A major factor in maintaining homeostasis. *The Northup Book. A Memorial Tribute to Thomas L. Northup, D.O.* The American Academy of Osteopathy, Chicago.

Pascual-Leone, A., Cohen, L.G. and Hallett, M. (1992) Cortical map plasticity in humans. *Trends in Neuroscience*, 15(1) 13–14.

Payan, D.G., Levine, J.D. and Goetzl, E.J. (1984) Modulation of immunity and hypersensitivity by sensory neuropeptides. *The Journal of Immunology*, 132(4) 1601–4.

Pert, C.B., Ruff, M.R., Weber, R.J. and Herkenham, M. (1985) Neuropeptides and their receptors: a psychosomatic network. *The Journal of Immunology*. 135(2) 820s–826s.

Pottenger, F.M. (1984) *Symptoms of Visceral Disease*. Sixth edition. C.V. Mosby Company, St. Louis.

Rand, M.I. (1992) Nitrergic transmission: nitric oxide as a mediator of non-adrenergic, non-cholinergic neuroeffector transmission. *Clinical Experiments in Pharmacology and Physiology*, 19, 147–69.

Rasch, P.J. and Cole, W.V. (1960) Role of the gamma system in posture. *The Journal of the American Osteopathic Association*, 60, 277–80.

Robinson, B. (1910) *The Abdominal and Pelvic Brains*. Frank Betz, Hammond, IND.

Rouvière, H. (1929): Sur les lymphatiques des ganglions sympathetiques cerviceaux. *Ann. Anat. Path.* 6, 222–3.

Ruszynák, I., Földi, M., and Szabó, G. (1967) *Lymphatics and Lymphatic Circulation*. Pergamon Press, Oxford.

Sasaki, K. (1990) Arterial supply to the lumbar lymph nodes in man. *Journal of Anatomy*, 168, 229–33.

Sherrington, C.S. (1894) On anatomical constitution of nerves of skeletal muscles; with remarks on recurrent fibres in ventral spinal nerve roots. *Journal of Physiology*, 17, 211–58.

Shichijo, K., Ito, M., Taaniyama, K., and Sekine, I. (1993) The role of sympathetic neurons for low susceptibility to stress in gastric lesions. *Life Sciences*, 53, 261–7.

Snyder, S.H. (1992) Nitric oxide: first in a new class of neurotransmitter? *Science*, 257, 494–6.

Speransky, A.D. (1933) How the theory of neuro-trophism arose. *Archives of Biological Sciences*, Parts 5–6, 629–41.

Speransky, A.D. (1944) *A Basis for the Theory of Medicine*. International Publishers, New York.

Spiegel, E.A. and Adolf, M. (1920) Beiträge zur Anatomie und Pathologie des autonomen Nervensystems. I: Die Ganlien des Grenzstranges. *Arb. Neurol. Ins. Univ. Wein*. 23, 76–117.

Sprafka, S. *et al.* (1981) What characterizes an osteopathic principle? Selected responses to an open question. *The Journal of the American Osteopathic Association*, 81(1) 81–5.

Stein, J.F. and Glickstein, M. (1992) Role of the cerebellum in visual guidance of movement. *Physiological Reviews*, 72(4) 967–1017.

Stekel, D.J., Parker, C.E. and Nowak, M.A. (1997) A model of lymphocyte recirculation. *Immunology Today*, 18(5) 216–21.

Still, A.T. (1910) *Osteopathy, Research and Practice*. Published by the author. Kirksville, MI.

Strong, L.V. (1940) Thoughts on the autonomic nervous system: Part II. *The Journal of the American Osteopathic Association*. 40(1) 5.

Szentivanyi, A. (1989) The discovery of immune-neuroendocrine circuits in the fall of 1951. In *Interactions among CNS, Neuroendocrine and Immune Systems* (eds J.W. Hadden, K. Mašek and G. Nistico). Pythagoras Press, Rome.

Toulmin, S. (1990) *Cosmopolis: The Hidden Agenda of Modernity*. The University of Chicago Press, Chicago.

Van Buskirk, R.L. (1990) Nociceptive reflexes and the somatic dysfunction. *The Journal of the American Osteopathic Association*, 90(9) 792–809.

Vasiliu, D.I. (1932) Reflex auriculo-uterin. *Spitalul*, 52, 396.

von Euler, U.S. and Gaddum, J.H. (1931) An unidentified depressor substance in certain tissue extracts. *Journal of Physiology*, 72, 74–84.

Warwick, R. and Williams, P.L. (1978) *Gray's Anatomy*. 35th British edition. Longman, London.

Wells, J.P., Fisk, R.M. and Finn, W. (1980) Proceedings of the Twenty-fourth Annual Osteopathic Research Conference: Part 2. Functional anatomy of human locomotion and posture – A symposium. *The Journal of the American Osteopathic Association*, 80(4) 276–89.

Williams, J.M., Peterson, R.G., Shea, P.A. *et al.* (1981) Sympathetic innervation of murine thymus and spleen: evidence for a functional link between the nervous and immune systems. *Brain Research Bulletin*, 6, 83–94.

Further reading

Kamosinska, B., Nowicki, A., Szulczyk, A. and Szulczyk, P. (1991) Spinal segmental sympathetic outflow to cervical sympathetic trunk, vertebral nerve, inferior cardiac nerve and sympathetic fibres in the thoracic vagus. *Journal of the Autonomic Nervous System*, 32, 199–204.

Martin, P. (1997) *The Sickening Mind*. Harper Collins, London.

Porter, R. (1987) Image and illness: The body politic. In *The Connected Body*. Eds R. Allsopp and S. deLahunta. Amsterdam School of Arts, Amsterdam.

Strand, F.L., Rose, K.J., Zuccarelli, L.A., Kume, J., Alves, S.E., Antonawich, F.J. and Garrett, L.Y. (1991) Neuropeptide hormones as neurotrophic factors. *Physiological Reviews*. 71(4) 1071–46.

Thomas, R.B. (1952) Man the unit: an osteopathic philosophy. *The Journal of the American Osteopathic Association*. 52(3) 155–9.

CHAPTER 7

Psychology

'The majority of men lead lives of quiet desperation.'

Henry David Thoreau

'Only the body and its desires cause war, civil discord and battles, for all wars are due to the desire to acquire wealth, and it is the body and the care of it, to which we are enslaved, which compel us to acquire wealth, and all this makes us too busy to practise philosophy.'

Plato – Phaedo, *The Last Days of Socrates*

Psychology is well within the historical domain of osteopathy. As with all specialities it has changed and has been given up to the allopathic model of today. Osteopathic psychology is not a combination of osteopathy and psychology, it approaches a psychological dysfunction with the same principles as it would a twisted ankle. This does not mean that the psychology of today is wrong but an osteopathic approach shows an attempt, historically, to present the mind-in-the-body (including the head) rather than just the mind-in-the-head.

What constitutes osteopathic psychology? This can be answered without any change in the general principles of osteopathy. Osteopathic psychology can be described as the appreciation of the myofascioskeletal system in the expression of emotion. As cited in John Martin Littlejohn's *Lectures in Psycho-physiology* (1899)

'the physiologists have largely limited their investigations to the separate parts of the central nervous system without attempting to formulate any plans of systematic action on the part of the system as a whole. This has produced in physiology a tendency to overestimate the importance of specialisation of function, overlooking the fact that there is solidarity and unity of action on the part of the entire system. It is probable that every active operation of the nervous system affects the whole human system; in this way there must be constant activity on the part of the nerve cells. This forms the basis of "the continuity of conscious experience." Behind consciousness, at least, from a morphological standpoint there lies the anatomical structure of the nervous system; but as yet no one has been able to solve the problem of their relations. The region of consciousness has been gradually moving upwards with the development of physiological theories until, as one physiologist has said, it has had to take refuge in the only remaining region after the sensory and motor areas have been localised, namely, in the anterior portion of the grey matter of the cortex.'

The history of psychology

Historically there are three ways of approaching the mind–body problem: monism, dualism and trialism:

Monism

Materialistic monism has its roots in the distant past of Greek philosophy. Records show that one of its first suggestions can be claimed by Leucippus, 440 BC and Democritus, 420 BC. Their idea was that everything was made of atoms, hence the earliest atomic theory. This idea developed the concept that these atoms were in motion and their interactions were a factor in outcomes of life.

Dualism

The concept of dualism as the soul or mind and body like monism originates back to the earliest recorded times of Western thought. The Greeks accepted it in the fifth century BC with their materialistic monism with the earliest records attributing dualism to Empedocles and Anaxagoras. This mode of thinking in Western consciousness, philosophy and science is now accredited to Socrates, Plato and Aristotle. Aristotle for example wrote about the soul and mind being separate from the body. Ever since the time of the Greek philosophers the concept of dualism has been brought into present times by the works of Saint Augustine, Thomas Aquinas and in particular Descartes.

Trialism

In the trialistic theory the world is divided into minds, bodies, and also mind-bodies, i.e. entities in which the two substances are one (Cottingham, 1986).

Development of the mind–body relationship

The mind–body distinction in Western culture is attributed to its origins among the ancient Greeks. We know that the dualism of soul or mind and body was present in the fifth century BC. Anaxagoras and Empedocles (fifth century BC) were the first to be accredited with the concept of dualism. It was not until the works of Socrates, Plato and Aristotle that dualism became established into Greek philosophy. Equally important, if not more, was the contribution of Aristippus of Cyrene, a friend of Socrates. Aristippus believed in pleasure at all times, particularly a pleasure of the moment. This concept, generally known as *hedonism*, was not to be advocated without self-control. Aristippus insisted that friendship was the safest of all social pleasures and he disapproved of sexual intercourse as part of pleasure's expression.

It was not until the work of René Descartes that the first real systematic treatise on the mind–body relationship came into its own. As we have seen in the philosophy section Descartes was responsible for the final dead end non-humanistic approach to philosophy (Toulmin, 1990). This philosophy also affected psychology: 'The new-found meaning had significance in many ways, not least in its repercussion upon a young philosopher, Descartes, from whom modern psychology may be said to start' (Sherrington, 1946). Since Descartes was a mathematician he was acutely aware of the order and certainty of mathematics and the apparently controversial manner of philosophy. He believed that nature could be ordered in the same way as mathematics. His publications included the first works on physiological psychology in *De Homine*. Unfortunately, it was not published until after his death, because Descartes suppressed its publication on hearing that Galileo had suffered at the hands of the Inquisition for publishing new ideas.

In *De Homine* Descartes submitted the first mechanism for an automatic reaction response to the outside world. He proposed that the motions in the outside world affected the nerve fibrils, displacing the central ends. As these central ends are displacing there is a rearrangement of the pattern of the interfibrillar space directing the flow of animal spirits to the appropriate nerves. Due to this description it was Descartes who has been accredited with the foundation of the reflex arch theory.

In addition to the above work he began to look at mind–body interaction. His idea was that the rational soul, an entity separate from the body but nevertheless making contact with the body at the pineal gland, may or may not develop an awareness of the ebbing outflow of animal spirits brought about by the constant rearrangement of the interfibrillar spaces. When awareness did take place then you became conscious of yourself and surroundings. In voluntary action the soul may affect the outflow of the animal spirits before the bodily action is made; mind/soul could also affect the body. By working on the mathematical basis of truth and certainty Descartes made epistemology, the understanding of the relationship between mind and the world, a starting point in philosophy. It was his separation of mind and body that epitomises the dualistic concept in health care. Cartesian logic has had its time. Devlin (1997) reminds us that 'so deeply rooted has Descartes's dualist view become in present-day science – and indeed in much of our present-day world view – that it is widely believed that it is only a matter of time before familiar looking, mathematical sciences of reasoning, language, and communication are developed. Furthermore, any theory – of cognition, language, society, or whatever – that does not fit the expectations of Cartesian science runs the risk of being dismissed, at least by many scientists, as not completely respectable.'

Modern origins

The modern origins of psychology can be traced as far back as the seventeenth century where the main psychotherapists were the clergy. This counselling by members of the clergy was the main way of talking or narrating personal problems (Thomas, 1971). It was a form of confession about the way in which you led your life to that point in time and is why the original term for psychology was *moral philosophy*. The Protestant church influenced the exchange of the word soul for the word mind and the soul could not be in the body, therefore it ascended to the head. This demonstrates that the original ascending of the mind to the head was not the result of any experimentation or research but was due to the continuing influence of the church on the academic development of psychology. As with all professional developing sciences this also meant secularisation and specialisation. Fortunately this was not universal.

Groups of 'underground' academics and scholars believed in the unity of body and mind. They were not popular and continued to work even under the threat of blasphemy and incarceration. Few men and women opposed the church but those that did included Erasmus Darwin (grandfather of Charles Darwin), Percy Bysshe Shelley and Mary Shelley. Darwin and others opposed the mind-in-the-brain group of psychologists who were later labelled the 'cerebralists' or defenders of the soul. This did not mean that the mind was not part of the brain, but it was not isolated to the brain. As with most definitions time slightly warps them. One of the earliest definitions was for *a* brain rather than *the* brain as, 'an apparatus capable of reception, reorganisation and emission of nerve forces or impulses' (Robinson, 1907).

Numerous written works on the unity of body and mind had to be disseminated covertly and poetry was one of the best methods of presenting the body–mind unity movement. This thought can be found in the words of 'meta-poets' such as William Wordsworth. From a literary aspect one of the most famous works representing the underground psychology of unity of body and mind was Mary Shelley's *Frankenstein*. She cleverly gave this psychology the form of a gothic tale (and thus invented the science fiction novel). Her analysis of a being who was admittedly depraved was hugely successful, despite hostile reviews (Reed, 1997). Society is still under the influence of the church in the way that it practises psychology, so much so that few even recognise Mary Shelley's work for what it really is. It was only after the printers refused to be told what they could and could not print that many of these works made it into the public domain. The popularity of such works increased into the late nineteenth century until the academics under the church compromised by calling everything below the 'mind' (and head) the subconscious. Can we ever escape the influence of the church? Historian Lynn White, Jr., (cited in Zajonc, 1998) puts forward the mechanical clock as an icon of Christian theology. Within 150 years this mechanical clock was used as an attribute of the principle of virtue of fifteenth century temperance. The human body and the soul required regulation by reason, life was no longer regulated by the sun by day and the stars by night. Man was free from nature. White reminds us that 'human life no longer adapts the mechanism to its need; mankind is in some measure shaped by a machine which it adores'.

We in Europe have defined the academic discipline of 'psychology'. The present practice of psychology and all its derivatives is Eurocentric, has no regard for other cultures and is basically a precipitation, over time, of cultural imperialism (MacDonald, 1998). The modern biological, rather than cultural, psychology has its roots in physiology. The original works of Robert Whytt in the 1740s, Sir Charles Bell in 1811 and François Magendie in the 1820s suggested that the dorsal side of the spine was a sensory (input) side and the ventral a motor (output) side. This led quickly to the idea that the brain received and interpreted only the results of what had already been actively processed by the spinal cord (Reed, 1997). We are now well aware that the spinal cord is not a passive relay station but an active processor of the majority of sensations, and therefore interpretations, that ascend into the brain. Even towards the end of the twentieth century, experiments, as analytical as ever, are finding memory traces in the spinal cord (Wolpaw and Carp, 1990). With the work of Bell in particular came the origin of the *sixth sense*, muscle. It was Bell who developed the idea of muscle as a sixth sense and gave it a clear physiological relationship with the rest of the organism. As an added interest the term *Muslesinn* was used to describe a sense before 1790 by certain German philosophers (Carmichael, 1926).

Aspects of the nervous system and the relationship with muscle have in the past been seen as the physiological origins of both mind and memory. With memory comes the development of our own belief systems. Belief is a cultural and moral development reflecting our social development and makes its contribution to mental health. So depression, for instance, quite obviously a medical condition, is also inextricable from your self, the person you imagine yourself to be. In other words, it involves an element of choice: that depressives are not simply having something happen to them, they are also doing something. And they are aiming to get some profit out of what it is that they are doing. What does this mean? It is not as straightforward as saying that people 'choose' to get depressed. It simply means that every emotion you experience is connected to a belief. Beliefs are constructed not only out of reason but out of need, a need for psychological self-defence, need for a sense of personal significance, the need to maintain a sense of certainty, however high the cost (Lott, 1999). This false model of certainty is part of our Cartesian–Newtonian analytical cultural consciousness originating after the Thirty Years War when Europeans were looking for certainty. It makes us search repeatedly for small absolutes in a world that is dynamic and to a greater extent unpredictable.

Today there are changes in psychoanalysis, at least in its more doctrinaire form. Rumour has it that even the Americans are looking in a different direction. Here in the UK, Pavlov has been rediscovered so that behaviour therapy has become fashionable. Despite this, psychotherapy is a medicine to which many psychiatrists as well as their patients are undoubtedly addicted (Trethowan, 1979). What is the difference between the Cartesian–Newtonian model of physics and the model of psychoanalysis? In reality, there is very little. The psycho-analytical theory of man was fashioned after the causal–deterministic model of classical physics. Attention is drawn to the principle of physical determinism to human affairs which Karl Popper aptly termed 'historicism'. The psycho-analytical theory of behaviour is, therefore, a species of historicism. Historicism is a doctrine according to which historical prediction is essentially no different from physical prediction (Szasz, 1984). Maslow (1970) wrote that

'our first proposition states that the individual is an integrated, organised whole. In good theory there is no such entity as a need of the stomach or mouth, or a genital need. There is only a need of the individual. It is John Smith who wants food, not John Smith's stomach. Furthermore satisfaction comes to the whole individual and not just to a part of him. Food satisfies John Smith's hunger and not his stomach's hunger.'

The story of Phineas Gage

'At the same time, while it is essential to reduce the nervous system to its parts in order to understand its detailed mechanisms, such analyses provide only a partial and, if taken in isolation, a misleading picture of the nervous system; ultimately we are dealing with an immensely structured, integrated and coherent network which is itself a functional unity rather than merely a com-plicated assembly of individual components.'

Gray's Anatomy: The nervous system (Thirty-fifth edition)

Littlejohn (1899) was acutely aware at the end of the nineteenth century of suggestions of localisation carried out in the intermediate parts of the brain and that this indicated the possibility of localisation in the cerebrum. The doctrines of localisation were not yet more than a quarter of a century old. Earlier attempts met with little or no success, and the fact that large parts of the brain could be lost without any appreciable loss of sensory or motor functions assisted in discrediting any attempts to localise. The great physiologists of the first half of the nineteenth century decided against localisation, claiming that the different parts performed their own functions in relation to the entire brain. Paul Broca (1824–80) was the first to suggest localisation in connection with articulation associated with the frontal lobe. The experiments of Eduard Hitzig (1838–1907) and Gustav Fritsch (1838–1927) marked the first positive advance in the science of localisation.

Phineas Gage is probably the most famous patient to have survived severe damage to the brain. He was the foreman of an American railway construction gang working for the contractors preparing a trackbed for the *Rutland and Burlington rail road* when, on 13 September 1848, the accidental explosion of a charge he had set blew his tamping iron through his head. The tamping iron was 3 feet 7 inches long, weighed $13\frac{1}{2}$ pounds, and was $1\frac{1}{4}$ inches in diameter at one end, tapering over a distance of about 1 foot to a diameter of $\frac{1}{4}$ inch at the other end. The tamping iron went in point first under his left cheek bone and out through the top of his head, landing about 25 to 30 yards behind him. Gage was knocked over but may not have lost consciousness even though most of the front part of the left side of his brain was destroyed. Seven months later, he felt strong enough to resume work. But because his personality had changed so much, the contractors who had employed him would not give him his place again. Before the accident he had been their most capable and efficient foreman, with a well balanced mind and was looked on as a shrewd businessman. He was now fitful and grossly profane, showing little deference for his men and was also impatient and obstinate, unable to settle on any plans he devised for future action. Gage never worked as a foreman again. According to his physician, Dr Harlow, Gage appeared at Barnum's Museum in New York, worked in a livery stable and drove coaches and cared for horses in Chile. In about 1859, after his health began to fail he went to San Francisco to live with his mother. He began to have epileptic seizures in February 1860, and we know from the funeral and cemetery records that he died on 21 May 1860.

Littlejohn (1899) was very much aware of the Phineas Gage incident calling it the 'American crow bar case'. On the subject of this case and the ever increasing trend towards localisation of the central nervous system he went on to say

'this suggests the fact that all the defenders of localisation lay emphasis solely on cases that favour their theories of localisation without attempting to consider these negative cases that oppose their theories. This does not, however, destroy the work done in localising such regions. It has already borne fruit in modern surgical cases, for in a number of cases lesions have been removed by the aid of our imperfect knowledge of localisation.'

A unifying consciousness

> 'Men are disturbed not by things but the views which they take of them.'
>
> Epictetus

The problem of understanding mental health, and all disease, may be deeper than just scientific technique; the root may be in our language and its construction. Our ability to externalise and relate in an analytical mode of thought may be another problem. This is not wrong but it may be an obstruction and may lead us to make explanations reflecting our mode of thinking. We can give explanations for things we do not understand, but the closer we come to understanding the harder it becomes to explain in an analytical mode of consciousness. Languages composed of *iconic* signs, symbolisation dependent on a similarity between object and the sign used to represent it, lend themselves to and are suited mainly for classification on the basis of manifest (e.g. structural) similarities. On the other hand, logically more complex languages, for example those using conventional signs (words), permit classifying diverse objects and phenomena on the basis of more hidden (e.g. functional) similarities. Complex language systems, for example those composed of words or mathematical symbols, lend themselves to the formation of increasing levels of abstraction (Szasz, 1984). We have developed a form of Cartesian linguistics where children are taught that a 'noun' is the 'name of a person, place or thing', that a 'verb' is 'an action word', and so on. Today all that should be changed. Children should be told that a noun is a word having a certain relationship to a predicate. A verb is a certain relation to a noun, its subject (Bateson, 1979).

Our analytical consciousness develops in conjunction with our experience of perceiving and manipulating solid bodies. The internalisation of our experience of the closed boundaries of such bodies leads to a way of thinking which naturally emphasises the distinction and separation. Since the fundamental characteristic of the world of solid bodies is externality – i.e. everything is external to everything else – then this way of thinking is necessarily analytical, sequential and linear. For this reason the mode of consciousness associated with logical thinking is necessarily analytical (Bortoft, 1996). This is illustrated by the use of words such as 'war' and 'battle' in relation to finding a cure for mental illness. What is needed is a paradigm shift or, even more beneficial, is the ability to move consciously between paradigms. (A paradigm shift in the true sense – i.e. turning everything inside out – would lead to a total change in our mode of consciousness and we would see through all material bodies, but this would be too uncomfortable and distasteful.) A stepping stone or bridge between the analytical and organic is desirable. We will stick to the use of language and propose a word that already possesses some form of symbolism in the concept of bringing things together. This word should represent wholeness as a mode of consciousness and an analytical mode as an approach, as it is impossible to approach a solid body holistically. The body and its mind have to be brought back together in such a way that even our mode of consciousness and language does not allow for separation. We can use the first two letters of body and the last two letters of mind and use the BOND Principle©. It also allows for re-empowerment of both patient and practitioner. This could help to bring us closer to understanding *oneness* of form and its expression and is an attempt at a compromise between the modes of consciousness. We can now practise moving between the analytical and organic without losing a consciousness of either. This approach has to be practised as we have analytically since childhood. If we are to understand osteopathic psychology from a unifying perspective we have to practise understanding the oneness proposed by Andrew Taylor Still. It is not a reciprocal process in the normally functioning human and has to become the Weltanschauung or world view of the practitioner. This will be the foundation or principle of the practitioner's response to the patient's problem.

The osteopathic concept of psychology

Eventually the whole of our intellectual effort will be devoted to studying yesterdays. We are told that 'if you do not learn the lessons of history, you are doomed to repeat them'. We could just as well reply: 'If you *do* learn the lessons of history you are doomed to repeat them'. For in a changing world, the old lessons may be misleading. Generals are always fighting the last battle, not the current one. There are three basic aspects of thinking: 'what is'; 'what may be'; and 'what can be'. We are totally obsessed with 'what is'. We underestimate the extremely valuable contribution that 'what may be' has made to progress. We do very little about 'what can be' – even though our future depends entirely on this aspect (de Bono, 1997). This is consistent with the thoughts of Golo Mann when he said 'man is always more than he can know of himself; consequently his accomplishments, time and time again, will come as a surprise to him'.

Littlejohn's *Lectures on Psycho-physiology* was published in 1899 when he was then professor of physiology and psychology at the American School of Osteopathy, Kirksville, Missouri. Littlejohn recognised that 'while the body is a machine, it is not a machine that is wound up and capable of going for a number of years wholly under external influence'. He understood that the body is an internally organising system making its adjustments to demands over time. It is poor adjustment that we see as an external disturbance to all systems. 'If such emotions become chronic, how is it possible to have a perfect nutrition system?' This may be today what our secularised health system labels irritable bowel syndrome.

Within the past few years there has been an ever-increasing development in the 'new' field of psychoneuroimmunology. Littlejohn wrote

'Physiological chemistry has demonstrated that such a chronic condition produces toxic substances that interfere with every normal body process. So long as these exist, health is impossible, and there cannot be physical immunity from disease, because the system, is laid open to all kinds of germicides.'

Still (1899) emphasised that man exists as a total functioning unit and that one of the major factors in the protection of that unit is the stability of the mind and its components. He called for us to approach psychosomatic disorders just as we approach any other disturbance in the total economy of the body. The psychological part of the person is a unifying component as are all aspects of normal function. Emotional upset does not necessarily cause psychological illness. It is the summation of stressing factors in a particular direction that lead to a so-called breakdown of the individual. Patients with what appear to be psychosomatic disorders seem to be reacting to emotional stresses and strains no greater than those of other individuals who are clinically healthy. The psychologically ill patient would have to have been 'triggered' into that state by his or her inability as a unifying system to adjust to external demands that are in the main building over long periods of time (Northup, 1963). The increased cortical activity resulting from anxiety and self-conflict set up an increased flow of impulses in the descending spinal tracts, this may cause increased tone in the paravertebral and other somatic structures – especially those related to lesioned segments – and thus take part in lesion production (Haycock, 1955).

We can regard the osteopathic approach to the psychiatric patient as being psychosomatic at all times. It was always believed in osteopathy that treatment of psychological problems without physical treatment was open to failure (Dunn, 1948). This is important as the pioneers of the osteopathic approach to health and disease always considered the body as an integral unit and a self-organising system. In us anxiety is the start of all psychosomatic conditions. In time this leads to an increase in the resting tone of myofascial tissue and a disturbance in range and quality of joint function. The role played by receptors is paramount in the understanding of the development and expression of a psychological state. Littlejohn recognised the receptor and in particular the condition of the tissue in which the receptor was found. This interface between receptor and tissue should be considered from a physicochemical aspect.

Littlejohn wrote

'In connection with the motor fibres we find the terminals in muscles, glands and electrical bodies. The nerves branching among the fasiculi of the muscles divide and subdivide, forming numerous ramifications, the single delicate fibres ending in muscle fibres. Losing the medullary sheath the axis cylinder is divided into minute fibrils. The axis cylinder passes through the sarcolemma, the neurilemma becoming continuous with it. As these fibres surround the disc shaped bodies inside the sarcolemma they form motor end plates. The form and structure of these vary in different muscles, the terminal characterising the particular muscle. Thus we see the close and inseparable relation of the nervous mechanism to the muscles, bones and ligaments, indicating the close relation of mind and the mental phenomena to the delicate structure of the body, so that the mind is localised in the body rather than in the neural mechanism.'

The above demonstrates that by the end of the nineteenth century osteopathic medicine was teaching officially that the mind was in the substance of the body and was not localised to the brain. Osteopathic psychology, with its sense of unity of body and environment, emphasises the role of the myofascioskeletal system in the expression of the person. It is essentially the principle of moving and thinking forward. All distress, emotional or physical, involves the initial shock, a defence mechanism, arousal and memory. An osteopathic approach to an emotional disturbance is the same as to a sprained ankle.

Any emotional presentation represents a disturbance of homeostasis compromising the body's ability to function as an adjusting unit. Allopathic psychology regards expressions of the soma as 'mental'. The patient is not regarded as a unit and the structural somatic disturbances are not considered in the main. Psychologists recognised in the 1890s in Europe that some women developed anaesthesia in their hands and forearms, and a new kind of back pain localised in one of the thoracic vertebrae. This vertebra then turned into a *hysterogenic zone*, 'in which every pressure on the spot produced either an attack of ructus or a fainting fit without convulsion'. Even the most famous of psychologists realised that there was a somatic component. In 1895 Sigmund Freud (1856–1939) was treating a Mrs K. for 'cramplike pains in her chest'. 'In her case,' he told his friend Wilhelm Fliess, 'I have invented a strange therapy of my own: I search for sensitive areas, press on them, and thus provoke fits of shaking which free her' (Shorter, 1992). Korr (1986) reminds us that 'startling the subject or including mild anxiety caused exaggerated and prolonged muscle responses in the dysfunctional segments' related to already chronic facilitated segments of the motor neurone 'pool'. In addition we have seen that the vasomotor (sympathetic) chain of ganglia does not stop at the neck but reaches far into the head joining both sides as the ganglion of Ribes. All psychological expressions of ill health are psychosomatic including the body; as are all broken legs including the mind.

We talk of a person being unstable mentally, in fact osteopathically the opposite is true. The aspect of looking at a person as being mentally balanced is incorrect. By choosing to use the word 'balance' we have developed this consciousness of duality representing something tipping from left to right in response to emotional demands. Under extreme cases of outside influence this balanced person shows signs of extreme stability. This imagery or analogy is part of the problem of our understanding. Stability is death in any living organism. It is because the person is stabilising in relation to a dynamic environment and its demands that the problems begin, just as could be said for a soft tissue problem.

Patients stand still emotionally when they are becoming anxious or depressed. The word emotion, *psychosomatic* is derived from the Latin *emovere* meaning to move away. These patients have lost their ability to adjust, or even run away, as our evolutionary neurohormonal form demands. Instead of psychology developing into a system of understanding the whole expression of the nervous system through the myofascioskeletal system it has become a victim of an ever-increasing amount of 'pop psychology' in the form of soap operas reflecting Shakespearean dialogues (Bloom, 1999). Bloom demonstrates the essence of language development and as we have seen this is a major contributor to our mode of consciousness. Akin-Ogundeji (1991) reminds us that 'psychology is an expansive field. But psychology tends to be what psychologists make of it. In our research and research reporting (in Africa) we have so far held to this notion that we have forgotten the essence of psychology, which is relating meaningfully to human values, social realities and whole-life issues.'

We should remember what the philosophical basis of osteopathy is. In each of the three couples of body/mind, structure/function and brain/thought, the first term governs the second: the first is the foundation of the second. There is no mind without body, no function without structure, no thought without brain. Only in myths are there minds without bodies, functions without structures, thoughts without brains. But there can be bodies without minds, structures without functions, brains without thoughts. A corpse is a body, and has a structure and a brain; but it has no mind, no function and no thought (Podmore, 1993).

Allopathic physicians tend to look to rule out only organic disease as a primary cause of mental illness. If there is no organic disease the patient is medicated to 'control' his or her expression of illness. Organic disease is not always present in most ill health and the brain is regarded in the main as the seat of the problem. Osteopathic principles teach us that the body is a unit and in particular we have seen earlier that the enteric nervous network contains as many neurones as the brain itself, if not more, and does not need the brain or spinal cord for continued function (see the section on the autonomic nervous system on p. 100). The response of a patient to any illness is a total body response. Academically we can look at the aetiology of the psychologically ill or dysfunctional patient in four major areas: somatic predisposition; sociopsychological predisposition; psychological precipitating causes; and somatic precipitating factors.

Our main interest is in the somatic predisposing and precipitating factors. Osteopathic considerations of importance are with somatopsychic problems.

(1) Altered visceromotor functions and myofascial contractures, with or without consequent altered vertebral or joint relationships.

(2) Vertebral, peripheral joint and myofascial structural changes producing symptoms identical with the clinical presentations of psychosomatic illness.

(3) Those pre-existing vertebral, peripheral and myofascial contractures leading

to organ or other sections of the body through which anxiety will be expressed.

(4) The reciprocal influence through the autonomic nervous, immune and hormonal systems.

Historically, there is a tendency to look at behavioural expression as a mental 'thing' and a disturbance of neurotransmitters as the cause. As Marano (1999) reminds us, 'regarding depression as "just" a chemical imbalance wildly misconstrues this disorder. Depression is not just a disorder from the neck up but a disorder involving many systems.' It is well documented that other body systems can express dysfunction well before so-called mental disease is diagnosed. And stress factors precipitate around 50% of depression cases. In women suffering from depression it has been shown that there is a close association with a decrease in mineral bone density (Michelson and Stratakis et al., 1996). Parkinson himself in 1817 first described constipation in the context of Parkinson's disease. Parkinson found that constipation is one of several gastrointestinal dysfunctional precursors characteristic of the disease. More careful examination of the enteric ganglion cells in a patient with idiopathic Parkinson's disease and acquired megacolon showed the myenteric plexus neurons containing numerous Lewy bodies in both pigmented and non-pigmented cells. This suggests that in some patients with the disease, there is primary involvement of the enteric nervous system as well as of central nervous system neurons (Appenzeller and Oribe, 1997).

Lesioned areas, it is believed, determine the organ or avenue through which the personality will find somatic expression for unresolved conflicts. Osteopathically there are findings of altered vertebral, shoulder girdle and pelvic girdle mechanics in most patients with clinical diagnosis of psychoneurosis and hysteria. Denslow (cited in Dunn, 1950) states that his investigations led him to conclude that the presence of lesion pathology is sufficient cause for the production of muscular and visceral changes which result in the symptom picture known as *neurasthenia*. This is confirmed by the historic work of Speransky (1944) who realised that the primary source of dysfunction could be in the viscera or any body part far from the spinal cord. A relatively minor disorder could initiate a change in the physiological state of the nerve cells associated with the spinal segment or segments and, as we now know, the cord lesioned state will stay the same after the original cause has disappeared, thus the facilitated segment. The resulting chronic facilitation, or lowered spinal cord threshold, eventually may bombard higher centres with noxious impulses over time initiating plasticity changes in those higher centres. Well before the individual is conscious of these impulses, structural change has taken place. Adjustments in the patient's reflex visceromotor and motor adjustments are initiated, only finally recognised at a cortical level. Subtle changes in personality are the beginning of the expression of this neural plasticity. The patient does not know where it is coming from, but will be aware of tensions in the body, anywhere from the head to the feet.

Historically it is relevant to show that the Still-Hildreth Osteopathic Sanatorium surveyed 1000 cases of schizophrenia for frequency of spinal lesions, the results are in Table 4 below. We should remind ourselves that vertebral joint levels are named as landmarks (like the stars in ocean navigation) in a 'sea' of body tissue and are not related purely to bone or joint levels.

Table 4 Lesion Frequency in Schizophrenia. (cited in Dunn, 1950)

Lesion	Frequency
Cervical 1	37.6%
Cervical 2	66.0%
Cervical 3	41.2%
Cervical 4	6.7%
Cervical 5	1.7%
Cervical 6	1.0%
Cervical 7	1.2%
Dorsal 1	18.2%
Dorsal 2	25.3%
Dorsal 3	32.3%
Dorsal 4	54.5%
Dorsal 5	74.6%
Dorsal 6	67.6%
Dorsal 7	41.3%
Dorsal 8	18.7%
Dorsal 9	7.2%
Dorsal 10	21.4%
Dorsal 11	30.5%
Dorsal 12	36.2%
Lumbar 1	12.3%
Lumbar 2	3.2%
Lumbar 3	1.0%
Lumbar 4	0.7%
Lumbar 5	2.7%

An osteopathic consideration of the autonomic nervous system

Of paramount importance in osteopathic considerations is an understanding of the role of the autonomic nervous system (ANS) and the true role of psychosomatic problems. As we have seen above, all problems are somatopsychic being various degrees of the same body and mind expression. We are aware of the ganglions of Ribes and Impar, reflecting the unification and extent of the paravertebral sympathetic ganglionic cycle and the enteric system from the prevertebral ganglia as a self-reliant region. It is due to the extent of the autonomic nervous system that all anxiety results in the development of somatopsychic expression. In particular the ANS begins the defence mechanisms resulting in contracture of adipose, muscular and fascial tissue. We are more aware of the high resting tone of the skeletal muscles in the states of acute anxiety and the thickening fibrosis in more chronic states. On examination these muscle tissue changes are always found in the paravertebral muscles.

Aberrant reflex phenomena always lead to the development of visceromotor disturbance. This is expressed as constipation and/or diarrhoea, depending on the contracture of circular or longitudinal muscles, respectively, irritable bowel syndrome, colitis and even anorexia nervosa. Any visceromotor disturbance affects the whole body due to the range of its sympathetic and parasympathetic communication. As the disturbance increases in intensity and/or continues over a period of time the whole body contracts in a natural biological attempt by the body to defend itself. The initial muscles to contract are those that share the same spinal cord segments as the disturbed viscera. This protective contraction occurs even before the next protective reaction, development of pain, occurs (Dunn, 1948).

This finding of contracted and fibrotic paravertebral muscles is always associated with vertebral joint disturbance. The resulting vertebral joint complex receptor disturbance is as important as the soft tissue changes in maintaining the flow of neural impulse disturbance to the entire nervous system. These joint receptors are the closest to the spinal cord and their resulting lowered threshold contributes to the development of facilitation of the spinal cord and associated levels of the autonomic nervous system. This maintained vertebral articular disturbance, as part of an osteopathic lesion, is initially receptor, sensory, dependent developing into a reciprocal motor-sensory disturbance. This increases the adjustments of self-defence leading to a disturbed cycle within the entire nervous system. The motor neurone pool in the spinal cord becomes excitable at various levels. Impulses in these sensitive areas within the motor neurone pool summate, ascending the spinothalamic sensory tracts and travelling along afferent pathways from the muscle spindles along the posterior columns of the spinal cord to the brain. We now know that lesioned areas occur outside of the spinal cord in the enteric division of the autonomic nervous system. These ganglia in the enteric system act as small 'spinal cords' relaying impulses back into the gut.

These spinal cord and autonomic lesioned areas can be added to the descending impulse bombardment of the higher centres of the brain. Impulses descending the reticulospinal tract excite the already sensitive regions of the spinal cord. The areas first to be affected are those of the lowest threshold segments, where impulses are more intense and prolonged in duration, even in states of 'rest'.

It is these lesions that are major predisposing and maintaining factors in the expressive neurological disturbance that we call psychology. Each patient has their own pattern of lesions and further lesion development. This would explain why some patients develop individual initial symptoms, for example, cardiac, dermal or gastric and others may develop combinations. We should primarily be concerned with the following:

(1) predisposing quality and range of hypertonic paravertebral muscle and vertebral joint disturbance
(2) the findings and range of hypertonic paravertebral muscle and vertebral joint disturbance in the presenting disturbed patient.

Development of somatopsychic disturbance leading to disturbed emotional expression is not limited to the axial structures. Limb trauma can be an initial source of spinal cord disturbance with its associated pain and disfigurement affecting the patient's self-confidence and precipitating anxiety resulting in visceral disturbance.

Anxiety, self-conflict and muscle tone

'Anxious man in real life brings to each new challenge old ones, unresolved.'
H.G. Grainger, DO

Major distinct pathways are always involved in the increase of muscle tone resulting from anxiety and self-conflict. This increase in resting muscle tone includes a combination of neural pathways. These preferred pathways of the body are those of lowest thresholds in essentially a stress response.

Anxiety and/or self-conflict is the response to the meaning we place into any situation. This is usually based on a combination of past experience, expectation and anticipation with varying degrees of threat and excitement. Thinking seems to be the main initiating factor. The more we think the more we hold on to an impression, real or imaginary. This interpretation leads to an arousal of the autonomic nervous system and the development of an anxiety–self-conflict neurosis. Previous facilitated (low threshold) areas of the nervous system as a whole will augment any anxiety response. In the muscle the physiologically reacting area is the muscle spindle. The muscle spindles combine with the spinal cord resulting in the gamma system response or loop. This loop becomes self-sustaining and contributes to aberrant impulses bombarding the central nervous system disturbing and adding to the sensitivity of the motor neurone pool.

A condition of arousal and/or self-conflict leads to bombardment and sensitivity of the reticulospinal tract in the lateral column of the spinal cord; this we could consider as a starting point in the cycle of anxiety and muscle tone. This descending pathway of aberrant impulses will exit the spinal cord towards the muscle tissue along the gamma (γ)-cell efferent motor pathway. The initial γ-cell pathways followed will be those of a lower threshold anywhere in the spinal cord and exiting the spinal cord along anterior efferent fibres. An increase in impulse rate and intensity leads to a contraction of the muscle through the gamma motor neurone within the intrafusal muscle fibres.

Contraction activates the spindles and muscle bundles. As a consequence there is an increase in sensitivity of the alpha (α) cells raising the resting tone of the muscle in preparation for physical and/or emotional action. Responses involve the addition of any previously facilitated (lower threshold) areas of neural tissue. Initial reticulospinal discharge initiating a gamma cell response is only one way of producing the efferent–afferent tone in resting muscle tissue. The nervous system is bi-directional and nervous tissue reaches all areas of the body, therefore all nervous tissue, particularly the receptors and the tissue in which they lie, initiate and establish a way of 'feeling' (Fig. 12).

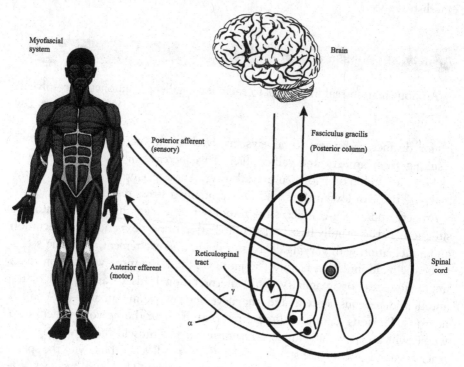

Fig. 12 The gamma-gain or 'feeling' system.

The pain related to the summation of previous experiences and responses that is not related directly to tissue damage, may be regarded as *symbolic* pain. It is real to the patient and is related to fear and defence against any real damage. Symbolic pain will also be involved to a degree when the tissue damage is minor and the emotional response is out of proportion to this damage. Again this is a defence mechanism and is usually based on the meaning the patient places in relation to information assumed, read or hearsay.

An osteopathic approach to psychiatry

Dunn (1949) developed an osteopathic approach to psychiatry, which he described as 'holistic' due to its interrelationship of four basic categories as aetiological factors in psychic disorders. These categories were grouped as heredity, environmental, somatic (or physical), and psychic (or mental). The ideal was that a person would have a good representation of these four factors by being dynamic (constantly off balance) and flexible to outside demands and the meaning they placed into them.

He went on to say that the resultant forces of these dynamic forces meet the pressure of the milieu. They are at the same time strengthened or diminished as need be by the constitutional stability factor of the personality, so that the personality maintains its adjustment and balance in its particular milieu at that moment. Thus with the aid of the stability factor, the personality maintains its functional level above its own minimum hedonic level even under adverse circumstances, drawing when necessary upon its reserves of resistance, its somatic, or its psychic factors.

This approach of Dunn's emphasises the importance of a complete case history. Psychological factors interpreted by the body can stress the homeostatic functional levels if they are below the hedonic minimum. Accumulative increasing tone of somatic components over years or sudden onset of trauma, emotional or physical, can be a major factor in the expression of behavioural disturbance. Speransky (1944), Pottenger (1944) and Gershon (1998) remind us that the most obvious place for the beginning of psychological (stress) disturbance is the gut. As we shall see the expression and interpretation of the autonomic nervous system is paramount in the osteopathic approach to patient care.

Adaptive capability and osteopathic care

What factors could be at work that contribute to our adaptive capability? This has to be looked at in a *biosocial* context. The *bio* aspect involves the anatomicophysiological complex, development and makeup, while the *social* aspect includes experience, experiment, exposure and a developing response to events. Unfortunately, again, this is an artificial breakdown of what is essentially one process going forward in time. At the level of the person in the environment we can talk of *tissue plasticity* (neural, lymphatic, muscular etc.) as the person changes in the environment. This is a good example of the internally organising nature of the body and cannot be reduced to just neurotransmitter action.

We tend to look at the person/patient in a combination of the basic three ways.

(1) *Primarily emotional*: this is obviously osteopathically impossible by definition. Since osteopathic observation is central to the diagnosis, if one osteopath cannot find a disturbed somatic pattern it may be obvious to another.
(2) *Abnormal physical expression expanding emotional stimuli*: it is possible that the slow development of structural change will only allow the person a small amount of adjustment capability. This may not be seen so much in the surgery or practice. It is during the time spent outside the surgery that the neuroendocrine reserves of the patient are being taxed. It will be under the

conditions of everyday life that their baseline of arousal and adjustment capabilities is under strain. This is the most common condition where adrenalin exhaustion becomes apparent.

(3) *Emotional expression from pure physical distress:* here the patient is not really psychologically ill but tends to show signs of poor coping in the face of information and sensations regarding their physical state. Long-term emotional distress can develop due to expectations, unqualified and qualified information.

References

Akin-Ogundeji, O (1991) Asserting psychology in Africa. *The Psychologist*, January, 2–4.

Appenzeller, O. and Oribe, E. (1997) The enteric nervous system. In *The Autonomic Nervous System: An Introduction to Basic and Clinical Concepts*. Elsevier, Oxford.

Bateson, G. (1979) *Mind and Nature: A Necessary Unit*. Flamingo, London.

de Bono, E. (1997) Away with the Gang of Three. *Guardian*, Saturday, January 25.

Bloom, H. (1999) *Shakespeare: The Invention of the Human*. Fourth Estate, London.

Bortoft, H. (1996) *The Wholeness of Nature: Goethe's Way of Science*. Floris Books, Edinburgh.

Carmichael, L. (1926) Sir Charles Bell: a contribution to the history of physiological psychology. *Psychological Reviews* 33, 188–217.

Cottingham, J. (1986) *Descartes*. Blackwell. London.

Devlin, K. (1997) *Goodbye, Descartes: The End of Logic and the Search for a new Cosmology of the Mind*. John Wiley and Sons, New York.

Dunn, F.E. (1948) The osteopathic management of psychosomatic problems. *The Journal of the American Osteopathic Association*. 48(4) 196–9.

Dunn, F.E. (1949) Some thoughts on the etiology and interrelationships in psychiatric disorders. *The Journal of the American Osteopathic Association*. 49(3) 166–8.

Dunn, F.E. (1950) Osteopathic concepts in psychiatry. *The Journal of the American Osteopathic Association*. 49(7) 354–7.

Gershon, M.D. (1998) *The Second Brain*. Harper Collins, London.

Haycock, W. (1955) The expanding concept of osteopathy. *The John Martin Littlejohn Memorial Lecture, 1955*. The Osteopathic Publishing Co., Ltd.

Korr, I.M. (1986) Somatic dysfunction, osteopathic manipulative treatment, and the nervous system: a few facts, some theories, many questions. *The Journal of the American Osteopathic Association*. 86(2) 109–14.

Littlejohn, J.M. (1899) *Lectures on Psycho-physiology*. E.G. Kinney, Kirksville, MI.

Lott, T. (1999) Story of the blues. *Life, The Observer Magazine*, 21 February.

MacDonald, T.H. (1998) *Rethinking Health Promotion: A Global Perspective*. Routledge, London.

Marano, H.E. (1999) Depression: beyond serotonin. *Psychology Today* April, pp.30–76.

Maslow, A. (1970) *Motivation and Personality*. Harper Collins, New York.

Michelson, D., Stratakis, M.D., Hill, L., Reynolds, J., *et al.* (1996) Bone mineral density in women with depression. *The New England Journal of Medicine*. 335(16) 1176–81.

Northup, G.W. (1963) The psychic component. *The Journal of Osteopathy*. September, 41–8.

Podmore, W. (1993) The philosophy of osteopathy. *British Osteopathic Journal*. XII, 30–1.

Pottenger, F.M. (1944) *Symptoms of Visceral Disease*. C. V. Mosby Company, St. Louis.

Reed, E.S. (1989) Theory, concept, and experiment in the history of psychology: the older tradition behind a 'young science'. *History of the Human Sciences*. 2(3) 332–56.

Reed, E.S. (1997) *From Soul to Mind. The Emergence of Psychology from Erasmus Darwin to William James*. Yale University Press, London.

Robinson, B. (1907) *The Abdominal and Pelvic Brain: With Autonomic Visceral Ganglia.* Frank Betz, Hammond IND.

Sherrington, C. (1946) *The Endeavour of Jean Fernel.* Cambridge University Press. Reprinted 1974, Dawsons of Pall Mall, Folkestone and London.

Shorter, E. (1992) *From Paralysis to Fatigue. A History of Psychosomatic Illness in the Modern Era.* Free Press, Oxford.

Speransky, A.D. (1944) *A Basis for the Theory of Medicine.* International Publishers, New York.

Still, A.T. (1899) *Philosophy of Osteopathy.* Published by the author, Kirksville, MI.

Szasz, T.S. (1984) *The Myth of Mental Illness.* Paladin, London.

Thomas, K. (1991) *Religion and the Decline of Magic.* Penguin Books, London.

Toulmin, S. (1990) *Cosmopolis: The Hidden Agenda of Modernity.* The University of Chicago Press, Chicago.

Trethowan, W.H. (1979) From straightjackets to soma. *World Medicine.* June 16, 26–8.

Wolpaw, J.R. and Carp, J.S. (1990) Memory traces in spinal cord. *Trends in Neuroscience.* 13(4) 137–42.

Zajonc, A. (1998) Light and cognition. In *Goethe's Way of Science: A Phenomenology of Nature.* Eds. D. Seamon and A. Zajonc, Chapter 13. State University of New York Press, New York.

Further reading

Brigham, F.M. (1970) Masks as a psychotherapeutic modality: a hypothesis. *The Journal of the American Osteopathic Association.* 69, 51–7.

Darwin, C. (1872) *The Expression of the Emotions in Man and Animals.* Reprinted 1998, Harper Collins, London.

Lott, T. (1999) *The Scent of Dried Roses.* Observer Culture Shop, London.

Williams, B. (1978) *Descartes: The Project of Pure Enquiry.* Pelican Books, London.

Wilson, M. (Ed) *The Essential Descartes.* Mentor Books, New York.

CHAPTER 8

Health and Disease

'What the public wants, therefore, is a cheap magic charm to prevent, and a cheap pill or potion to cure, all disease. It forces all such charms on the doctors.'

George Bernard Shaw, *The Doctor's Dilemma*

The word health originated from the goddess who watched over the Greeks in Athens, Hygeia. Being a Greek goddess she was a concept rather than a real person. The belief in Hygeia eventually led to the belief in the god of healing, Asclepius (Asklepios), from the fifth century onwards. According to legend Asclepius was the first Greek physician, the son of Apollo and the nymph Coronis. He lived around the twelfth century BC and was renowned for mastering the knife and recognising the curative value of plants. Asclepian medicine was a form of healing known as temple incubation involving belief in the healing powers of a god and relying upon knowledge of dreams. Due to his success Hygeia was relegated to a member of his retinue, usually as his daughter, sometimes as his sister or wife, but always subservient to him (Dubos, 1979). The other goddess, daughter of Asclepius, relegated to a similar position was Panacaea (Panakeia) and as the sister of Hygeia, Dubos suggests, she 'became omnipotent as a healing goddess through knowledge of drugs either from plants or from the earth. Her cult is alive today in the universal search for a panacea'.

These myths represent two major aspects of the philosophy of medicine. Hygeia is represented as the goddess of the aspects of nature in the form of preventive or environmental medicine, holism, whereas Panacaea is the specialisation in the use of drugs orientated towards the disease, the 'magic bullet' (Waldron, 1978). Physics, as a basic discipline and as a speciality, is central to the development of biomedicine. We have begun to accept that what we see is the sum of smaller parts and the more we know about small parts the more we shall understand Nature. As Bortoft (1998) reminds us 'we tend to think of the large-scale universe of matter as being made up of separate and independent masses interacting with one another through the force of gravity. This viewpoint that emerges from modern physics is very different from the traditional conception. It is now believed that mass is not an intrinsic property of a body, but in fact a reflection of the whole of the rest of the universe in that body. Einstein imagined, following Ernst Mach, that a single particle of matter would have no mass if it were not for all the rest of the matter in the universe.'

The reductionist techniques of biomedicine (allopathic medicine) deliberately reduce all aspects in an attempt to understand how things work. This is where the problems began with the biomedical understanding of health. Their methods assume that a deeper, reductionist, understanding of illness will lead to an understanding of health or cure of disease. But 'health' is most certainly not an appropriate subject for reductionist techniques. Interpreting health requires a holistic approach, an approach that looks at how the variables interact without attempting to see some 'independent' and some 'dependent'. The interconnections are far too complex for that (MacDonald, 1998). As Calnan (1987) suggests, ' "middle class" women often define health as "being fit", "being active", and "taking exercise"; in contrast "working-class" women often perceived health as "never being ill" and being able to "get through the day".' This is consistent with the teachings of A.T. Still: 'anyone can find disease. . .'. Osteopathic medicine tends towards the Hygeia belief rather than that of Panacaea, but neither can exist in total isolation.

Due to the influence of Greek culture on Western philosophy it is impossible to reduce the definition of health, or disease, to simple anatomical, physiological, or mental criteria. In addition health cannot be described as just the absence of illness or disease. Individuals describe themselves and others as 'being healthy' depending on their own experiences. Therefore, for the sake of some structure, health could be described as

- A reserve: we all know people who get ill but recover quickly; or never get a hangover.
- A behaviour: the healthy lifestyle; he or she has never smoked and is a marathon running vegetarian.
- Physical fitness: this person has always been exercising and at 60 looks no older than 45.
- Energy and vitality: he or she wakes up early, seems always ready to go, and possesses a 'drive'.
- A social relationship: he or she always talks to other people and seems to enjoy life.
- A function: an overall aspect; people who can still work despite their age.

- A psycho-social well-being: a combination of energy, social relationships, and function.

(from Baxter, 1990.)

The osteopathic approach to health regards the splitting of physical and mental health as purely educational rather than biological. Unfortunately the volumes of literature on mental health rarely make this point. We fear the mentally ill more than the physically ill, tending to forget that there is no mental illness without physical structural change. There is no mind without body. We are culture bound towards the fear of a 'body' without a rationalising mind, whereas in reality it is the body that expresses itself as 'mind'.

In Still's *The Philosophy and Mechanical Principles of Osteopathy*, 1902, he wrote

'In Nature we look for good machines in form and action. We have learned to know that Nature does no imperfect work, but, on the other hand, does its work to perfection, and perfection is its watch word in all its parts and functions. The wise man has long since learned that no suggestions he can offer can do any good, but, as a rule, are vastly harmful. He often kills or ruins the machine to such a degree that it fails in part or in whole to do its work. He finds his supposed helps have disabled his man or woman even to death. The drug-giver is not satisfied that God has quite the wisdom necessary to make a machine that will do the work that all daily demands require. He hopes to do something to have life do better work. He sees only one thing in which to begin and end all his labours, "drugs".

The idea of God in history seems to have been derived from the need for a primary mover of the heavens and earth (Koestler, 1989a).

Frost (1918) discussed the osteopathic approach to health being more of a biological philosophy rather than a social approach. 'By reason of this intensive study (on membranes) of one of the physiological processes he (J.S. Haldane in *Organisms and Environment as Illustrated by the Physiology of Breathing*) justifies an assumption that other functions are controlled in a somewhat similar manner, and that there is a very delicate interplay of adjustment and readjustment in the various functions of the body which tends to maintain the "internal environment" in as stable a condition as possible.' Haldane goes on to say (cited in Frost, 1919)

'the organs and tissues which regulate the internal environment are themselves centres of nutritional activity, dependent from moment to moment on their environment. They are constantly taking up and giving off material of many sorts, and their 'structure' is nothing but the appearance taken by this flow of material through them.'

We have heard on numerous occasions that health is not simply the absence of disease. Osteopaths at the end of the nineteenth and the beginning of the twentieth century were quite sure what they meant by health: *structural integrity, the ability to adjust* and *conservation of energy*, basically the principles of osteopathy. McConnell (1919) wrote,

'conservation of energy is no small thing to be attained whether in disease or health. Indeed even here may be the starting point of disease processes, for repeated loss and lessening of strength depletes the chemical forces, irritates the nervous system, over-taxes the heart, lessens the tone and lowers the resistance. This disturbance of balance between energy production and dissipation with a resultant accumulation of waste products and a tendency toward structural impairment and probable infection is not infrequently of prime importance. . . . If freedom from over-fatigue, worry, debilitating habits, impure air, poor food, etc., are essential factors in the retainment of health they are then essential fundamentals in its attainment.'

Health does not 'include' mental aspects and physical aspects, they are not even different aspects of the same process. They are the same processes.

Holism, holon and the holographic paradigm

Holism is not concerned with the nature of parts, but the relationship of parts. Holism suggests that possibility of integration, of feeling that all parts of ourselves belong to the same essential person and have meaning in relation to one another. Holism has almost religious connotations, suggesting that the whole person can be found and that, when it is, the individual will be healed (Coward, 1990).

Koestler (1989b) demonstrates an analytical mode of consciousness even when applied to wholes by suggesting that 'a "part", as we generally use the word, means something fragmentary and incomplete, which by itself would have no legitimate existence. On the other hand, a "whole" is considered as something complete in itself which needs no further explanation. But *"wholes" and "parts" in this absolute sense just do not exist anywhere*, whether in the domain of living organism or of social organisations. What we find are intermediary structures on a series of levels in an ascending order of complexity: sub-wholes which display, according to the way you look at them, some of the characteristics commonly attributed to wholes and some of the characteristics attributed to parts. The members of a hierarchy, like the Roman god Janus, all have two faces looking in opposite directions: the face turned toward the subordinate levels is that of a self-contained whole; the face turned upward toward the apex, that of a dependent part. One is the face of the master, the other of the servant. This *"Janus effect"* is a fundamental characteristic of sub-wholes in all types of hierarchies. But there is no satisfactory word in our vocabulary to refer to the Janus-faced entities: to talk of sub-wholes (or sub-assemblies, sub-structures, sub-skills, sub-systems) is awkward and tedious. The term I would propose is "holon", from the Greek *holos* = whole, with the suffix *on* which, as in pro*ton* or neutr*on*, suggests a particle or part.'

At this point it should be realised that Koestler assumes a hierarchical system within nature, which is a good example of the mathematical style and organically cannot be so.

J. Curtis-Lake (1998) goes on to say:

'although human embryological development appears to happen in broad principles, there is enough evidence to show that this model of linear development does not satisfactorily answer many of the questions found within the human process. For example why do some individuals with severe developmental damage in one area, develop normally in other areas? Also why, with two apparently similar individuals, from one family or group structure, should they each develop differently? They may express themselves in two different characters who have very different views of reality. This shows a paradox within the linear paradigm, especially when the experience of the two has apparently been the same. To gain some insight into this phenomenon, it is necessary to look at other ideas on the patterns of development. The most promising theory of these is that of the *holographic paradigm*.

To understand the holographic paradigm, it is first necessary to look at the properties of a hologram. The hologram is a development of modern science. It is an image formed when a large number of laser beams strike an object and are projected, without a lens, onto a photographic plate. The projection forms a three-dimensional image from which all aspects of the image can be viewed at once or in its dimensional parts. The conceived image depends where the viewer places himself. The viewer will form an image of the projection depending where his position is in relation to the image. In other words the viewer will perceive an image which conforms to his own position of reality. It is a property of the hologram that any part or particle of the image may be taken and projected as the whole. This in turn means that each part of the image contains the whole. Each part though will not show the whole in the same detail as the complete image. The amount shown will depend on which particular facet of the image is focused at the time of the projection.

Taking this paradigm we can then say that each particle of the whole reflects the whole but to appreciate the completeness of the whole it is necessary to see the complete image. This of course from the point of view of the viewer is impossible, as he also will have his/her point of viewing. *Therefore only a part of the hologram can be in focus at any one time.* If the viewer is capable of moving around the projected static image, he will be able to see and appreciate much more of the image in its entirety. If also the hologram is capable of moving, a shifting matrix of reality of the image is apparent to the viewer. Computer science is now able to construct a package or program which allows the operator to change his terms of reference. By revealing more of the stored information within the program, he can change and extend the reality of the projected image. In effect the operator can extend the reality of a two-dimensional image into the reality of a three-dimensional figure. Providing that the operator has the terms of reference needed to recognise the perceived information, he will be able to recognise the whole object as it is, rather than as his imagination or previous knowledge would want it to be.'

This demonstrates the true and original meaning of the word *evolution*.

Lifestyle

'There is no "blueprint" for the behaviour in the brain, or in the genes – no more than there is a blueprint for flocking in the head of the bird.'

Andy Clark, *Being There*

There is almost no agreement either in theory or practice as to what constitutes a 'lifestyle'. The term 'lifestyle' is taken to mean a general way of living based on the interplay between living conditions in the wide sense and individual patterns of behaviour as determined by sociocultural factors and personal characteristics (World Health Organisation, 1993).

As you can see by the definition above the implications of lifestyle as a health factor are very convoluted, broad, relative and subjective. Due to this I have chosen, below, to look at one of the most modern trends in lifestyle, in particular cholesterol. This will allow for further discussion and show that the reductionist techniques of finger pointing is not a realistic issue in 'normal' everyday life. It is also very easy to blame individuals for their actions and apparent disregard in the face of all the 'healthy' information around them, otherwise known as victim blaming. Society implements degrees of acceptability with regard to the actions of individuals or groups. An example is the use of drugs. All drugs are poisons. As Daly (cited in Porter and Teich, 1996) reminds us, it seems that the phrase 'drug abuse', used to mean 'illegal drug use', was first used in the United States to express disapproval of the use of cocaine by Southern blacks. As so often happens, the phrase was, and is, used to condemn the user and his group rather than the drug itself. Coward (1990) suggests that,

'we live in a society which believes that the individual is ultimately responsible for whatever happens to her in society, whether she succeeds or fails. This is the legacy of Protestant Christianity with its belief that the salvation of the individual depends on his or her own actions.'

Well into the middle of the nineteenth century Protestant theology gave us moral philosophy, a way of living or conducting our lives, later to be known as psychology.

Cholesterol

A day does not go by where we are not reminded of the benefits and destructive capabilities of different types of lifestyle. Now to make things even worse you have the added disadvantage of being bald and stocky. Dairy products are now bad, with margarine being as bad as butter. If you live in Glasgow or eastern Finland it is not worth getting up in the morning especially if you have a Type A behaviour, do not take your daily aspirin or beta-blocker and are jobless. All this is before they find your genetic disposition. With all these combinations to worry about it is no wonder you are at risk from a heart attack. The 1993 Fifth International Montreux Congress on Stress listed 300 risk factors of heart attacks. Naturally confusion about what constitutes 'risk factors' was the result.

Confusion continues with the amount of alcohol that we are supposed, or not supposed, to consume in one week. This gets worse when we are told that red wine is good for you and will protect your heart, then white wine is just as good if not better. Obviously too much is bad for you. The result of research at Johns Hopkins University showed that a 176 lb male would need to drink 7 oz of 80° proof hard liquor, 23 oz wine, or more than five cans of beer daily in order to prevent a heart attack. It is realised that there is an association between cigarettes and coronaries, but the Framingham data suggest that ex-smokers have fewer heart attacks than people who have never smoked, and pipe and cigar smokers have less than half the rate of non-smokers (Rosch, 1993). Should we now advise our patients to smoke cigars, hit the bottle, start napping, consider a hair transplant, or get out of Glasgow?

The dominant diet–cholesterol–heart disease theory has risen to its position due to the fact that it is the easiest way to visualise a mechanism for the development of atherosclerosis in arteries. As you can see by the name, cholesterol belongs to the alcohol group. It is also a large molecule that is inert and impossible to dissolve in water. The importance of cholesterol to us lies in the fact that is essential for the structure and function of living cells, by being part of the wall of cells. This waterproof characteristic is vital in the structure and function of nerve cells and the highest concentration of cholesterol is present in the entire nervous system. Due to its waterproof characteristics cholesterol is transported in our blood inside lipid-protein particles, known as *lipoproteins*. The outer water-soluble protein cover allows the cholesterol to move throughout the body with ease.

The two most common types of combined molecules, based on density, are the high density lipoproteins (HDL) and low density lipoproteins (LDL). HDL transport cholesterol from peripheral tissues to the liver and LDL transport cholesterol from the liver to the peripheral tissues, e.g. vascular tissue. They move in opposite directions. The majority of serum (in the blood) cholesterol is LDL or the 'bad' cholesterol and this is between 60 and 80%. The HDL or 'good' cholesterol makes up around 15–20%. Serum cholesterol levels have been shown not to rise after ingestion of animal fats. As a result there has never been any positive proof of atherosclerosis and links with cholesterol levels, in the comparison of cultures (Gore *et al.*, 1959 and Resch *et al.*, 1969). What has happened is an association between coronary heart disease (CHD) and increased levels of LDL. There is no proof of linear causation between serum cholesterol and CHD.

We now have to distinguish between univariate and multivariate methods of statistics. A univariate approach will take into account the high LDL but ignores all other factors in the link to CDH. Multivariate methods 'adjust' to other factors such as number of people, as well as smoking and weight. The result in a multivariate approach is that the more variables you adjust for the less reliable your results become. The difficulty arises when you consider the real life situation that involves being overweight, smoking, inactivity, high blood pressure and stress. In real life we cannot isolate any one of these factors, least of all a high LDL level. Trials have shown that in patients treated with diet and drugs the numbers of fatal heart attacks fell slightly; in other trials, the number actually rose (Muldoon *et al.*, 1990 and Ravnskov, 1992).

Before 1940 in Africans of Kenya and Uganda blood pressure did not rise with age and essential hypertension was rarely seen; it is now a common disease. Obesity was almost unknown in 1930 when Julian Huxley noted with amazement that almost the only fat women he saw in Africa were in the Nairobi brewery; the towns of East Africa now contain many fat upper class Africans and their leaders are often grossly obese. In Kenya in the 1930s, diabetes was rare in Africans but not in Europeans and Indians; today there are large diabetic clinics in all town hospitals. This is consistent with the thoughts of Erasmus Darwin in the early 1800s (McKeown, 1983).

Since the 1950s a new ideology has been spreading: its main aspect is that illness is related to our behaviour (i.e. smoking, lack of exercise, unsafe sex etc.). This is classic victim blaming, and could be classified as an example of 'lifestyles of the rich and postpositivist' (Turshen, 1989). It is known today that diseases are determined before birth due to structure and interrelated function. Dietary changes had the most important effect on the incidence of coronary heart disease – much more than did changes in smoking (Smith, 1982).

Smoking

Again we have to look at the rationale for the reductionist and linear causation view that smoking 'alone' is the major cause of lung cancer. The author does not in any way condone smoking but the issue here is the reason for the lung damage and the relationship to smoking, passive or active. Stress, habituation and poor nutrition, for instance, combined with smoking are a recipe for disaster. What is socially unacceptable is one thing; what is supposedly a medical fact is another.

In the United States around 3000 adolescents take a drag on their first cigarette every day (Schwartz, 1996). The American Cancer Society has labelled smoking a 'paediatric disease'. There are more than 50 million smokers in the United States, 39% of adult men and 29% of adult women. The chemical nicotine stimulates the heart, nervous system and slightly raises the blood pressure. The tar in the cigarettes is definitely carcinogenic and the carbon monoxide competes for oxygen. In chronic smokers there are definite myofascial changes that may lead to premature osteoarthritis, fibromyalgia and cervical joint damage due to repeated neck extensions when dragging on a cigarette. Goethe often expressed himself severely about smoking, and compared tobacco with the things he hated most in the world. We see in his *Venezianishe Epigramme*, 'Many ills can I bear with, and most of the things that displease me. Quietly, bravely I meet, bowed by the will of a God. Yet are there some that I hate, that are worse than the venom of serpents, Four: tobacco the first, bugs then and garlic and...' This temper was naturally reflected in Goethe's attitudes toward his friends, according to whether they were smokers or non-smokers (Corti, 1931).

There is no simple linear causation between cholesterol and heart disease, as there is no linear causation between smoking and lung cancer. If this were the case then maggots are just as much the cause of death as germs are the cause of disease.

Let's leave the last words to Paul J. Rosch (1983), 'Association never proved causation ... Why we smoke, eat rich food, have high blood pressures and serum cholesterol levels may be much more important than the mere observation of such stress-related statistics.'

Environment

In the late nineteenth and early twentieth centuries, impressive declines in mortality also took place before either effective medical therapies or prophylactic treatments had been developed, and occurred largely as a result of social and environmental change intended to improve the quality of life and enhance economic production (McKeown, 1976 and Tesh, 1981 and 1982). As is generally the case the real cause of the change in health status is not written about. The main instigator of improved health in cities was Sir Joseph Bazalgette who planned and developed the sewerage systems of Manchester and London.

Beliefs in health

Health beliefs affect both the public and the practitioners. Beliefs cover the areas of cause, prevention and the cures for ill health. Otherwise known as 'ethno-medicine' it has been defined as:

'those beliefs and practices relating to disease which are the products of indigenous cultural development and are not explicitly derived from the conceptual framework of modern medicine.'

Hughes (1968)

The health-belief model is a social psychological perspective first developed to explain preventative health behaviour (Conrad, 1985).

'Feed a cold, starve a fever.'

Possibly the most common of all Western health-belief models, 'feed a cold, starve a fever' is the folk model where the patient's perceived disequilibrium is regarded as an illness and which is perceived as changes in body temperature – either 'hotter' than normal or 'colder'. These changes, in general, are purely subjective; they bear little or no relation to the biomedical model of 'normal' body temperature around 98.4°F or 37°C measured with an oral clinical thermometer. There are two important principles underlying the folk classification of 'illness-misfortune': (1) the relation of man with *nature*, i.e. the natural environment, in colds and chills, and (2) the relation of man to man, which exists within human *society*, in fevers. (Helman, 1978). This 'feeling' or heating up is similar to hot flushes and may be an autonomic conditioned response, the same as 'feeling' cold. The system is responding to some kind of life event or combination of events. There is an overlap between the germ, life style and environmental theories of real life. The biomedical model does not fit the experience of patients e.g. sore throats caused by cold draughts.

'The bruising has to come out.'

This concept is ancient and like many beliefs has its roots in the religious frame of exorcising an evil spirit or expulsion. In normal function body fluids circulate. A patient will say, about bruising, 'it's getting better, because the bruising is coming out'. Other phrases include, 'my blocked up nose is better, because it is running', 'my bowels clear out regularly' in the case of diarrhoea.

Members of the medical profession do not escape beliefs. Their beliefs and values are often influenced by cultural factors which help to define not only how health and illness are perceived and treated, but also how health research is conducted (Payer, 1989). The medical professions have to meet the public half-way. If a practitioner's description and explanation is too extreme and the patient does not understand then the patient will be confused and will feel they have no part in the health process. The position osteopathic practitioners hold in the community is important for the empowerment or re-education of health beliefs. One of the major advantages is that osteopaths are not hospital based and are empowering and treating in the 'real' environment as the old doctors used to practise. It is important, therefore, that osteopaths become part of the community in which they practise.

Compliance and non-compliance

Compliance has been defined as 'the extent to which a person's behaviour (in terms of taking medications, following diets, or executing lifestyle changes) coincides with medical or health advice' (Haynes, Taylor and Sackett, 1979). It is easy to relate poor compliance to the patient and the doctor may complain that 'the patient does not seem to want to understand'. This poor communication can lead to problems including the GP removing a patient from his or her list, due to 'a lack of communication', or at worst the patient taking the wrong medication. Compliance is always practitioner based, as the wishes of the practitioner are the centre of the intended action.

Why do some patients follow the doctor's wishes while others do not? There are four basic ways of looking at compliance and non-compliance.

(1)   *Previously held patient beliefs.* We must assume that the patient acts upon our information based on already held health or illness based beliefs. This has the effect of the patient filtering out our information until they form a model that is consistent or at least similar to their already held beliefs. Unfortunately, they may filter out some important elements and in other cases add some elements. How many times have you heard a patient say 'oh, I thought this is what you meant, I have always done it this way in the past.' This is still the doctor's perspective of non-compliance.

(2)   *Patient as a more active participant.* We can see the patient as a more active agent in the treatment rather than 'passive and obedient recipients of medical instructions' (Parsons, 1951). The patient's experiences and inter-pretations of their illness are important, even if they differ from those of the professional (Morgan, 1991). This means meeting the patient halfway and taking time to explain what is required. Obviously, this makes life easier for the patient and reduces the risk of misunderstanding. Patients may well have some preconceived idea of what treatment and prevention entails. This may be different to the practitioner's idea.

(3)   *Sources of beliefs.* Information received by the patient from relatives,

friends, magazines, informed sales staff (health food stores), people in the exercise industry and other health professionals will influence the health belief model, especially if it has had some degree of effect in the past.

(4) It is important that the practitioner facilitates the illness experience of the patient within the *context* of the cultural and socio-economic status of the patient. Afro-Caribbean, Indian, European cultures etc., have different beliefs, and there are regional differences within the U.K. With respect to socio-economic status it is of little help telling a self-employed painter with four children, a partner, a mortgage and a bank manager to look after to lie in bed for six weeks with a back problem unless it is really necessary. Anybody in this position would rather have treatment every day than stop work.

The less the practitioner meets the basic components of the compliance model, the less cooperation will he get from the patient.
  Non-compliance factors include:

- practitioner's rigid implementations
- too much information in a short period of time
- strongly held beliefs on the part of the patient
- unrealistic socio-economic demands on the patient.

It should not be forgotten that the environment in which osteopathy developed was close to that of present third world countries. Many children, in third world countries, die within a few years of birth and a majority are dead before maturity. One of the most common natural hazards, the pathogens, kills a considerable proportion of children within a few years of birth. Oral hydration, improvements in water supply, in excreta disposal, and in domestic and food hygiene (McKeown, 1989), not heroic use of drugs are needed to prevent the transmission of diarrhoeal pathogens.

Health education and promotion

Health education implies a hierarchical setup in which someone who knows the facts (a teacher) dispenses them – possibly even in a simplified form – to less qualified people (MacDonald, 1994). This creates the same dependency attitudes that would characterise patient/doctor relationships, in which the patient hands over ownership of his body to the doctor and relinquishes personal responsibility for it (Lever, 1977). In health promotion there must be active involvement of the people in what actually constitutes health and how they can obtain it. Essential to health promotion is 'empowerment' of the person or organisation. Therefore to become a health promotion initiative the people involved must promote both an understanding of what their health objectives are and how they intend to obtain them (Navarro, 1975).

The osteopath, being outside of the mainstream of medical services, tends to be approached by the patient in a different way from the local GP. Patients feel, in the main, that they can 'talk' to the osteopath more than they can to their allopathic physician. This does not imply that the osteopathic practitioner is a better talker but it does have a basis in the time available to both practitioner and patient. Information about the details of exercise, diet etc. can be conveyed and discussed even when the patient is being treated. These discussions empower the patient to make decisions, choices and have some control over their health. A subsequent visit to the osteopath facilitates further discussion and possibly some fine tuning with regards to the patient's actions. This should equip the patient with the basic tools to shape their own, and their community's, future. It is osteopathy's link with empowerment that renders it a natural expression of health promotion (MacDonald, 1994). Increasing evidence is being placed upon the beneficial nature of the interpersonal relationship between patient and practitioner and the rights of the patient as consumer (Department of Health, 1991). This empowerment results in less indecision (cognitive dissonance) and therefore less stress (Totman et al., 1977).

With health as the issue, I will finally include chronological development of the British National Health Service with some significant events that have taken place:

5 July 1948 Establishment of the NHS.
1949 First prescription charges.
1950 Ceiling on NHS spending imposed.
1951 Charges for dental and eye tests introduced.
1954 First kidney transplant.
1955 First ultrasound in obstetrics.
1956 Polio vaccine introduced.
1960 Tranquillisers introduced.
1961 The Pill. Thalidomide disaster.
1963 First liver transplant.
1966 Measles vaccine introduced.
1967 Abortion legalised.
1973 Health service ombudsman appointed.
1974 Reorganisation.
1975 CT scans introduced.
1979 Winter of discontent.
1980 World eradication of smallpox.
1982 First reported case of AIDS.
1986 First reported case of BSE in cattle.
1988 MMR (measles, mumps, rubella) vaccine introduced.

1989 Winter beds crisis.
1989 Flu epidemic.
1990 Introduction of Care in the Community.
1991 NHS internal market launched by Conservatives.
1991 Patients' Charter introduced.
1992 Targets for health introduced.
1995 Scares over the Pill and cancer.
1996 Funding crisis.
1996 Combination therapy for AIDS introduction.
1997 Record waiting lists.
1998 Labour White Paper on NHS reform.
Source: *Observer*, 1998.

'Health is centred on happiness – hugging people, connecting, loving your family, clowning and celebrating, loving your work, and connecting ecstatically to nature and the arts. Happiness cannot happen without intimacy.'

Patch Adams MD

Disease

'Nature spontaneously keeps us well. Do not resist her!'

Henry David Thoreau

The language used in the description of disease causes us to visualise the process as if they were autonomous entities, predatory in nature and always awaiting the opportunity to attack. For example, we speak of the 'natural history' of this or that disease, as though it were a free-living organism, and we argue as to whether this or that combination of signs and symptoms represents a 'real entity' (a species?). One speaks of fighting disease ('the war against cancer') and of increasing an individual's resistance to disease as though it were indeed an adversary threatening from without. One hears and reads, in various versions, that the physician must treat the patient as well as the disease, as though it were possible to treat a disease *except* through the patient. Physicians do treat the patient whether they like it or not. It is the patient that suffers the side effects, or gets better, not the disease. The term 'disease' has been defined within the context of the biomedical model and pathological processes 'on the basis of deviations and malfunctions of the chemical and physiologic systems of the body' (Fabrega, 1975).

The dominant Newtonian–Cartesian model

However we think and talk about diseases, the fact is that nobody has ever seen one. All that is evident are persons who are sick in various, more or less patterned, ways. The unfortunate consequence of the focus on disease, their natural history, causes and cures, is inevitably a de-emphasis of the person who is said to 'have' the disease. Patients who share the same or similar patterns are 'filed' into the same category, are implicitly 'victims' of the same 'causes,' and are candidates for the same 'cures.' Their differences as human beings become irrelevant or, at best, become of secondary interest and the patients see themselves as victims. This is Goethe's multiplicity in unity or diversity in unity.

It is fair to say that a large part of the structure of the allopathic or biomedical model is built on the germ theory of disease. Allopathic theory implies that physical illness or disease which cannot be attributed directly to psychological or physical trauma, congenital defects, poisons, and dietary deficiencies must be caused by organisms, microscopic and macroscopic. Each disease, or group of diseases, is believed to be the product of a specific organism. Modifications of this theory have gone on to involve the immune system and our ability to 'fight' these evil organisms. Disease is believed to occur when organisms from the outside invade the body destroying the parts or the entire person. When a person comes into contact with a 'pathogenic', disease-producing, organism its contribution to the disease depends on certain factors:

(1) the virulence of the organism, the exact extent of which is not known
(2) the individual's susceptibility to colonisation in general and his immunity to that infection in particular
(3) extreme circumstances beyond the individual's control, that is to say whether the organism reaches a point in the body where it can establish itself and do harm
(4) the ability of the body to stand the general strain of adaptation to the organism's colonisation and surviving it, if it succeeds in establishing itself in the body.

Allopathic or biomedical protocols of treatment are a response to this theory of infection. They seem to form a logical approach, at first sight. They promise to achieve some of the following:

(1) killing all 'disease producing' organisms which can be found both inside and outside the body
(2) building up resistance and specific immunity by general measures and by specific vaccine and serum treatment
(3) helping the body to ride the crisis by adopting measures which are believed to combat symptoms which appear to be dangerous
(4) removing the actual or supposed seat of the problem, or at least the debris of the battle, by means of surgery.

The germ theory of disease is in some ways plausible and attractive in that it seems to provide an explanation of certain phenomena that undoubtedly occur, but it will be seen on closer examination that there are many events and facts which it finds difficult to explain. It is natural therefore to take a look at the foundations on which this germ theory was built.

The following includes some of the work of Proby (1939) in approaching the problem of the germ theory. It is best to start with the facts about which there is general agreement. It is generally known that Homo sapiens is subject to diseases of various kinds. Such diseases have roughly been divided into acute and chronic. Acute diseases tend to be short and violent in their course and to be accompanied with fever. They usually end quickly either with recovery or death. Chronic diseases are less violent and less immediately dangerous, but recovery, if it occurs at all, is slow and uneventful. It can be seen that many of these diseases, especially the acute ones, are communicable to various degrees, i.e. one person in a community contracts the infection and others tend to follow. Since the discovery and development of the microscope it has been demonstrated that many diseases, acute and chronic, are generally associated with the presence of organisms in or on the body of the patient. The form and habits of these organisms have been extensively studied and it has been found that certain organisms are commonly associated with particular sets of clinical symptoms.

Assuming that the above facts are generally true several questions are raised.

(1) Why do people get these acute and chronic diseases?
(2) When diseases are communicable, how, why and under what conditions are they so?
(3) Where do the organisms, which often accompany diseases, come from?
(4) What is the relation of these organisms to the diseases, that is to say are they causes, results or merely symptoms?

The germ theory answers these questions by saying that the organisms are the causes of the diseases, that they enter the body from outside, being either communicated directly or carried through the air, and that they are parasitic in character.

Louis Pasteur (1822–95) (who we now know exercised a little creative licence in his papers for fame and fortune) is the great exponent of this theory in its original form. During his development of the germ theory he attracted the attention of scientists towards the problem of fermentation. It was observed that many organic substances of vegetable and animal origin when left exposed to the air at ordinary temperatures chemically changed, ultimately destroying them or at least altering essential characteristics. It was noted by various scientists, including Pasteur, that these changes occurred in the presence of minute living organisms which derived nourishment from the organic material, absorbing it and excreting some kind of excess that it did not need. These living organisms – or fermented bodies – were not themselves soluble and they were only able to live on the organic material and break it up by excreting soluble ferments that fulfilled the same functions as the digestive juices of man and animals. They observed that the organisms that brought about these changes came, to a large extent, from the air, apparently full of living bodies which were capable of producing fermentation, or at least of germs of such living bodies. It was discovered that such well known processes as the making of wine and beer, which had been long practised but little understood, were due to the action of these organisms. In these cases the organisms (yeast etc,) were often artificially introduced by man into the substance to be changed. These conclusions came to be generally accepted and have not since been seriously challenged. There are two main points in connection with this theory that should draw our attention.

(1) All substances which were found to undergo alteration in this way were of organic origin, but they had all ceased to be a functioning part of a living animal or plant. In some cases they were dead animals and plants, in others they were parts removed from animals and plants and in others substances were derived from animals and plants such as sugar, starch, milk or urine.

(2) It was agreed that the changes in these substances usually took place as the result of the action of the germs coming from outside and in many cases could only take place in that way. Some scientists maintained that certain substances were capable of undergoing fermentative and putrefactive change even if they were completely isolated from outside germs. Most notable among the scientists who held this view was the Frenchman, Antoine Béchamp. He drew careful distinction between non-living substances of organic origin, such as sugar and starch, which he called 'proximate principles' (*principes immédiats*), and 'natural organic substances' (*matières organiques naturelles*) which had once been actual parts of living or animal tissue. On the subject of the introduction of germs, like anthrax, into animals Béchamp asked many colleagues when was the last time they caught a disease by injection.

Antoine Béchamp was born in 1816 and died penniless in Paris in 1908. He started his career as a pharmacist but later took his degree in medicine. All through his professional life he was attached to medical schools as a professor and was in close touch with clinical work. Pasteur, on the other hand, was not trained as a physician and had no real grounding in physiology or pathology. He was primarily a chemist and produced, without a doubt, many discoveries in his field in his early days. Unfortunately, he was a self-publicist and realised early on the commercial possibilities of his theories. His lack of ethics even went as far as ridiculing Béchamp, who was sitting at the back of one of Pasteur's lectures in front of other professionals (Geison, 1995). Pasteur has since been exposed as a fraud by examination of his papers relating to the development of the germ theory. These he did not want released into the public domain. Interestingly enough, he allegedly denounced his own work on his death bed: he said, ' it was the terrain', the soil or environment, that was the cause of disease not the microorganism. But we have conveniently forgotten this (Inglis, 1981).

Cecil Helman (1991) wrote of a *germism* in modern society. The use of the word 'germ' has become symbolic conjuring up memories and meanings of ways of being. Everyday we use the words 'germs', 'viruses', 'bugs' and bacilli' interchangeably as if they were the same thing. This age of germism, Helman interprets, is arising into the modern age from the days of Pasteur. The middle of the nineteenth century was not only a time of hot and cold wars in Europe and North America but more importantly a time of massive social change and disorder.

'For many now living, the Age of Germism has seen the decline of religion, and of much of its explanatory power, while in its place have flourished the cults of Science and of Medicine. This Gerministic way of thinking places the blame for our misfortunes on powerful, capricious "forces" that are said to rule over our lives – just as they were once ruled by devils, or Divine grace or punishment.'

Helman (1991)

Invasion by germs, with the so-called spread of infection, is seen as a metaphor for sudden social change.

The gerministic approach is Eurocentric and a simple way out for our culture rather than having to deal with the complexities of real life. Helman goes on to say 'Using the impoverished models it has borrowed from bacteriology, its insights are limited by its constant imagery of war and attack, by its relentless search for invisible enemies and scapegoats, by its ignorance of economics and structure of society, and by the meagre slices of life visible to it on the microscope slide.' We have developed a victim culture in which the doctors will save us. 'Things they (people) used to cope with and take responsibility for become things beyond the reach of their responsibility. They become illnesses. The world is awash with new syndromes and disorders, all kitted out with alarming technical names that carry with them the authority of science' (Humphrys, 1999). Unfortunately, after years of issuing antibiotics the medical profession has now come clean about their uselessness. They have no new drugs for the ones they had been giving that were 'unknowingly' useless. The antibiotic is not the first wonder drug to fall foul of the marketing power of the pharmaceutical industry, Prozac is right behind the antibiotic. Le Fanu (1999) has seen this as the beginning of the end for the monopoly of health and disease care by the biomedical system. An example is the medical record recently published in The *Observer* showing how little things have changed in the East End of London:

- death rate: 14% above the national average
- illness: 27% above the national average
- hospital stays: 28% are for mental illness
- infant deaths: high, with many low birth weight babies
- diabetes: twice the national average, increasing the risk of disability
- main causes of illness: heart disease and mental illness.

(Source: Revill, 1998.)

The public is ignorant, being entertained and led further along the path of germism by 'health issues' in glossy magazines, television commercials and Pavlovian conditioning. Medical science is, in the main, composed of 'warriors' in a military hierarchy who are the epitome of the 'double seeing son':

Father 'Son, you are seeing double.'
Son 'Father, if I were seeing double then when I looked up I would see four moons.'

One of the greatest campaigners for an alternative to the monopoly of the medical profession was Brian Inglis. In *The Diseases of Civilisation*, 1981, Inglis wrote about the role played by illness in our society. The public is unaware of the hidden agenda in our society interwoven with economics, commercialism and the main legacy from the past, that of the Roman Catholic church. With particular emphasis on colds and flu Inglis wrote

'Whether a patient has a cold or flu can be ascertained in the laboratory, but in the great majority of cases the decision whether a patient's symptoms should be attributed to one or to the other is made by rule of thumb. Although the rule varies from household to household, the general assumption is that the symptoms – sore throat, aches, shivering, running nose, and general malaise – qualify as flu only if they are severe, particularly if there is a temperature of over 100°F. If there happens to be a flu epidemic, however, the symptoms of what would be ordinarily be regarded as a cold may achieve promotion.'

The model of the evil micro-organism became so powerful, within the fast growing economy of the industrial revolution, that even the instigator of the new germ theory, Louis Pasteur, could not stop it. Inglis continued, 'On his deathbed, according to a friend who was with him, he reiterated that Bernard had been right: "The germ is nothing; the terrain is everything." To Claude Bernard, pathogens were like seeds described in the New Testament parable of the sower: some falling by the wayside, some on stony ground, some among the thorns, and only those falling on fertile ground taking root, and bringing forth the fruit. Pathogens, Bernard argued, obeyed the same rules; they could flourish only where the host was accommodating.' Osteopathic medicine has always recognised disease as a two-way patient–micro-organism relationship.

Eubrotic medicine

Eubrotic medicine is defined as the 'medicine of man in health'. It was first mentioned by Iago Gladston MD in his 1949 publication, *Medicine in the Changing Order* (cited in Becker, 1949). In discussing eubrotic medicine Gladston wrote

'We are so dazzled by the achievements in modern medicine that we forget to look behind and beyond.... We sort of naively believe that the patient having been cured of his disease – by the sulfas, penicillin, or some other antibiotic – will live happy and healthy "forever after".'

It is significant that Dr Still spoke of the avoidance of structural upsets in maintaining health and the relationship of the individual to the environment. Out of understanding this need for the maintenance of health grew the later development of the addition of osteopathic manipulative therapy. Gladston continues

'... during the last century, medicine was a backward and indeed disreputable science ... Modern (medicine) has not been modern very long. In effect for not more than three-quarters of a century.... From the time of Paracelsus or last century the practice of Sydenham down until the end of last century the practice of medicine was impotent and disreputable – and that for a very good reason: because the physician in this intervening period forgot or did not learn how to treat the patient and did not yet know how to treat the disease. During the last seventy-five years and more particularly during the last three decades, we have learned very effectively how to treat the disease.'

Antibiotic means against life.

Eubrotic medicine, the medicine of man in health, is therefore, according to osteopathic philosophy, of paramount importance in osteopathic medicine. This is why Dr Still emphasised the education of students to include anatomy, physiology, chemistry, surgery and obstetrics (Still, 1902). We are aware of the contribution of I.M. Korr to the understanding of the basic physiologic concepts of the practice of osteopathic medicine. On the subject of the association between eubrotic medicine and osteopathy Korr (1948) wrote

'Although chronic and degenerative disorders are spoken of as diseases of maturity or of middle and late life, it is not adequately appreciated that often they have their beginnings in youth and childhood ... Today the osteopath is the only one sufficiently broad and sufficiently unitary in outlook, upon which a *system* of practice can be based, that is capable of encompassing all these diseases. Today osteopathy is the only system of practice which has preventive potentialities with respect to these diseases.'

Of major importance to the osteopathic physician is the fact that if Korr and his fellow workers are correct and the nervous system is the organiser of disease, then the pathogen would be the specific irritant setting up the neurodystrophia. In this case osteopathic treatment would be directed at the restoration, to a greater or lesser degree, of homeostatic vascular/neural function. This would give at least some symptomatic relief. *Haemophilus influenzae* and *Streptococcus pneumoniae* may be the dominant pathogens in chronic bronchitis, although the available evidence indicates that infection of the bronchi is secondary to some dysfunction of the bronchi themselves. Haemophilus influenzae can persist in the sputum in spite of the patient's more or less marked clinical improvement. It is possible that a bacteria or virus is secondary to some dysfunction of the bronchi themselves. This is Speransky's dystrophia of the bronchi due to chronic neurodystrophia.

This discrepancy of a clinical cure in the absence of a bacteriologic one and of the common rapid relapses of infection has been a subject of debate over many years, and it is of interest to speculate just what role the endogenous anaerobes might play in this somewhat obscure scenario. The patient thinks they are better but the 'lesion' has not been reduced. The result may be a rapid relapse. Earlier workers remarked at length on the discrepancy between clinical cure and the persistence of *H. influenzae* (Willis, 1984).

Causes of disease

Historically, causative factors of illness have been attributed to some of the following:

- the sins of the individual or ancestor
- the curse of a jealous rival
- the humoral or miasmal effects of the environment (considered in more detail below)
- micro-organisms from the environment
- childhood experiences and family relationships.

The miasma theory

The origins of disease are environmental in a very broad sense according to this theory. Disease is caused by bad smells resulting from putrefaction, poor sewage, etc. Disease can be prevented by altering the environment without the need of detailed knowledge of pathogenic mechanisms. The resulting improvement in sanitation led to an unparalleled effect on the health of the city population, even though the rationale for the sanitation was incorrect (Donaldson and Donaldson, 1993; Jones, 1994). The one disease that comfortably fitted the miasmal theory was malaria. The word is derived from *mala aria*, foul air.

Job Lewis Smith (1827–97) served as a physician in the slums of New York City where the 'summer diarrhoea of infants', known as 'cholera infantum' was a major cause of infant mortality. He described its cause in the first edition of his text:

'One of the chief causes of (cholera infantum, the summer diarrhoea of infants) is, doubtless, residence in an atmosphere loaded with noxious vapours, especially gases arising from animal and vegetable decomposition, or an atmosphere rendered impure by overcrowding and by personal and domiciliary uncleanness. It is therefore much more common in tenement houses and parts of the city occupied by the poor than in cleaner and less crowded apartments.'

Yankauer (1994)

The humoral theory

The origins of this theory probably arose as far back as Hippocrates and later Galen. In the humoral theory the body was seen as a reflection or microcosm of the world. It would go even further to reflect the entire universe or macrocosm. The elements of Nature, which were earth, fire, air and water, would correspond to the four body humours. These humours are melancholic (black bile), phlegmatic (phlegm), choleric (yellow bile) and sanguine (blood). In addition these four humours had particular qualities: wet, dry, hot and cold.

More germs

Long before Pasteur, others had speculated about germs. F. Harrison, Principal Professor of Bacteriology at Macdonald College (Faculty of Agriculture, McGill University), Quebec, Canada, who wrote a historical review of microbiology, published in *Microbiology* writes of

'Geronimo Fracastorio (an Italian poet and physician, 1483–1553) of Verona, published a work, *De Contagionibus et Contagiosis Morbis, et eorum Curatione* 1546 in Venice, which contained the first statement of the true nature of contagion, infection, or disease organisms, and of the modes of transmission of infectious disease. He divided diseases into those which infect by immediate contact, through intermediate agents, and at a distance through the air. Organisms which cause disease, called seminaria contagionum, he supposed to be of the nature of viscous or glutinous matter, similar to the colloidal states of substances described by modern physical chemists. These particles, too small to be seen, were capable of reproduction in appropriate media, and became pathogenic through the action of animal heat. Thus Fracastorio, in the middle of the sixteenth century, gave us an outline of morbid processes in terms of microbiology.'

Florence Nightingale (1820–1910) wrote letters attacking the idea of the germ theory in 1860. She said of 'infection'

'Diseases are not individuals arranged in classes, like cats and dogs, but conditions growing out of one another. . . . Is it not living in a continual mistake to look upon diseases as we do now, as separate entities, which must exist, like cats and dogs, instead of looking upon them as conditions, like a dirty and a clean condition, and just as much under our control; or rather as the reactions of kindly nature, against the conditions in which we have placed ourselves?

'I was brought up to believe that smallpox, for instance, was a thing of which there was once a first specimen in the world, which went on propagating itself, in a perpetual chain of descent, just as there was a first dog, (or a first pair of dogs) and that smallpox would not begin itself, any more than a new dog would begin without there having been a parent dog. ... Since then I have seen with my own eyes and smelled with my own nose smallpox growing up in first specimens, either in closed rooms or in overcrowded wards, where it could not by any possibility have been 'caught', but must have begun. ... I have seen diseases begin, grow up, and pass into one another. Now, dogs do not pass into cats. ... I have seen, for instance, with a little overcrowding, continued fever grow up; and with a little more, typhoid fever; and with a little more, typhus, all in the same ward or hut.

'Would it not be far better, truer, and more practical, if we looked upon disease in this light (for diseases, as all experience shows, are adjectives, not noun-substantives):

- True nursing ignores infection, except to prevent it. Cleanliness and fresh air from open windows, with unremitting attention to the patient, are the only defence a true nurse either asks or needs.
- Wise and humane management of the patient is the best safeguard against infection. The greater part of nursing consists of preserving cleanliness.
- The specific disease doctrine is the grand refuge of weak, uncultured, unstable minds, such as now rule in the medical profession. There are no specific diseases; there are specific disease conditions.'

Looking back into biomedical history it will be seen that the ideas for aetiology for disease existed before Pasteur's famous 'germ theory', it will be noticed that Pasteur did not discover anything. What he did use was another man's hard work and adapted it for his own purposes as a 'discovery'.

The germ theory places the responsibility for health on the health professionals. Payton Rous, working with chickens at the Rockefeller Institute, produced the first clear demonstration that viruses are implicated in malignant tumour formation, a discovery that won him a Nobel prize in 1966. In 1933 Richard Shope, also with the Rockefeller Institute, isolated a tumour virus from rabbits; and three years later, J.J. Bittner discovered an oncogenic virus in rats with breast cancer. The excitement these discoveries and other published works on cancer viruses caused between 1911 and 1940 died down during the Second World War. Today research continues in the field of genetics looking for the cancer gene. Interestingly, with all the advanced laboratory equipment we have today there has been no isolation of a cancer virus in a human (Andrewes, 1970 and Goodfield, 1975). The real issue here is that if a virus is isolated then an anti-viral drug can be developed. This would naturally reduce fear and disability for patients and society.

Two issues arise here. Firstly, there is the issue known as the species barrier, where viruses and bacteria behave differently in different species. Even in the same species the reactions to the same virus or bacteria are not the same. We are today well aware that in the extremes one animal can continue on healthily while another will die from the administration of the same micro-organism. Secondly, if there is a cancer virus, would it not be infectious?

Viruses, requiring a living cell for energy, exhibit creative adaptability in reaching their target cells through a barrage of antibodies and host chemical defences. This influxion is often achieved through minor mutations in envelope chemical structure sufficient for the core molecule to penetrate antibody protection and complete another reproductive cycle. Of the hundreds of viruses that are recognised, and after millions of doses of virus vaccines, smallpox is the only virus that has been boxed into the laboratory freezer by human efforts. The heroic efforts of a multitude of dedicated and creative scientists have not yet extinguished a single bacterial or viral species from the earth (McIntyre, 1991).

'But while certain facts lend support to the bacteria theory, certain other facts show, in my opinion, that there must be some other cause of diphtheria which is distinct from the bacteria. In the intervals of epidemics, and in localities where diphtheria has not occurred, or has occurred rarely, the microscope discloses the existence of bacteria, which seem to be identical with those found in diphtheric inflammations ... bacteria, which seem to be identical with those of diphtheria, are frequently found upon the gums, between the teeth in a state of health, where they produce no perceptible irritation.

'It is evident that the truth regarding the relation of bacteria to diphtheria lies in one of two hypotheses – either that these parasites are the specific virus, and therefore cause the disease; or that the cause is something more subtle not yet discovered, which also alters the tissues and the blood that they become a indus in which the bacteria are early and quickly developed, so that from being few and innocuous in the system, they occur in myriads. My own belief is more and more confirmed that the latter is the true theory and that a consequence (has been mistaken) for a cause.'

(Job Lewis Smith, cited in Yankauer, 1994)

Research indicates that the model of biomedicine at general practitioner level is different from that at consultant hospital level. The general practitioner treatment is the result of more 'negotiation' and has a closer resemblance to the folk model (Helman, 1978). Unfortunately, this means there is a decreasing effectiveness of the model at the greatest point of contact. The biomedical model is diluted at the point of delivery. The point of delivery is not the same as the textbook or lecture presentation. This may be due to the fact that the control imposed on the patients in hospitals is not realistic in the community. In the hospital they can reduce the patient to a disease and treat them as a disease. In osteopathic training we start and begin with the patient and their social needs: they have to work or be mothers. Osteopathy deals with the commonest problems, back pain etc. This is why doctors tend to have problems dealing with many illnesses as they have no control of their patients, which they need, to have any degree of success. The biomedical model is unrealistic in real life. For the amount of effort put in its returns are minimal. 'Patients suffer "illness"; physicians diagnose and treat "disease"' (Eisenberg, 1977). Cassell (1976) had a more holistic view of ill health 'use the word "illness" to stand for what the patient feels when he goes to the doctor, and "disease" for what he has on the way home. Disease, then, is something an organ has; illness is something a man has.'

Epidemics

'Most disease is the result of change in our environment, behaviour, or both.'
Spokesman for the Pasteur Institute

New epidemics come into existence, change, and vanish. Most disease is the result of change in our environment, behaviour, or both. Moreover, the triumph of scientific medicine over epidemic disease is not the clear victory commonly supposed. The great plagues of Europe disappeared long before the emergence of bacteriology (McNeil, 1976).

The Black Death

A good introduction to epidemics is a brief history of the Black Death, showing the complexity of disease as a social, behavioural and biological phenomenon.

The Black Death ranked as one of the three worst catastrophes in history, and marked the start of the second plague pandemic. Successive epidemics kept the European population low until 1470 and life expectancy fell dramatically.

The plague first hit Europe in 541. There were three major varieties: bubonic, pneumonic, and septicaemic, all caused by *Yersinia Pestis*. Bubonic plague was transmitted by fleas and proved fatal in 50%–60% of cases. Pneumonic plague is transmitted person to person and is fatal in 95%–100% of cases. Septicaemic plague is not as well understood. Humans are not the first choice of insect carriers and tend only to be affected as a result of environmental changes.

During pandemic conditions, plague strikes every 2–20 years. *Yersinia Pestis* is native to Central Asia, Siberia, the Yunan region of China, Iran, Libya, Arabian Peninsular, and east Africa.

The plague lasted from 541–750 AD, spreading from East Africa via the Nile, to strike 'world wide' (apart from central Asia). One of its political effects was the prevention of the Byzantine empire from reconquering Europe. The plague killed 50–60% of the population of the Mediterranean basin.

Until the Black Death Europe was largely epidemic free. Between the tenth and thirteenth centuries the population rose 300% to 75–80 million, the highest in 1000 years. This followed 700 years of population stagnation (more or less), which had been caused by new agricultural techniques and disease pool equilibrium.

Environmental changes

The environmental changes which preceded the Black Death were as follows.

The weather improved between 750/800 and 1150/1200 (this is vouched for in glacial evidence), and a trend began towards milder winters and drier summers (there was a 1° Celsius average temperature change). Then temperatures went down again, causing glaciers and peat bogs to expand. The new cold conditions even caused the Baltic sea to freeze in 1303 and in 1306–7. The River Thames froze 12 times between 1400–80.

At the same time farming yields went down three-fold between 1209–1300 to pre-population explosion levels. By 1300 Europe was in a classic Malthusian crisis. Due to the low disease rate, the population continued to rise. Wheat was planted more and more as being the most efficient crop. Regular famines occurred from the 1290s to 1343. Despite this, little population decrease occurred, although the general standard of living went down. The tripartite nature of society based on the aristocracy, the clergy and the peasantry was also starting to decline.

Beginning of the plague

There are alternative theories about the origins of the Black Death: (1) that it was spread from Yunan by Mongols, and (2) that environmental changes caused Mongols and Turks to move to greener pastures which also caused rodent migrations.

The significance of Mongolia in the plague is certainly considerable. Tribesmen connected plague with rodents, but there was no trapping of marmots which will have contributed to the spread of the disease. Slow-moving animals were regarded as untouchable; and some rodent furs were forbidden.

With these favourable conditions, the plague erupted in the Gobi desert in the late 1320s. As the Black Death, it reduced China's population from 125 million to 90 million. In 1345 plague hit the Crimea; and in 1346 it hit Azerbaijan.

The Black Death reached Europe in two ways: (1) rodent migrations; and (2) via the trade routes, (this vector was contributed to by peace being declared with the Mongols. Plague caused 25%–50% fatalities in the Western world and had other wider side effects. In particular, it led to anti-Semitism and a general breakdown in law and order.

Consequences

The Black Death had many consequences, some of them still recognisable today. There was a psychological shock, similar to World War One. But humans are resilient, and this was important particularly bearing in mind the repetitive nature of plague.

A sense of epicurian individualism developed, engendered by a sense of urgency, a wish to live life for the here and now. This, however, involved an overall change of mood from optimism to pessimism. The influence of Islam decreased as religious leaders struggled to deal with the disease and its aftermath; although the Ottoman conquest of the Balkans had taken place, the invaders failed to colonise the territory. Islamic leaders likened death from plague to death in combat.

Christian leaders fled from plague, and the influence of the Catholic church waned. In government, bureaucrats died, so causing chaos while the influence of kings increased, as lesser nobles couldn't cope. Three-quarters of the English aristocracy were left without a male heir for two generations. The decreased population caused labour rates to rise, and the manorial system to decrease, while real wages rose to their highest level until the twentieth century: wages increased five-fold between 1347 and 1350 in England. Society began a change from being land based to labour based, and an increased sense of class identity developed. Several pro-king/anti-aristocracy revolts occurred. Most of these changes were not caused but accelerated by the plague.

Later, the Great Plague of 1665 reflected the environment that developed the *new philosophy of rationality*. This was the rationality of Newton and Descartes. Contrary to popular belief, the development of theory-based science did not develop in an era of prosperity, but from an era of desperation. This was after the Thirty Years' War (1618–48). Life in the seventeenth century could not have been any worse. Economies had collapsed and there was a pan-European destabilisation of the Protestants and Catholics. In England it led to civil war and the demise of Charles I. The development of modern concepts are linked to disease, war and famine. Rational modern scientific development came out of despair and a need for certainty and stability, not out of logical scientific methodology (Toulmin, 1990).

Influenza and cognitive dissonance

The word 'influenza' comes directly from the Italian word for influence. It was thought that earthquakes and volcanic eruption caused the influenza. This has naturally been dismissed by medical science, but modern experience shows that natural disasters are often precursors of influenza outbreaks which spread rapidly.

On 17 January 1995 at 05.46 an earthquake of 7.2 on the Richter scale took place 20 miles south of Kobe, Japan's sixth biggest city with a population of 1.5 million people. The ground moved an average of 7 inches horizontally and 4 inches in a vertical direction. In the ensuing chaos there were no blankets, and electricity, gas and phones were cut off. The night temperature dropped to $-2°C$ and naturally people did not want to return to buildings due to aftershocks, they slept in the parks and streets. Running water was still not available in Kobe and the surrounding cities of Nishinomiya and Ashiya by 18 January. This affected an estimated 2.3 million people. Within the first week there was an outbreak of influenza due to what has been medically termed *cognitive dissonance* (Fig. 13).

Sir Christopher Andrewes described in his book *The Common Cold* that 'colds, turned out to be "by no means a very infectious kind of disease" – a verdict which has been confirmed by other trials' (cited in Inglis, 1981). Inglis described an experiment designed by psychologists from Oxford and the Common Cold Unit to find out if cognitive dissonance was involved in the transference of the disease. The results were interesting where the answer was yes, and they found that 'stress levels were a better predictor of the severity of the colds than antibody levels.'

A flu epidemic in 1969 disrupted the UK's postal and telecommunications service, and immunisation was offered to 400 000 employees. The immunisation programme was deemed to have prevented the epidemic from getting worse. But on closer inspection of the figures there was little or no effect; in fact it showed the power of the placebo. Inglis went on to state that 'If, as the *New Scientist* claimed in its reports of the experiment, it shows that "psychological factors play a large part in deciding whether or not we can stop cold viruses multiplying".'

The influenza pandemic 1918–9

In the influenza pandemic of 1918–19 an estimated 555 000 American people died. The most recent research places global mortality as a result of the pandemic at around 30 million or more (Brown, 1992 and Davis, 1999). The disease swept through whole countries in a matter of weeks. In Nigeria 10 people infected an entire port. Research shows that India had the highest mortality with between 42 and 67 deaths from influenza per 1000 population. In this respect the United States of America was particularly lucky, with a mortality rate at about 5.2 per 1000. Even though it was called 'Spanish flu' (coded A(H1N1)), evidence showed that it started in the USA on March 8, 1918, in Camp Funston, Kansas. This scientists are confident that it began due to a sudden and dramatic genetic 'shift' in the virus. Subsequently the virus underwent a second 'shift' on the Western

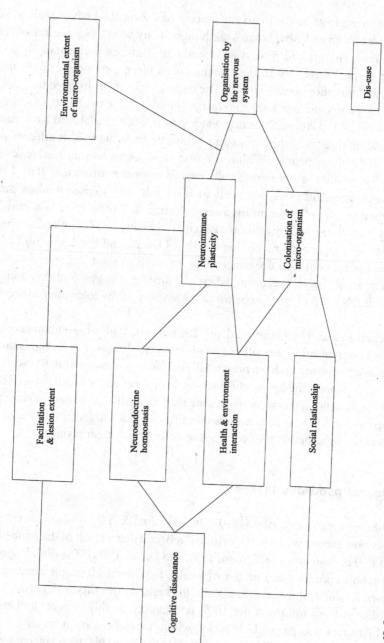

Fig. 13 Cognitive dissonance.

Front making the virus even more lethal. It was this second strain that spread around the world, leading to the pandemic having a mortality rate in the millions. Strangely, there was another outbreak in 1976, in an isolated incident, of the same 1918 virus in a soldier at Fort Dix, New Jersey.

The influenza and pneumonia pandemic in the USA gave osteopathic medicine one of its greatest opportunities. The USA did not have a specific anti-toxin to allow them to kill the 'germ' causing the infection. What osteopaths knew was how to produce a physiological phagocytosis, manipulatively increasing the production of white blood cells. When the osteopaths did this, more than 99% of cases treated recovered. During the epidemic there were more than 500 licensed osteopathic physicians in the Army and Navy doing the work of privates. They were never asked to make a contribution towards the health of the thousands of servicemen and women who were dying of the disease. Why not? Because their degree was a DO instead of an MD. In the bases at Camp Grant, Camp Benjamin Harrison, Camp Sherman and hundreds of other camps in the USA, service personnel were dying at a rate of 34 out of every 100 from pneumonia. Outside the camps osteopathic physicians were working hard. If approximately 330 or 340 out of every 1000 pneumonia cases died under medical care and approximately 100 out of every 1000 cases died under osteopathic care, who was responsible for the additional 240 deaths in every 1000? A major contributing factor was the administration of drugs, in liquid form, which reduced the patient's ability to cough; essentially they drowned.

A further and very interesting feature of these reports is the fact that so many of the osteopathic physicians reported that practically none of their patients, who just preceding and at the time of the epidemic had been having osteopathic treatment contracted these diseases. In their opinion, the resistance of these patients was up to such a level that they were able to withstand the infection of the epidemic (Riley, 1919).

The evidence of the effectiveness of the osteopathic physicians in the 'flu epidemic has in the most part been considered anecdotal. This is primarily from the American osteopathic profession's interpretation of a questionnaire sent out to osteopathic physicians and its results (Peterson, 1980). Evidence-based information is weak but as Korr repeatedly requests, we need a paradigm shift with a focus on outcomes and common denominators.

The following extract from Hildreth (1942) is reproduced in full due to its historical importance:

'Along with this reference to the yielding of pneumonia to osteopathic care, it is interesting and gratifying to recount the comparative results obtained by drug medication and osteopathic treatment in the great pandemic of pneumonia and influenza at the time of the World War in 1917–19. In order to make this comparison, I sent requests for reports on the number of cases of influenza and pneumonia and the number of deaths from each, to every State Health

Commissioner and to all the City Health Commissioners, in cities in the United States of 40,000 population and over. One hundred and forty-eight replies were received.

'Sufficient data was received in the replies and reports of those one hundred and forty-eight Health Commissioners coupled with the estimates of the National Census Bureau and the several Insurance Companies to warrant the ultra-conservative estimate of five per cent of fatalities in influenza cases and 33 per cent of fatalities in pneumonia cases under medicinal care, the latter running, in some larger centres of population, as high as 68 and 73 per cent. Up to the date of the survey, the official compilation of fatalities, in epidemic pneumonia in our Army Camps, amounted to $34\frac{1}{2}$ per cent. Such experiences under medicinal care naturally made me wonder what were the results obtained under osteopathic care.

'I sent report blanks to all practicing osteopathic physicians in the United States and Canada for data on all cases of influenza and epidemic pneumonia. Strict instructions were given to report only well developed cases, and to report all such with all fatalities. All told, 2445 osteopathic physicians reported. These 2445 reports representing every section of the country and Canada, the small towns as well as the large cities, cover 110 122 cases of influenza with only 257 deaths, or a mortality of less than one-fourth of 1 per cent. They also reported having cared for 6258 cases of epidemic pneumonia with only 635 deaths, or a pneumonia mortality of only 10 per cent. Some fifty of these deaths occurred within twenty-four hours after the osteopathic physicians were called. This is a sufficient number of cases to warrant intelligent and conservative conclusions and comparisons.

The following table gives, in brief, the comparative results:

MORTALITY IN INFLUENZA

Under	Cases	Deaths	Percentage
Medicinal care in	1000	50	5
Osteopathic care in	1000	2.25	$\frac{1}{4}$ of 1

MORTALITY IN PNEUMONIA

Under	Cases	Deaths	Percentage
Medicinal care in	1000	350	35
Osteopathic care in	1000	100	10

In addition to these splendid results, this survey disclosed another most gratifying one: There was not an osteopathic physician among all those who treated these cases who could not stand before his fellowmen with chest up, head erect, eye beaming, and a consciousness that not one in all that army of 116 380 patients had become a drug addict through any professional act of his, while bringing them through those dreadfully anxious hours during their influenza or pneumonia illness.'

'The actual questionnaire sent out is as follows:

(1) What kinds of lesions were found?
(2) Where?
(3) How corrected?
(4) What general manipulations were given for bedside treatment?
(5) What was the *average time* used per patient for osteopathic treatment?
(6) How frequently were patients treated?
(7) Did you observe any unfavourable reactions from too long too thorough a treatment?
(8) *How many days* were patients under treatment?
(9) Did patients who had been drugged respond as well as others to osteopathic treatment?
(10) What regulation of diet was prescribed for (a) influenza alone? (b) Pulmonary complications? (c) Bowel and stomach complications? (d) Nervous complications?
(11) Did you use any substances like Antiphlogistine, Dionol or other local applications? If so what?
(12) What methods were used to keep the bowels active? (a) If enema, what kind, how much, how often? (b) If manipulations, what kind and how? (c) If laxative, what kind and how?
(13) What method used to keep kidneys active?
(14) Did you sweat the patient? If so, how and at what stage of disease?
(15) Did you use cotton jacket for pulmonary complications?
(16) What about ventilation, that is, much or little?
(17) What was average temperature of room?
(18) Were any means used to reduce temperature of patients? (a) If manipulation, where, what kind, and how applied? (b) If baths, what kind, how often? (c) Enemas? What kind?
(19) Were any means used to overcome cough? If so, what?
(20) Were any means used to stimulate the heart? If drugs were used, mention them and quantity used? If not used, *state so definitely.*
(21) (a) How many cases of influenza did you treat? (b) How many deaths? (c) How many cases of pneumonia? (d) How many deaths?
(22) How many patients were you able to treat a day during the great rush?
(23) Cases reported herein were of the epidemic of 1918–19_____ 1920_____. (Do not report both together)
(24) Sign your name and address and date your report.

Here are two of the replies:

Lucius M. Bush, DO, Jersey City, N.J.
170 cases of flu and 15 of pneumonia; no deaths.

(1)   Muscular, ligamentous and bony specially. Bronchial and intestinal.

(2)   Upper dorsal and cervical mainly. Lumbar region contracted. Severe pain at sacroiliac joint in some cases.

(3)   Relaxation of contraction first usually through bony correction. All done with patient lying down.

(4)   Stretching, rotation, exaggeration of lesions and corrections.

(5)   Twenty minutes.

(6)   Twice a day usually in bad cases. Some over three or four times a day. Light cases once a day.

(7)   No. The oftener treated the quicker the results.

(8)   Average four to five days. Longest two weeks in bed. No treatment over seven days.

(9)   No. The case was prolonged.

(10)   Liquid diet and fruit juices in influenza; the same only less in pulmonary complications; the same in bowel or stomach complications if no distress was indicated; nothing but water if a severe case. In nervous complications, the same.

(11)   Antiphlogistine in pulmonary cases.

(12)   Occasional enemas; abdominal manipulation. Every treatment was to free gases and lift intestines and colon. Work on sides of abdomen, mostly toward center.

(13)   Plenty of water. Lower dorsal treatment.

(14)   Yes, at first. Water and hot lemonade and plenty of covers. Also if strong enough a hot bath and glass of cold water drunk in it.

(15)   Occasionally.

(16)   As much as possible, without draft, keeping temperature about 60 degrees F.

(17)   60 degrees F.

(18)   Cold packs where fever was above 103 degrees.

(19)   Cough drops in some cases. Inhibition 1st to 3rd dorsal.

(20)   No drugs. Osteopathic treatment only.

Marcus E. Brown, DO, Sioux City, Iowa
216 cases, no deaths.

(1) Osseous and muscular.
(2) Mostly cervical and dorsal in those cases that bordered on typhoid lumbar.
(3) Extension, flexion and inhibition.
(4) A thorough relaxation in the cervical and dorsal region.
(5) Ten minutes.
(6) From one to five times in 24 hours.
(7) Experience has taught me to give such cases thorough extension of spine. Spine stretched by my taking hold of the patient's head having assistants hold feet and stretching patient until I feel the spine relax; then I inhibit the cervical and dorsal regions (dorsal mostly) until I felt patient relax. I have a piece of heavy webbing (saddle girt) 4 inches wide and 13 feet long that I put on the patient's head and wrap around the bed post and I take hold of feet when there is no one to assist me.
(8) From three to thirty. When they come or called me in the early stages and had no drugs, one treatment reduced temperatures of 104 and 106 degrees.
(9) Most emphatically no.
(10) Rhubarb sauce, pineapple, pears, peaches, baked apple, Mellen's food. Three hours between any two kinds of food. A glass of water every hour, Colfax preferred.
(11) Hot water bottles, hot sand and salt bags.
(12) In very high fever cold saline enema. One was usually enough; if not, another, in 24 hours. 4 quarts. Relaxation of lumbar inhibition of splanchnic nerves. No laxatives used.
(13) Abundance of water.
(14) Hot water bottles, hot sand and hot salt bags.
(15) No; put a strip 7 or 8 inches wide, 4-ply down the spine.
(16) Abundance of fresh air. Cheese cloth over window when necessary.
(17) 60 degrees.
(18) Thorough relaxation over the kidney area. Inhibition cervical and splanchnic areas. Cold enema. No baths.
(19) Heat, upper dorsal. Thorough stretching of intercostal muscles anterior and posterior.
(20) Stimulation to cardiac nerves. Stimulation of ganglia impar in severe cases. As I am an osteopathic physician no drugs were needed.

(Source: Peterson, 1980)

Common modern causes of mortality

A review of the *World Health Report 1996*, (cited in Manning, 1996) says approximately 52 million people died from all causes in 1995. Of these, infectious diseases killed more than 17 million people. The greatest mortality resulted from acute respiratory infections, including pneumonia; diarrhoea related diseases such as cholera, typhoid and dysentery; tuberculosis; and malaria. The report outlined other major concerns published by the World Health Organisation regarding the position on global health; it goes on to look at two particular areas.

- Drug-resistant strains of microbes that cause tuberculosis, malaria, cholera, diarrhoea and pneumonia are having a deadly impact. Some bacteria are resistant to 10 different drugs. Resistant bacteria are responsible for up to 60% of hospital acquired infections in the USA.
- Cancer of the stomach, cervix and liver are associated with viruses and bacteria. More than 1.5 million of the 10 million new cancer cases a year could be avoided by preventing infections associated with them.

The report included the categories ten biggest killers, ten most common infections and new diseases.

The ten biggest killers

(1) Acute lower respiratory infections such as pneumonia killed 4.4 million people; around 4 million were children.
(2) Diarrhoea related disease such as cholera, typhoid, and dysentery, which were spread mainly by contaminated water or food, killed 3.1 million, mostly children.
(3) Tuberculosis killed almost 3.1 million, mostly adults.
(4) Malaria killed 2.1 million people; this includes 1 million children.
(5) Hepatitis B infections killed more than 1.1 million people.
(6) HIV/AIDS killed more than 1 million children.
(7) Measles killed more than 1 million children.
(8) Neonatal tetanus killed almost 460 000 children.
(9) Whooping cough (pertussis) killed 355 000 children.
(10) Intestinal worm diseases killed at least 135 000 people.

(Source: *World Health Report*, 1996.)

The ten most common infections

(1) Diarrhoeal diseases – about 4 billion episodes in 1995.
(2) Tuberculosis – about 1.9 billion carry tuberculosis bacilli; there were 8.9 million new cases in 1995.
(3) Intestinal worms – about 1.4 infected at any given time.
(4) Malaria – up to 500 million new cases in 1995.
(5) Hepatitis – about 350 million hepatitis B chronic carriers, and about 100 million hepatitis C chronic carriers.
(6) Acute lower respiratory infections – about 395 million episodes in 1995.
(7) Sexually transmitted diseases – at least 330 million new cases in 1995.
(8) Measles – 42 million total cases in 1995.
(9) Whooping cough – 40 million total cases in 1995.
(10) Meningococcal meningitis – about 3.5 million new cases in 1995.

(Source: *World Health Report*, 1996.)

New diseases

The following are some of the 'new diseases', causative agents, and diseases associated with them, in chronological order of their identification:

1973: Rotavirus, a major cause of infantile diarrhoea world-wide.
1976: *Cryptosporidium parvum*, a parasite that causes acute and chronic diarrhoea.
1977: *Legionella pneumophila*, the bacterium that causes potentially fatal Legionnaire's disease.
1977: Ebola virus, which causes haemorrhagic fever – fatal in up to 80% of cases.
1977: Hantaan virus, which causes potentially fatal haemorrhagic fever with renal syndrome.
1977: *Campylobacter jejuni*, a bacterium that causes diarrhoea.
1980: Human T-lymphotropic virus I (HTLV-1), which causes lymphoma-leukaemia.
1982: *Escherichia coli*, 0157:H7 strain of bacteria, which causes bloody diarrhoea.
1982: HTLV-2 virus, which causes hairy cell leukaemia.
1983: *Helicobacter pylori*, the bacterium associated with peptic ulcer disease and stomach cancer.
1983: Human immunodeficiency virus (HIV), which causes AIDS.
1988: Hepatitis E virus, which causes epidemics of jaundice in hot climates.
1988: Human herpes virus 6, which causes fever and rash.
1989: Hepatitis C virus, which causes liver cancer as well as liver disease.
1991: Guanarito virus, which causes Venezuelan haemorrhagic fever.

1992: *Vibrio cholerae*, 0139, which causes epidemic cholera.
1994: Sabia virus, which causes Brazilian haemorrhagic fever.
1995: Human herpes virus 8, associated with Kaposi's sarcoma in AIDS patients.
(Source: *World Health Report*, 1996.)

Osteopathic therapeutics in infectious diseases

Edgar S. Comstock, DO of Chicago wrote the following study in the Journal of the American Osteopathic Association in 1920. It provides a succinct and practical comparison of the osteopathic and medical approaches to disease.

'The osteopathic conception of aetiology of disease is quite at variance with the usual medical conception, and so our viewpoint of the causation of the infectious disease does not entirely coincide with that of other systems. Therefore the osteopathic interpretation of symptomology differs from that of the medical. The osteopathic aetiology carries the mind back to the fundamental, or primary, factors that underlie the disease; while the usual medical aetiology pays particular attention to the immediate, or exciting, cause. It is only in very recent editions of medical practice that a cursory attention given to the predisposing causes that underlie the susceptibility of the patient to the infectious disease. Formerly the underlying factor was passed over as 'lowered resistance', with practically no intimation of the cause of the lowered resistance.

Indeed, medical literature of the past has often belittled the possibility of exposures to dampness, sudden temperature changes and draughts as being at all possible as a factor in lowering body resistance. Particular stress was nearly always placed upon the micro-organism as the cause of these diseases, little or no explanation being given as to why some individuals were more susceptible than others. In the very recent medical textbooks, however, we are beginning to find allusions to the effects of 'neurotic heredity, exposure, fatigue, diet and draughts' in lowering resistance.

The osteopathic physician considers aetiology on a dual basis, studying the predisposing factors quite as much as the exciting causes; in fact, giving the predisposing factors first consideration. It is certainly evident from osteopathic clinical experience that infectious disease can be prevented, and frequently even aborted if the predisposing factors are removed, though the patient has been directly exposed.

There are many extrinsic causes of those structural changes which the osteopathic physician finds; these are the lesions that he considers the predisposing factors. Some of these extrinsic causes are fatigue; overuse and abuse of function; violence (either severe or sudden, or less severe and applied for a considerable period of time); dietetic errors; exposure to dampness, sudden changes in temperature; and many other environmental conditions which alter the functions of the body structures. These structural changes are the fore-runners of the lowered resistance, which must exist to make the body susceptible.

What, then, is lowered resistance? Lowered resistance implies an imbalance of, or obstruction to, the vital fluids and forces of the body. These fluids and forces are the blood and lymph streams and the nervous energy. It is through these fluids and forces that Nature protects the body, by means of the products of the body's 'auto-protective mechanism'. These products are carried in the blood and lymph streams, and their activity is directed by the nervous system.

Nature has endowed the body with vital-chemical substances or properties, manufactured by various cells and glands, and with vital-physical organisms, which are carried by fluids and directed by inherent forces. These vital-chemical substances and vital-physical organisms ensure that the fictive infectious organisms are destroyed and their toxic products neutralise it. The body is thus immunised from infections.

The cause of this imbalance of, or obstruction to, these vital fluids and forces is structural in Nature and is due to the environmental, or extrinsic, conditions above mentioned. The tissues of the body readily respond to environmental changes, and if the changes are too sudden, or of too great violence, the soft tissues do not then fully react to these environmental influences or forces and remain in a state of contraction or even contracture.'

Comstock, 1920

References

Andrewes, C. (1970) *Viruses and Cancer*. Weidenfeld and Nicolson, London.

Baxter, M. (1990) What is health? In *Health and Lifestyles*. Tavistock-Routledge, London.

Becker, K. (1949) Osteopathy and 'eubrotic medicine'. *The Journal of the American Osteopathic Association*, 49(1) 15.

Bortoft, H. (1998) Counterfeit and authentic wholes: finding a means for dwelling in nature. In *Goethe's Way of Science: A Phenomenology of Nature*. Eds D. Seamon and A. Zajonc, Chapter 12. State University of New York Press, New York.

Brown, D. (1992) It all started in Kansas. *Washington Post Weekly Edition*. 9(21) March 23–30.

Calnan, M. (1987) *Health and Illness – The Lay Perspective*. Routledge, London.

Cassell, E.J. (1976) *The Healer's Art: A New Approach to the Doctor–Patient Relationship* (pp. 77–94) Lippincott, New York.

Comstock, A. (1920) Osteopathic therapeutics in infectious diseases. *The Journal of the American Osteopathic Association*, 20(2) pp. 111–13.

Conrad, P. (1985) The meaning of medications: another look at compliance. *Social Science and Medicine*, 20(1) p. 29–37.

Corti, Count (1931) *A History of Smoking*. Translated by Paul England. Bracken Books, London.

Coward, R. (1990) *The Whole Truth: The Myth of Alternative Health*. Faber and Faber, London.

Curtis-Lake, J. (1998) *Development. A Holographic Experience*. Unpublished work. Head of Children's Clinic, Personal communication, The British School of Osteopathy, London.

Dally, A. (1996) Anomalies and mysteries in the 'war on drugs'. In *Drugs and Narcotics in History*, eds R. Porter and M. Teich, pp. 199–215. Cambridge University Press, Cambridge.

Davis, P. (1999) *Catching Cold: 1918's Forgotten Tragedy and the Scientific Hunt for the Virus that Caused it*. Michael Joseph, London.

Department of Health, UK (1991) *The Patient's Charter*. HMSO, London.

Donaldson, R.J. and Donaldson, L.J. (1993) *Essential Public Health Medicine*. Kluwer, London.

Dubos, R. (1979) *Mirage of Health*. Harper Colophon, New York.

Eisenberg, L. (1977) Disease and illness: distinctions between professional and popular ideas of sickness. *Culture, Medicine and Psychiatry*, 1, 9–23.

Fabrega, H. (1975) The need for an ethnomedical science. *Science*, 189, 969–75.

Frost, H.P. (1919) Biological philosophy. *The Journal of the American Osteopathic Association*, 18(2) 78–80.

Geison, G.L. (1995) *The Private Science of Louis Pasteur*. Princeton University Press, Princeton, NJ.

Goodfield, J. (1975) *The Siege of Cancer*. Random House, New York.

Gore, I., Hirst, A.E. and Koseki, Y. (1959) Comparison of aortic atherosclerosis in the United States, Japan and Guatemala. *American Journal of Clinical Nutrition*, 7, 50–4.

Haynes, R.B., Taylor, D.W. and Sackett, D.L. (eds) (1979) *Compliance in Health Care*. Johns Hopkins University Press, Baltimore.

Helman, C.G. (1978) 'Feed a cold, starve a fever' – Folk models of infection in an English suburban community, and their relation to medical treatment. *Culture, Medicine and Psychiatry*, 2, 107–37.

Helman, C. (1991) *Body Myths*. Chatto and Windus, London.

Hildreth, A.G. (1942) *The Lengthening Shadow of Dr Andrew Taylor Still*. Second edition. Published privately by Mrs A.G. Hildreth and Mrs A.E. Van Vleck.

Hughes, C.C. (1968) Ethnomedicine. *International Encyclopaedia of Social Sciences*, Vol. 10, pp. 87–93. Free Press/Macmillan, New York.

Humphrys, J. (1999) *Devil's Advocate*. Hutchinson, London.

Inglis, B. (1981) *The Diseases of Civilisation*. Hodder and Stoughton, London.

Jones, L. (1994) *The Context of Health and Health Work*. Macmillan, London.

Koestler, A. (1989a) *The Sleepwalkers*, Arkana/Penguin Books, London.

Koestler, A. (1989b) The holon. In *The Ghost in the Machine*. Arkana/Penguin Books, London.

Korr, I.M. (1948) The emerging concept of the osteopathic lesion. *The Journal of the American Osteopathic Association*, 48(3) pp. 127–38.

Le Fanu, J. (1999) *The Rise and Fall of Modern Medicine*. Little, Brown and Company, London.

Lever, A. (1977) Medicine under challenge. *The Lancet*, I, 353–5.

MacDonald, T. (1994) Osteopathy as health promotion: a semantic analysis. *British Osteopathic Journal*, XIV, 30–2.

MacDonald, T. (1998) *Rethinking Health Promotion*. Routledge, London.

McConnell, C.P. (1919) Dr McConnell's discussions. *The Journal of the American Osteopathic Association*, 19(6) 351–6.

McIntyre, R.V. (1991) On the germ theory of disease. Editorial. *Journal of Oklahoma State Medical Association*, 84 October 495–6.

McNeill, W.H. (1976) *Plagues and People*. Anchor Press/Doubleday, Garden City, NJ.

McKeown, T. (1976) *The Role of Medicine*. Nuffield Provincial Hospital Trust, London.

McKeown, T. (1983) A basis for health strategies. A classification of disease. *British Medical Journal*, 287, 594–6.

McKeown, T. (1989) The road to health. *World Health Forum*, 10, 408–416.

Manning, A. (1996) The rise and fall of infectious diseases. *USA Today*, May 20.

Morgan, M. (1991) The doctor–patient relationship. In *Sociology as Applied to Medicine* (ed. G. Scambler) third edition pp. 47–64. Baillière Tindall, London.

Muldoon, M.F., Manuck, S.B., and Matthews, K.A. (1990) Lowering cholesterol concentrations and mortality: a quantitative review of primary prevention trials. *British Medical Journal*, 301, 309–14.

Navarro, V. (1975) The industrialization of fetishism: A critique of Ivan Illich. *International Journal of Health Services*, 5, 351–71.

The *Observer* (1988) *In Sickness and in Health*. 5 July, p. 17.

Parsons, T. (1951) *The Social System*. Free Press, Glencoe.

Payer, L. (1989) *Medicine and Culture*. Victor Gollancz, London.

Peterson, B. (1980) Time capsule. A little survey on flu. *The DO*, January pp. 31–6.

Proby, J.C. (1939) *Essay on the Relation of Micro-organisms to Disease*. Printed by the author, Oxford.

Ravnskov, U. (1992) Cholesterol lowering trials in coronary heart disease: frequency of citation and outcome. *British Medical Journal*, 305, 15–19.

Resch, J.A., Okabe, N. and Kimoto, K. (1969) Cerebral atherosclerosis. *Geriatrics*, November, 111–32.

Revil, J. (1998) A year on and nothing has changed, Minister. *Evening Standard*. West End Final, Monday 3 August, pp. 8–9.

Riley, G.W. (1919) Osteopathic success in the treatment of influenza and pneumonia. *The Journal of the American Osteopathic Association*, 19(12) 565–9.

Rosch, P.J. (1983) Stress, cholesterol and coronary heart disease. *The Lancet*, 2, 851–2.

Rosch, P.J. (1993) Ridiculous risk factors and heart attacks: diet-cholesterol dogma versus stress. *Stress Medicine*, Editorial 9, 203–205.

Schwartz, J. (1996) Young smokers at risk. 5 million smokers expected to die of illness related to tobacco. *Washington Post*, 8 November.

Smith, T. (1982) Chestnuts, fats and fibre. *British Medical Journal*, 285, 117.

Still. A.T. (1902) *Philosophy and Mechanical Principles of Osteopathy*. Hudson-Kimberly Publishing Company Kansas City, MI.

Tesh, S. (1981) Disease causality and politics. *Journal of Health Politics, Policy and Law*, Fall, 6(3) 369–90.

Tesh, S. (1982) Political ideology and public health in the nineteenth century. *International Journal of Health Services*, 12, 321–342.

Totman, R. *et al.* (1977) Cognitive dissonance, stress, and virus-induced common colds. *Journal of Psychosomatic Research*, 55–63.

Toulmin, S. (1990) *Cosmopolis: The Hidden Agenda of Modernity*. The University of Chicago Press, Chicago.

Turshen, M. (1989) *The Politics of Health*. Rutgers University Press, New Brunswick, NJ.

Waldron, H.A. (1978) *The Medical Role in Environmental Health*. Oxford University Press. Oxford.

Willis, A.T. (1984) Anaerobic bacterial disease now and then: where do we go from here? *Reviews of Infectious Disease*. 6 (supplement 1) March–April, S293–9.

World Health Organization, Health Education Unit. (1993) *Lifestyles and Health. Health and Wellbeing: A Reader*. The Open University Press, Milton Keynes.

The World Health Report (1996) *Fighting Disease, Fostering Development*. World Health Organization, Geneva (E-mail: *publications@who.ch*).

Yankauer, A. (1994) Job Lewis Smith and the germ theory of disease. *Pediatrics*, 93(6) 936–8.

Further reading

Barker, D.J.P. (1992) *Fetal and infant origins of adult disease. British Medical Journal*.

Gadamer, H.-G. (1996) *The Enigma of Health*. Polity Press (in association with Blackwell Press), Oxford.

Hubbard, R. and Wald, E. (1999) *Exploding the Gene Myth*. Beacon Press, Boston.

Sontag, S. (1991) *Illness as Metaphor/Aids and its Metaphors*. Penguin Books, London.

Trowbridge, B. (1996) *The Hidden Meaning of Illness: Disease as a Symbol and Metaphor*. A.R.E.

CHAPTER 9

Pathology

'The functional abnormalities and the structural alterations which make up the signs, symptoms, and lesions of disease involve the expression of no new functional capacities which the normal body does not possess. These may be diminished or exalted; they may be perverted or abolished; or the cells may now and then revert to forms and to phases of activity which the body has long since outgrown or largely suppressed in its slow adaptation to conditions of life which now constitute the normal. But the body in disease manifests no new functions, develops no new forms of energy, reveals no new capacities.'

Francis Delafield and T. Mitchell Predden

Through the history of osteopathy it has been said that the osteopathic concept of disease has been obscured by a misconception of the use of the words 'manipulation' and 'osteopathy' and the presumption that these words are synonymous. Osteopathy was developed by Andrew Taylor Still as a philosophy, 'to give the world a *start* in a *philosophy* that may be a *guide* for the future' (my italics). It is important to realise that he wrote the words 'start', 'philosophy' and 'guide'.

Still was aware that the types of treatments used in his time killed more than they cured in the name of science and were more than useless. Even a century later we are aware of the uselessness of drugs, like antibiotics, that have been prescribed but are known not to work. Many drugs have a psychosocial and placebo effect, rightly or wrongly, and at best they are harmful if used in the long term.

With all the advances in medicine we are still today aware of the fact that the pathogenic agent is not the disease. A pathogen is not a complete disease entity inside or outside of the body. It may be a contributing factor or stimulus but it is not a disease. We cannot therefore make the simple equation 'pathogen = disease': this is far from the truth. The *Oxford English Dictionary* defines disease as 'a condition of the body, or of some part or organ of the body, in which its functions are disturbed or deranged; a morbid physical condition; a departure from the state of health, especially when caused by structural change'. Disease must involve the body.

So, the new equation can look something like, 'pathogen + organism = disease', which is more realistic. But again just mixing the two factors does not lead to a state of disease. Claude Bernard tried to convince the medical profession of the importance of the homeostatic mechanism of the body in infections and the prevention of disease. Pathogens obeyed the rules of the 'seeds in the New Testament parable of the sower: some falling by the wayside, some on stony ground, some among the thorns, and only those falling on fertile ground taking root, and bringing forth fruit'. There is the classic demonstration by Max von Pettenkofer with regard to Koch's bacillus as the cause of cholera: Pettenkofer swallowed a fatal amount of the bacilli yet suffered nothing more than mild diarrhoea with samples of the bacilli in his stools. Even Pasteur admitted on his deathbed that Bernard was correct saying 'the germ is nothing; the terrain is everything' (cited in Inglis, 1981). The type of bacteria and virus and its virulence are no real measure of the effect it may have on the organism. The disease is the expression of the receptor organism and not of the pathogen. Therefore it may be more realistic to have the final equation as 'pathogen + vulnerable organism = disease' and the real study of the disease is the organism or man.

As the osteopathic concept reminds us, to eradicate the micro-organism is not to eliminate disease. Further to this concept is the misunderstanding that to use manipulative therapy is the only way to cure disease. Due to the role of the myofascioskeletal system in health and disease, the use of osteopathic manipulative techniques has been called the single most powerful therapeutic modality in the reduction of the total somatic contribution to the disease process, but it is *not* the totality of the osteopathic concept. As mentioned earlier, Still said 'I do not instruct the student to punch or pull a certain bone, nerve or muscle for a certain disease, but by knowledge of the normal and abnormal, I hope to give a specific knowledge for all diseases'.

Osteopathic pathology

What is osteopathic pathology? This is the study and appreciation of the role of facilitation in the origin and maintenance of ill health and injury. To the medical practitioner, simple gastritis is a vastly different condition from a gastric ulcer. Within the mind of the osteopath, these conditions differ in degree, not in kind. The same organ, the same blood supply, the same nerves are all involved in both conditions, therefore we treat these structures. Our dietetic treatment takes account of the differing activity of the stomach, but our manipulative treatment does not. We apply the same method to all organs. Our manipulative therapeutics are based on structure more than function (Tasker, 1925). Osteopathic pathology describes the structural communicative similarities of health, dysfunction and disease.

Over 75% of the body is represented by the myofascioskeletal system. If we are to believe that man is a unit and therefore functions as a unit then all areas of the body are interrelated, especially with the myofascioskeletal system. Historically medicine has tended to ignore the role of the myofascioskeletal system in health and disease. I.M. Korr referred to this system, with its neurological components, as the 'primary machinery of life' particularly from an anthropological aspect. It is only through this system that we can express ourselves and act upon our environment, and structurally it binds us together. The act of motion at a macro and micro level is life itself. The nervous system is the drive behind the actions and the circulatory system is the nutritional exchange mechanism of the myofascioskeletal system. It acts on the interpretation of information it receives from the internal and external environments.

The demand for nutrition and the creation of waste is greatest from the myofascioskeletal system. So, from a structure–function relationship, not to mention a body–economy relationship, the myofascioskeletal system is of the utmost importance for survival. From a biological aspect it would seem that all other structures, especially the viscera, are secondary. Of primary importance is the role of the fascia. The fascia supports organs; myotendinous units could not function properly without the attachment to fascia and its connective tissue derivatives.

The osteopathic lesion

The osteopathic lesion in the historical and clinical contexts is paramount for the understanding and application of osteopathic medicine. At worst it is a restrictive theoretical definition of joint-somatic dysfunction; at best it is part of the osteopathic consciousness. Certainly the term osteopathic lesion is not descriptive, but neither are such terms as Parkinson's disease and Cushing's disease (Northup, 1972). Taking this into consideration the use, or thought, of the words osteopathic lesion should represent an understanding of total body unity with a consideration of the role of the dysfunctioning neuromusculoskeletal system at all times. Even if it is symbolic this in itself will represent a unity of thought preventing the reductionism or poly-reductionism of the body by the osteopathic student and practitioner. It must be understood that the concept of the osteopathic lesion is in the context of the patient's health. Correcting a 'lesion' will rarely alter the course of the patient's problem. The lesion or greater lesion complex must be in relation to the health of the patient; it is the musculoskeletal consideration of the total ill health presentation. A consideration of the myofascioskeletal system and of its contributing lesions to the health and illness of the patient is the osteopathic contribution to medicine. A partial lesion, i.e. a joint disturbance, is one thing; an osteopathic lesion, i.e. with accompanying vasomotor and trophic changes, is a continuation of the same phenomenon.

The *Oxford English Dictionary* defines a lesion as any morbid change in the exercise of functions or the texture of organs. Therefore, an osteopathic lesion, or somatic dysfunction, may be defined as an area of impaired function of related components of the musculoskeletal system (muscle, bone, fascia, ligament), and its associated or related parts in the vascular, lymphatic, and nervous systems (Rumney, 1975).

Denslow (1947) suggests the combination of chronic segmental facilitation and the osteopathic lesion come together as the following:

'(An) osteopathic lesion represents a facilitated segment of the spinal cord maintained in that state by impulses of endogenous origin entering the corresponding dorsal root. All structures receiving efferent nerve fibres from that segment are, therefore, potentially exposed to excessive excitation or inhibition.'

Haycock (1955) gives one of the best-understood descriptions of the osteopathic lesion as follows.

'The increased cortical activity resulting from mental and emotional strain, by setting up an increased flow of impulses in the descending spinal tracts, may cause increased tone in the paravertebral and other somatic structures – especially those related to lesioned segments – and thus take part in lesion production. It is clear from the foregoing that the lesion is not merely a positional disturbance of vertebrae to be adjusted by an appropriate mechanical procedure. It is an entity, produced and maintained in being by a wide variety of factors – paravertebral stress; hyperirritability of spinal cord cells, viscera and other tissues; and mental and emotional strain – all of which the practitioner must take into consideration when planning the campaign of treatment.'

He goes on to say, first, there are many factors, from every part of the body, and from its environment, which may contribute to the setting up of an osteopathic lesion. Second, the lesion may result in facilitation of related neural segments; all operative factors may react detrimentally on each other, even after the original source of irritation has been eliminated. The osteopathic concept of unity of disease considers of paramount importance the osteopathic spinal lesion in the development of disease processes and considers the osteopathic adjustive techniques vital in the disintegration of the disease-producing pattern.

Simply put, an osteopathic lesion may be described as a biophysical process that takes place through and within the myofascioskeletal system producing changes in articular, periarticular and visceral form and function (Fig. 14).

The causes and consequences of osteopathic lesions are important in two basic ways.

(1) Structural change and therefore functional adaptation of accessory movements are the results of injury, illness, and emotion. The change perpetuates a form–function cycle increasing the demand on the body economy.
(2) Upsets in the myofascioskeletal system can mimic the signs and symptoms of organs and other systems. By ignoring the myofascioskeletal system a

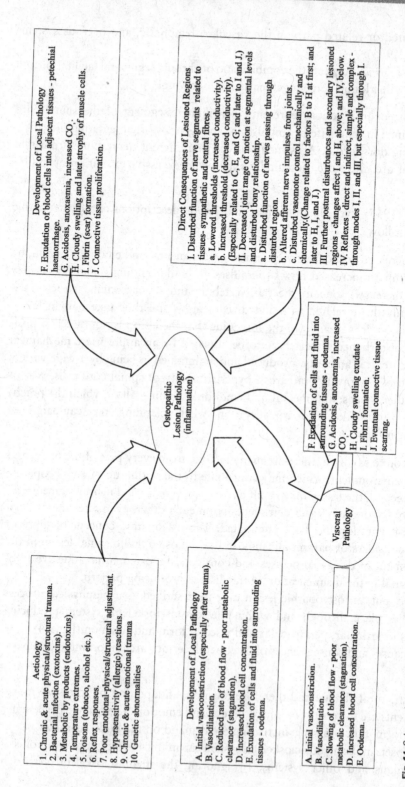

Aetiology
1. Chronic & acute physical/structural trauma.
2. Bacterial infection (exotoxins).
3. Metabolic by products (endotoxins).
4. Temperature extremes.
5. Poisons (tobacco, alcohol etc.).
6. Reflex responses.
7. Poor emotional–physical/structural adjustment.
8. Hypersensitivity (allergic) reactions.
9. Chronic & acute emotional trauma
10. Genetic abnormalities

Development of Local Pathology
A. Initial vasoconstriction (especially after trauma).
B. Vasodilatation.
C. Reduced rate of blood flow - poor metabolic clearance (stagnation).
D. Increased blood cell concentration.
E. Exudation of cells and fluid into surrounding tissues - oedema.

Development of Local Pathology
F. Exudation of blood cells into adjacent tissues - petechial haemorrhage.
G. Acidosis, anoxaemia, increased CO_2.
H. Cloudy swelling and later atrophy of muscle cells.
I. Fibrin (scar) formation.
J. Connective tissue proliferation.

Direct Consequences of Lesioned Regions
I. Disturbed function of nerve segments related to tissues - sympathetic and central fibres.
  a. Lowered thresholds (increased conductivity).
  b. Increased threshold (decreased conductivity). (Especially related to C, E, and G; and later to I and J.)
II. Decreased joint range of motion at segmental levels and disturbed bony relationship.
  a. Disturbed function of nerves passing through disturbed region.
  b. Altered afferent nerve impulses from joints.
  c. Disturbed vasomotor control mechanically and chemically.(Change related to factors B to H at first; and later to H, I, and J.)
III. Further postural disturbances and secondary lesioned regions - changes affect I and II, above; and IV, below.
IV. Reflexes - direct and indirect, simple and complex - through modes I, II, and III, but especially through I.

Osteopathic Lesion Pathology (inflammation)

Visceral Pathology

Development of Local Pathology
F. Exudation of cells and fluid into surrounding tissues - oedema.
G. Acidosis, anoxaemia, increased CO_2.
H. Cloudy swelling exudate
I. Fibrin formation.
J. Eventual connective tissue scarring.

A. Initial vasoconstriction.
B. Vasodilatation.
C. Slowing of blood flow - poor metabolic clearance (stagnation).
D. Increased blood cell concentration.
E. Oedema.

Fig. 14 Schematic representation of the intervertebral osteopathic lesion (adapted from the original work of Paul van. B. Allen, D.O. *Journal of the American Osteopathic Association,* Oct. 1935.)

number of medical tests are only recording the reflection of this system through organs. This is therefore important in differential diagnosis.

The osteopathic lesion is not a 'bone out of place' or a form of articular derangement, it is a functional disturbance that includes, to a greater or lesser degree, the myofascioskeletal system. This functional disturbance results in a resistance to motion and a decreased range of motion, no matter what the origin. The handling of vertebral bones (or any bones), in a manipulative procedure, should be purely a lever for application of manual forces.

Are the osteopathic lesions caused by organ disease or do numerous osteopathic lesions cause organ disease? Is the environment the cause of the osteopathic lesion and does it go on to precipitate an organ disease? If we are true to our system then we are looking at a dynamic model in a time frame. There cannot be any true isolated myofascioskeletal osteopathic lesion, just as there cannot be any true isolated kidney disease.

The characteristics of the osteopathic lesion classified by Pearson (1934) are:

- an improper venous–arterial balance producing a *relative acidosis*
- the lowered alkalinity becomes a chemical stimulation to the colloidal structures to take on additional water, so producing *oedema*
- oedema, being characterised by an increase in the water content within definite cellular limitations, results in an *increase in pressure*
- pressure from the oedema disturbs the capillary function and permits exudation of the capillary content into the tissue spaces, producing *haemorrhage*
- the exudation of this material, foreign to the tissue, sets up a protective mechanism, eventually demonstrating itself in *fibrosis*.

Pain in tissue is usually attributed to only stimulation of the nociceptors, just as we seem to think inflammation, disease and pain are the same (Leadbetter, 1993). Neither is true. Pain can occur through fear without direct nociceptor stimulation, diseases can progress without pain, and inflammation is not always present in painful presentations. Studies have shown that more than 30% of asymptomatic individuals have structural abnormalities, such as herniated discs resulting in impingement of neural structures and spinal stenosis (Turk and Okifuji, 1999; Jensen *et al.*, 1994 and Boden *et al.*, 1990).

The structures supplied by the nerves passing through the area of osteopathic pathology will have in themselves all the above phases of abnormality (providing the character of the tissue permits these changes) and in addition will show:

- lowered tensile strength
- lowered leukocytic activity
- lowered proteolytic activity
- degenerative changes
- round cell infiltration.

The syndrome of tissue changes characterises the areas of improper body mechanics, this results from the quantitative and qualitative changes in the rhythmical rate of flow of nerve impulses and axoplasmic flow through the factors of:

- relative acidosis
- pressure
- tissue tension
- retained metabolic products.

If the osteopathic lesion is permitted to exert its influence, both health and normal processes of recovery will be impaired. The osteopathic lesion is a potent factor in the alteration of the normal sympathetic–parasympathetic balance, the yardstick upon which all body processes are measured osteopathically.

Chronic segmental facilitation

The neuronal areas or motor neurone 'pools', within the spinal cord (segments), are related to somatic dysfunction and maintain a state of chronic facilitation (Denslow, 1944; Denslow et al. 1947). These areas are hyperirritable and will overreact to nerve impulses coming into the area from any part of the body. The areas of input include proprioceptors, cutaneous receptors, and every other sensory receptor including cerebral areas. Therefore the muscles innervated by these areas are maintained in a state of hypertonia. This is our alarm response that includes chronic *increases* in

- protein catabolism
- peripheral blood vessel dilatation
- lactic acid, ischaemia and *decreases* in
- metabolic clearance rate
- gut peristalsis and
- vascularity of lung tissue.

If the exposure to physical, environmental, nutritional, and emotional stimuli (irritation) continues, the sympathetic responses become exaggerated and prolonged. The spinal cord segments respond as though they are continually switched 'on'. This is a state of 'physiological alarm'. In this state, as we have seen above, there is disturbance of function – dysfunction (abnormal activity) in all organs and tissues in the entire body and nervous system, but the disturbance is greater in those target tissues and organs receiving information from those particular facilitated segments. Amplification of the problem becomes cyclic as a result of the person's lifestyle in relation to the above factors of poor nutrition, anxiety, physical and environmental stressors. The overall state of the sympathetic portion of the autonomic nervous system is known as *sympathiconia*.

Concepts in pathology

Over 50 years ago Korr (1948) brought together three basic concepts. Significantly these were developed on three different continents, thousands of miles apart. These concepts were (1) the osteopathic, (2) that of referred pain and associated phenomena and (3) the state of disease developed by A.D. Speransky from Leningrad.

Osteopathic concepts

The following are some of the most important osteopathic concepts.

- The body is a unit; all its parts function in the context of the entire organism.
- Disease is a reaction of the organism as a whole. Abnormal structure or function in one part exerts an abnormal influence on other parts and, therefore, on the total body economy.
- The organism has the inherent capacity to defend itself, to repair, and to resist serious upsets in equilibria.
- The nervous system plays a dominant organising role in the disease processes.
- There is a somatic component to every disease that is not only a manifestation of the disease, but an important contributing factor.
- Appropriate treatment of the somatic component has important therapeutic value in that it leads to improvement in the other components.

Referred pain and associated phenomena

Referred pain

An example of referred pain is where the pain of visceral disease is not felt in the organ itself, but is referred to the soma, that is, the skin, muscles, joints etc. Generally the somatic structures do not lie over or near the diseased viscera, they may be quite some distance away. The common denominator between the diseased viscera and the somatic site of referral is that they share a common segmental relationship, within the spinal cord. In addition it must be remembered that the segments are only educational not biological boundaries. Taking this into consideration it should always be appreciated that pre-existing areas of spinal cord excitability can amplify the primary pathways of referred pain spreading the disturbance over many spinal cord segments via ascending and descending tracts of low thresholds. This leads to a far more complex clinical picture as other somatic structures, previously unknown to the patient, reach a certain level of consciousness.

Examples of a primary pathway include angina pectoris, beginning in the myocardium and being referred to the chest wall, the back, shoulder, face, and arm; renal colic, with its flank pain covering an area from the low back to the groin. Sites of somatic presentation will be in the dermatome and/or myotome. Again they may present from different spinal cord or nerve root segments. Here it is important to recognise the difference between anatomical pathways and the more confused picture of clinical presentations. On the other hand, an area of hypertonia containing an upper rib or ribs on the left may irritate a spinal cord segment giving a clinical presentation in the true sense of the word *angina*, pain in the chest. Commonly this would lead to immediate cardiac investigations with the phenomena reflected in the disturbed function of the heart.

With a pathway similar to that of the reflex arc, at a segmental level, the route for a referred pain complex involves dorsal root (afferent) fibres with impulses converging from all tissues (somatic and visceral). Afferent impulses include touch, pressure, and stretch and tension receptors in muscles and tendons. The interneurons, located in the lateral horn cells of the spinal cord, mediate all impulses. Some will continue on into the anterior root (efferent), others will continue on into spinothalamic fibres to higher centres. The efferent impulses, out of the spinal cord, include motor neurons to skeletal muscles, sympathetic postganglionic neurons to blood vessels of the skin and muscle, to sweat glands and pilomotor muscles of the skin and the sympathetic postganglionic neurons to visceral smooth muscle, blood vessels and glands.

Hyperalgesia

The tenderness of somatic structures may be segmentally related to the diseased viscus. This may present as any of the following.

- Skin tenderness in the form of an oversensitivity due to pressure in the dermatome related to the common spinal cord segment of the diseased viscus.
- Muscular tone change, tenderness and oversensitivity to deep pressure.
- Tenderness of bony prominences, including the spinous processes. Over the years many physicians have placed great emphasis on tender spinous processes. As far back as 1912, Mackenzie found the following common findings: disease of the heart presented with tender spinous processes between T1 to T4; the stomach, T4 to T8; the liver, T8 to T11 and rectum and uterus, L5 to S2.

Motor phenomena

This is the spasm, sustained contraction, and rigidity in muscles segmentally related to the pathological organ, initially described by Mackenzie (1893).

With this pathway in view Mackenzie postulated the theory of the irritable focus. The irritable focus hypothesis states that irritation (stimulation) along an afferent path, from any viscera, excites many of the nerve cells in the same segment producing a state of hyperirritability. In due course all tissues and organs innervated from that level would be involved in the visceral pathology. In time this hypothesis was developed further and is now known as *facilitation*.

This irritation pathway is not only restricted to viscera. Any irritation of deep lying somatic structures leads to a triad of responses with the osteopathic lesion complex; these are:

- cutaneous hyperalgesia
- muscular hyperalgesia, and
- muscular rigidity.

From this we can see that the irritation or pathology of tissues or organs can initiate dysfunction in other tissues or organs local and/or distant. The complex patterns and development of health and the disruptive patterns of ill health are organised by the nervous system and especially by the spinal cord. Spinal cord reflex paths are complex and continual processes that are central to the principle of homeostasis.

These reflex pathways lead to irritation of secondary structures. Structural changes that develop in these secondary structures themselves become a source of irritation leading to an amplification and further establishment of the cycle of irritation. The intensity, duration and character of the irritation is organised by the spinal cord, not by the primary or secondary sources of irritation. Since this pattern is eventually cyclic, clinically we should be able to reduce the irritation contributed by the most accessible component of the osteopathic lesion complex – the somatic component. It is well documented that the pain of visceral disease can be relieved by local anaesthesia of the skin and somatic tissues where referred pain is presenting. In addition it has been shown that the pain relief outlasted the duration of the local anaesthesia (Weiss and Davis, 1928).

Sustained muscular contractions, which are part of the somatic component, due to referred mechanisms can be identified by palpation. Relaxation of these muscles relieves pain and reduces associated autonomic disturbances (Wolff and Hardy, 1947). The pain of myocardial infarction can be completely and immediately relieved by the infiltration of myofascial structures within the reference zone with dilute procaine hydrochloride. Those myofascial structures near the skin surface can be sprayed with ethyl chloride. The zone of reference includes the brain and spinal cord. Changes in these areas include an autonomic upset in the control of circulation. Aberrant neural impulses of high intensity produce continual vasoconstriction with partial ischaemia in localised areas in the brain, spinal cord or peripheral nerves.

Speransky's theories

In 1944 there was a translation and publication of Speransky's *A Basis for the Theory of Medicine*. Speransky and co-workers from what was then Leningrad unknowingly supported the osteopathic lesion theory. In the preface to the book Speransky wrote

'What is wrong then? (with medicine). An effort to answer this question leads inevitably to the conclusion that medicine has gradually and almost imperceptibly ceased to treat its subject matter in a synthetic form, substituting instead a comprehensive and often profound analysis of details ... Hence the question remains one of the search for the essential principles of union ... For a number of years past with my collaborators, I have been engaged in the genesis of various pathological processes ... The appraisal of these data led so often to a conflict with many existing views that very soon we perceived the necessity of giving up the study of isolated questions. By force of circumstances we were compelled to pass to a revision of the conceptions of the basic processes of general pathology, from the point of view of the nervous component in their origin and history.'

Summaries of the key points in Speransky's theories are as follows.

- The nervous system participates in every disease and plays a dominant role in the organisation of pathological processes.
- Chronic irritation, inflammation or any pathological change of muscles, skin, bone, viscera or nervous tissue will begin a process within the nervous system which leads to functional and organic changes. These changes are known as *neurodystrophy*. Once neurodystrophy begins it forms a cycle of irritation. From this point on the primary cause is no longer needed to maintain the cycle. Neurodystrophy will continue long after the primary disease or injury has gone.
- Neurodystrophy presents as pathological and trophic changes in tissues and organs, initially in the same segment of the primary pathology, then to related segments. Eventually the whole body is affected.
- The nature and expression of the neurodystrophy are chemically, physically and biologically *independent*. Biological agents, which include toxins, bacteria, viruses, etc., irritate the nervous system in the same way as the chemical and physical agents. These three agents simply set an independent process into action.
- The major role of the nervous system seems to be a much slower process than simple impulses for muscular action. This slow function is the movement of nutrients along the nerve axon (including impulses) known as the *trophic process*.
- Changes in the character of the nerves can be non-symptomatic for long

periods of time. The original signs and symptoms of the primary injury or pathology may have disappeared, but the effect of the primary process is still microscopically and functionally apparent as *neural plasticity*.

Haycock (1955) continues,

'we should now visualise the lesioned spine in terms of facilitation of the related neural segments. The cells of these segments are keyed-up and will discharge impulses more readily to the spinal cord tissues, the cerebral cortex, the spinal joint and paravertebral tissues and to related viscera and other tissues. Mental and emotional impulses travel from the cerebral cortex, along the descending spinal tracts, and continue outwards along the facilitated segments to related visceral and somatic tissues. Primary visceral, somatic and other tissue irritability will similarly cause an abnormal flow of impulses to the spinal cord, which will be relayed by the spinothalamic tracts to consciousness, and will touch off efferent neurones at the facilitated segments. Thus, no matter whether the irritation begins, as it probably most frequently does, as a result of a trauma or a postural disturbance at the spine, or at a viscus which has been abused or is assailed by disease, or at a hyperactive cerebral cortex, there is inaugurated a chain of actions and reactions, all detrimental to cellular welfare, and the organism's capacity to repair and defend itself. Furthermore, it is clear from reliable work from many sources that once this chain of action and reaction is established, it will continue, through the medium of the nervous system, long after the original insult has been eliminated. *The fact that the spinal cord is the central medium through which this disease-producing mechanism functions, and that the paravertebral tissues and spinal joint structures, which take part in it, are easily accessible, have resulted in the spinal structures being selected, by both osteopathic and non-osteopathic workers, as the site at which attempts should be made to break the vicious cycle* [my italics].'

Clinical presentations of osteopathic lesions

The following symptoms are observable where there is a lesion.

- in the zone of lesioned areas there is reduced alkalinity
- thickening and swelling of ligaments and muscle attachment points occur with associated thickening of periosteum
- thickening and swelling of synovial membranes of the associated lesioned articulation, accompanied by minor petechial haemorrhages resulting from diapedesis
- poor absorption of local fluids associated with thickening (hyperplasia) of connective tissue.
- local reduction in elasticity of connective and atrophy of cells

- muscle tissue, initially, appears normally contracted while sustained contraction by aberrant nerve impulses leads to poor vasomotor (sympathetic) control and resultant haemorrhaging into surrounding muscle (The haemorrhaging, by diapedesis, into surrounding tissue leads to replacement of the leaking cells resulting in fibrosis.)
- fascia and subcutaneous tissue, deep and superficial, haemorrhages by diapedesis in the lesioned area with reduced alkalinity.

Therefore the basic response of tissues in the area or associated with a lesion is the following:

- reduced alkalinity
- poor vasomotor (sympathetic) control
- leading to haemorrhaging by diapedesis
- oedema due to poor drainage, and
- local increase in metabolites.

Nerves associated with the lesioned area will undergo initial adaptive changes that with time may become pathological with the tissue they supply. Normal nerve function is sensitive to $_pH$ (potenz hydrogen) changes resulting from alterations in carbon dioxide and oxygen tension.

Changes leading to these disturbances usually begin with the following:

- oedema
- poor metabolite clearance
- impaired circulation
- reduced gaseous exchange and
- the reduction in pH.

The thicker the myelin sheaths the longer it takes to cause any disturbance. The non-myelinated nerve fibres, i.e. the sympathetic nerves, that supply blood vessels are usually the first to be disturbed.

These nerve changes include:

- a granular or hyaline appearance of the myelin sheath
- minor oedema of the nerve fibre and sheath
- an increasing sensitivity to the decreasing alkalinity

Lesioned areas and vasomotor disturbance

At no point is the following a 'hard-wire' relationship between cause and effect. Lesioned bone articulation levels are given as the most probable physical source area as part of the disturbance. From the view of any particular organ its source of supply, neural and vascular, is from many segments and areas that overlap and merge into zones. These levels are general guides from a combination of common clinical findings and anatomical variations. During this section various concepts will be re-introduced to allow the reader a more coherent visualisation of the dysfunction concerned. Bony levels are landmarks or beacons of reference for the osteopath; they are not the absolute cause or even contribution to the diseased state. These levels should never be taken out of context with the wider health or disease picture of the patient and all other contributing factors, stress, nutrition, drugs etc.

Occipito-atlantal lesions

Lesions result in pressure and reflex pattern disturbance. These disturbances affect arterial flow to the spinal cord and meninges, medulla, pons, cerebellum and part of the cerebrum. Due to its effect on these regions it has a root disturbance potential for all the cranial nerves. The disturbance of the sympathetic chain reaches as high as the ganglion of Ribes and as low as the Stellate ganglion. Facilitation of this range will increase the tone of blood vessels to the brain, face, throat, salivary glands and secretory membranes. The vertebral plexus vasomotor fibres to the vertebral artery and the muscles it supplies at this level, in the neck and throat, can show signs of disturbance. The author has decided to label this suboccipital area the 'gateway to the head'.

Axis lesions

Osteopathic practitioners generally regard the occipito-atlantal and axial lesions as one unit due to their close anatomical and functional relationship. Disturbances of this level contribute to vasomotor upset of the SCG, its communicating branches and cranial nerves nine, ten and twelve.

Third and fourth cervical lesions

Again these would follow some of the patterns of axis lesions including circulatory disturbance to the spinal cord and the trapezius, sternocleidomastoid and diaphragm muscles. Between the axis and third cervical vertebrae is the greatest level of potential disturbance of the SCG. When we consider that Littlejohn regarded the SCG as the major vasomotor connection between the head and body, the importance of this level cannot be underestimated.

Fifth and sixth cervical lesions

Vasomotor disturbance due to lesions of the fifth cervical vertebrae contributes to arterial upset of the lateral spinal, muscular and spinal branches of the ascending cervical and vertebral arteries. Patterns of circulation disruption can affect the brain, cervical portion of the spinal cord and the muscles of the neck. Vasomotor fibres supply the brachial artery continuing into the arm, the internal mammary artery as the ansa subclavia and the MCG onto the thyroid gland and general throat region.

Seventh cervical lesions

Disturbed arterial supply due to seventh cervical lesions includes those affected by the fifth and sixth with the addition of the superior intercostal artery. Any disruption of the ansa subclavia will naturally affect the arm, mammary glands and chest wall. Poor supply by the inferior thyroid artery will affect the oesophagus, trachea, larynx, deep muscles of the neck and the phrenic nerve. This level also affects the conduction through the ICG to the heart through its cardiac branches.

First thoracic lesions

Impulses from the first thoracic impart vasomotor effects to the head, neck, arms, shoulders and integument. In the head the ciliary nerve, from the upper thoracic region, supplies vasomotor impulses to the circulation of the orbit of the eye. Lesions disturb the subclavian artery continuing on to the superior intercostal and the lateral spinal arteries. Of even more importance clinically is that thoracic lesions begin to affect the lungs through the stellate ganglion, and accelerate the heart indirectly through the cervical ganglia or directly through the cardiac plexus. In addition there is supply to the thoracic aorta, coronary and brachial vessels and splanchnics.

Second thoracic lesions

As with the first thoracic, the second thoracic supplies the head, neck and arms including the subclavian and brachial plexuses. These vasomotor fibres accompany the somatic nerves to the thorax and arms. Vasomotor fibres pass to the ears and nasal tract, e.g. hayfever, in the head, to the pulmonary vessels, and the heart (acceleration) through the coronary plexus, in the thorax. There can be found a connection between the vagus and the upper thoracic ganglia which go on to become the motor supply to the heart. It should be noted here that stimulation of the cervical sympathetic nerves leads to contraction of the retinal blood vessels and stimulation of the upper thoracic sympathetic nerves leads to dilatation of these vessels.

Third thoracic lesions

Vasomotor supply from this level leads to the head, face, arms, lungs, heart, back muscles, spinal cord (and coverings), and motor impulses supply the heart. With regards to the head the third thoracic is part of a cilio-spinal complex associated with the vascularity of the eye. The third thoracic is considered a key factor in the treatment and control of asthma, even pressure applied laterally to the spinous process over the paravertebral muscles will help lessen an attack. This level seems to have been considered a general nutrition centre for the entire body influencing the trophic supply concerned with circulation to the heart, oxygenation of the blood and assimilation of digested nutrients.

Fourth thoracic lesions

Lesions of the fourth thoracic can affect the thoracic aorta and its branches, the pericardial, bronchial, oesophageal and fourth intercostal. These will lead to oedema of the areas supplied due to vasomotor inhibition. The sympathetic cords at this level communicate with the cardiac, coronary and pulmonary plexuses, therefore disturbance can affect the heart, its vessels and the lungs. With regard to the heart the effect can be clinically registered as arrhythmia, palpitations and tachycardia.

Fifth thoracic lesions

The main organ supplied by the fifth is the stomach. At this level neural communication is to the artery of the fifth intercostal and its muscular and spinal arteries. The fifth has a lesser contribution to the acceleration of the heart. The arms, abdominal blood vessels, liver, gall bladder, stomach and portal vein receive their vasomotor supply from the sympathetic greater splanchnic via the coeliac plexus. The parasympathetic supply is via the vagus.

Sixth thoracic lesions

There seems to be a greater influence on the circulation of the liver and gall bladder (stones) with lesions of the sixth thoracic. The nerve supply at this level communicates with the azygi and lateral spinal veins, the sixth intercostal, its branches and the thoracic level of the aorta and its branches. As with the fifth thoracic the vasomotor supply is via the greater splanchnic through the coeliac to the same abdominal vessels and the vagus as the parasympathetic.

Seventh thoracic lesions

As with the sixth, the seventh sends fibres to the greater splanchnic continuing on to the oesophagus and aorta.

Eighth thoracic lesions

The eighth seems to have a broad and general supply to the abdominal blood vessels. This includes the alimentary tract, portal, renal, splenic and the more superficial vessels due to supply of the intercostal branches. Lesions at the eighth have been regarded as the centre for diseases of the above viscus.

Ninth thoracic lesions

Vascular vessels affected by a ninth thoracic lesion include the intercostal nerves and its spinal and muscular branches. Through the greater splanchnic disturbance continues on to the abdominal aorta, liver, spleen, stomach, small intestines, pancreas, suprarenal capsule, ovary, testicle and kidney.

Tenth thoracic lesions

The vascular disturbance resulting from tenth thoracic lesions will contribute to disturbances of its intercostal artery and branches, renal, ovarian, spermatic, coeliac plexus and its branches, splenic, gastric, hepatic, superior mesenteric and azygi veins.

Eleventh thoracic lesions

The eleventh thoracic supplies vasomotor impulses to the small intestine, caecum, kidneys, ureter, testes, epididymis, ovaries, fundus of the uterus and fallopian tubes. Lesions of the eighth can contribute to constipation and appendicitis and more general disorders of the intestines, kidneys, and pelvic contents.

Twelfth thoracic lesions

Vasomotor disturbances through the lesser splanchnic and coeliac plexus contribute to the intercostal and branches, renal, ovarian and spermatic, mesenteric and iliac vessels.

First lumbar lesions

Disturbances at the first lumbar level contribute to disturbances of the abdominal aorta and branches, inferior vena cava, mesenteric vessels, ovarian and spermatic vessels, viceral, haemorrhoidal, uterine and vaginal vessels. At a deeper level there can be disturbance of the lumbar artery supply to the spinal cord.

Second lumbar lesions

The vasomotor supply is to the femoral artery; through the hypogastric plexus it communicates with the bladder, vas deferens, round ligament, rectum, uterus, genitalia and lower intestinal tract. Disturbances in this area can contribute to bladder infections, haemorrhoids and period pain.

Third lumbar lesions

The region of the third lumbar communicates with the lower bowel, bladder, ureter, vas deferens, testicle and uterus. These vasomotor fibres travel from the aortic plexus on to the inferior vena cava while other fibres continue on to the inferior mesenteric, hypogastric and ovarian or spermatic plexuses. Disturbances are similar to the second lumbar lesions.

Fourth lumbar lesions

Again the vasomotor supply is to the lower end of the bowel and pelvic contents. In addition there are supplies to the skin of the buttocks, general gluteal region and the upper thigh. Circulatory disturbance of this supply contributes to the poor health of the skin, pelvis and rectum.

Fifth lumbar lesions

The vasomotor supply tends to follow the main course of the sciatic nerve to the feet. Branches also communicate with the arteries of the iliac vessels and lower bowel from the aortic plexus. The iliac plexus supplies lower areas including the femoral and popliteal plexuses.

Sacro-iliac lesions

The arteries supplied from the area are the ilio-lumbar, itself supplying the spinal cord and ilium, the lateral sacral artery, which supplies the spinal membranes, and the gluteal arteries which communicate with the muscles of the pelvic cavity, pelvic bones, gluteus maximus, hip joint and its muscles. Poor circulation to the hip joint and pelvic bones is a precursor to weakness in the stability factors of soft tissue contributing to degeneration and instability of these structures.

Summary

- There is continuous communication via the spinal cord between both visceral and somatic structures: blood vessels, glands, smooth muscle, skeletal muscle, skin etc. This communication is always multi-segmental or patterned.

- Injury to or disease of any of these structures will establish a pattern of cyclic reference beginning a process of structural change. The area of the nervous system involved rather than the structure or character of the irritation determines the established cyclic pattern.

- As the structural changes continue patterns become established and the cycle becomes self-sustaining.

- Intervention of this cycle, for even the shortest time, reduces the possibility of the re-establishment of this cycle.

- Areas of myofascial and other somatic tissues become sources of continual afferent neural bombardment in the cyclic complex of spinal cord disruption. Reducing the somatic component in the cycle will lessen the summation of impulses and reduce pain.

- The somatic component is both more accessible than the visceral and therapeutically it reduces the cyclic reflex damaging impulses to the primary pathology.

- The spinal cord segmental model is exactly that, a model. Summation of neural processes involves the entire nervous system and its circulation at all times with varying intensity. This leads to remote changes from the primary source of irritation.

References

Boden, S.D., Davis, D.O., Dina, T.S., Patronas, N.J. and Wiesel, S.W. (1990) Abnormal magnetic-resonance scans of the lumbar spine in asymptomatic subjects. *The Journal of Bone and Joint Surgery*, March, 72-A(3) 403–408.

Denslow, J.S. (1944) An analysis of the variability of spinal reflex thresholds. *Journal of Neurophysiology*, July 7, 207–16.

Denslow, J.S., Korr, I.M. and Krems, A.D. (1947) Quantitative studies of chronic facilitation in human motorneurone pools. *American Journal of Physiology*, August 150, 229–238.

Haycock, W. (1955) The expanding concept of osteopathy. *The John Martin Littlejohn Memorial Lecture*, 16 October at the Mayfair Hotel, London W1. Published by the Board of Governors of the British School of Osteopathy.

Inglis, B. (1981) *The Diseases of Civilisation*. Hodder and Stoughton, London.

Jensen, M.C., Brant-Zwadzski, M.N., Obuchowski, N., Modic, M.T., Malkasian, D. and Ross, J.J. (1994) Magnetic resonance imaging of the lumbar spine in people without back pain. *The New England Journal of Medicine*, July 14 331(2), 69–73.

Korr, I.M. (1948) The emerging concept of the osteopathic lesion. *The Journal of the American Osteopathic Association*, November 48(3) 127–38.

Leadbetter, W.B. (1993) Basic principles of prevention and care. In *The Encyclopaedia of Sports Medicine* (ed. F.H. Renström), Chapter 23. Blackwell Scientific Publications, Oxford.

Mackenzie, J. (1893) Some points bearing on the association of sensory disorders and visceral disease. *Brain*, 16, 321–54.

Mackenzie, J. (1912) *Symptoms and their Interpretation*. Second edition. Paul B. Hoeber, New York.

Northup, G.W. (1972) Osteopathic lesions. *The Journal of the American Osteopathic Association*, 71, 845–865.

Pearson, W.M. (1934) An explanation of the results of osteopathic treatment in acute infectious disease. *The Journal of the American Osteopathic Association*, 33(11) 486–9.

Rumney, I.C. (1975) The relevance of somantic dysfunction. *The Journal of the American Osteopathic Association*, 74, 723–5.

Tasker, D.L. (1925) *Principles of Osteopathy*. (Fifth edition). Birkeley and Elson Printing Co.

Turk, D.C. and Okifuji, A. (1999) Assessment of patients' reporting of pain: an integrated perspective. *The Lancet*, 353, 1784–8.

Weiss, S., and Davis, D. (1928) Significance of afferent impulses from skin in mechanisms of visceral pain; skin infiltration as a useful therapeutic measure. *American Journal of Medical Science*, October 176, 517–36.

Wolff, H.G. and Hardy, J.D. (1947) On the nature of pain. *Physiological Review*, April 27, 167–99.

Further reading

Canguilhem, G. (1999) *The Normal and the Pathological*. Zone Books, New York.

Northrup, G.W. (1950) The osteopathic concept of disease. A critical evaluation. *The Journal of the American Osteopathic Association*, 50(4). Also published in *The Academy of Applied Osteopathy Yearbook 1962*.

Talbot, M. (1991) *The Holographic Universe*. Harper Collins, London.

CHAPTER 10

Practice

'For here it is not a question of causes, but of conditions under which the phenomenon appear; their consistent sequence, their eternal return under thousands of circumstances, their uniformity and mutability are perceived and predicted; their defined quality is recognised and again defined by the human mind.'

Goethe. Weimar, 15 January, 1798

'We say disease when we should say effect; for disease is the effect of a change in the parts of the physical body. Disease in an abnormal body is just natural as is health when all parts are in place.'

A.T. Still

Osteopathy can only happen in the present in the presence of the patient. Clinical osteopathy is the only osteopathy as it relies on the collective of its organic mode of consciousness as its philosophy, the holistic construct of its principles, the analytical application of its techniques and the spontaneous internally organising capacity of the patient. Hence the words *find it, fix it, leave it alone*, of Andrew Taylor Still and his recognition of this self-adjustment potential. Without the patient the self-adjustment capability cannot be considered and therefore there is no osteopathy. Descartes developed and furthered positivist science and philosophy into a series of dead-end searches for certainty. Sir Charles Bell recognised in his book *The Sixth Sense*, that the collective of nerve endings in the myofascioskeletal system forms a major part of our consciousness. Poor tissue relationship alters the consciousness and therefore the collective ability to adjust to otherwise simple moment to moment changes necessary for the expression of the form into the environment.

P.R. Hubbell wrote in The *Journal of the American Osteopathic Association*, (June, 1921) under the title Adjustment – the last word:

'There is a crew who have manned a ship, had a compass made like ours, and although they started after we did, and their equipment at present is limited compared to ours, nevertheless they already outnumber us nearly two to one, and their future is by no means disappointing. The public are demanding their services to such an extent that there are now in attendance in one of their schools 2600 students.

'Why this progress? There is but one answer. They have taken and kept our word. And this word is ADJUSTMENT. It is the one word which we have given to the healing world. Take it away from us and we as a profession have nothing left by which we could be identified. It is the keystone in the Arch of Healing. It is our compass. He who does not adjust has no work to do on the ship of osteopathy and the quicker he deserts the better for the rest of the crew.'

The autonomic nervous system

As we know the sympathetic division has its origin from all the thoracic and first three lumbar segments of the spinal cord reaching into all three body cavities. It is this system that is sympathetic, expressing into the environment. The parasympathetic arises from the cranial and sacral segments of the spinal cord. It should never be forgotten that these divisions, including the enteric, are in constant communication and are anatomically united. The next section is an adaptation of Waitely (1948).

The sympathetic system

The sympathetic system innervates every organ and all tissue of the human organism, supplying all blood vessels and, by its twofold action of vasoconstriction and dilatation, acting on or influencing all body tissues. It supplies structures that apparently have no parasympathetic innervation. The sympathetic division activates structures which the parasympathetic division inhibits, for example, the heart and the sphincters of the bowel and bladder. It has an inhibitory effect on parasympathetic action in the head and gastrointestinal tract.

Sensory fibres accompanying the motor fibres transmit impulses to the corresponding area of the cord. These impulses may be referred to neurones which in turn may influence other structures, causing signs and symptoms. These sympathetic reflexes (especially those of visceral origin) are of three basic types: two impulse-based, i.e. motor and sensory, and one non-impulse based, i.e. trophic.

The visceral motor reflex is the only real sympathetic reflex in the muscular tissue of the myofascioskeletal system. Skeletal muscles, as we know them, contract when a stimulus is carried over the sensory fibres of the sympathetics due to a motor response. If the aberrant bombardment of sensory impulses from the large bowel be sufficient in duration and/or intensity, the motor response in the skeletal musculature will produce a chronic contraction, with the outcome of the maintained contracture resulting in degeneration of muscle structure and limitation of normal spinal motion. Nerve cells which are subjected to long continued harmful stimuli are eventually impaired in function. Osteopathic lesions are not only maintained by this abnormal physiology, but they are most difficult to correct. A visceral cycle results, and further retrogression of physiologic bowel action is augmented by continued immobility. This very definitely interferes with sympathetic action of inhibition, which stabilises parasympathetic bowel activation.

The sensory nerve response from the large intestine does not influence the motor response to the organ directly. Rather, the sensory action is distributed to spinal musculature producing contraction and degeneration, resulting in disturbed function of the sympathetic nerves, which supply the gut.

Trophic changes are essentially nutritional disturbances of the impulse nerves. It is the nutrition of the tissues that is dependent upon the sensory and motor nerves which innervate it. Proper nutrition is essential to the normal function of all body cells. Thus, trophic change is a perversion of nerve function with the end result being an inadequate supply of nutrition to the cells. Nerve cells may be injured by mechanical stimuli which occur in osteopathic lesions. Nerve cells may not be harmed by a moderate number of these stimuli. The tissues supplied by these cells will undergo nutritional change.

To apply the osteopathic concept intelligently in regard to the treatment of human ailments, we must know what effect stimulation or irritation has on the sympathetic system. Pottenger (1984) listed among the effects of stimulation of sympathetics the following:

- lessened mucous secretion in the nose and throat
- lessened secretion in the gastrointestinal tract, manifested by retarded digestion and hyperchlorhydria
- lessened motility in the gastrointestinal tract with relaxation of intestinal musculature
- increase in pulse rate
- increase in glycogen content of blood (its being forced from liver)
- increase in body temperature and sweating (found in hyperactivity of both the sympathetic and parasympathetic).

The parasympathetic system

Technically the parasympathetic division has only two real areas of approach, namely the first, second and third sacral nerves and the vagus in the zone of the carotid.

According to Pottenger (1984) the parasympathetic stimulation produces some of the following:

- increased secretion of mouth, nose and pharynx
- increased bronchial secretion
- spasm of bronchi
- hypermotility and hypersecretion of gastric glands depending on degree of stimulation

- irritable bladder
- incontinence of urine and faeces.

Aetiology

Osteopathic aetiology of disease and injury differs from that of medical aetiology. The word aetiology originated from the Greek word *aitia*, for cause or reason. It was then moved to the Latin, *aetia*, combined with *ology*, the study of cause or reason. The osteopathic interpretation of signs and symptoms also differs. It is important in the osteopathic interpretation that we look back to the fundamental combination of primary factors that could be the basis for structural change, however small. The biomedical model tends to look at the immediate and more interesting possibilities, showing a characteristic of its system, impatience. Physicians should look at both the predisposing, long past history, and the more exciting recent contributions. The osteopathic concept of ill health is primarily that of lowered resistance and stress of the individual rather than the domination and presence of micro-organisms. Past combinations of emotional and physical demands upon the individual will set the anatomico-physiological basis for the poor adjustment of the individual and the expression of ill health. We should be developing an initial broad net of phenomena because it is clinically rare for one factor to be the cause of disease expression.

The origin of the use of the word *cause* can be traced back to Aristotle. Although its meaning then was not the same as today it is osteopathically significant that its original use was to describe *the being of anything* including its past experiences or the span of its experiences presenting in the present. White (1990) discusses the work of Mackie, amongst others, in an understanding of cause. Mackie used the analogy of the smoking cigarette butt being the cause of a fire. Even though the cigarette butt is a part of the sequence it cannot be taken in isolation or out of context. We also have to take into account the careless smoker, the flammable material close enough to the cigarette etc. A cigarette butt on its own is not enough to cause a fire. This is Mackie's INUS theory. The butt is an Insufficient but Necessary part of a scenario that is Unnecessary but Sufficient for a fire to occur. Finally, White brings to our attention a very important factor in practically all the papers he researched and that is 'causal identification will be constrained by beliefs about the sorts of things that can be causes (for example, if only events can be causes, then the condition of the road [in a car accident] will not be identified as the cause)'. This may reflect on the practitioner's and patient's relationship to 'what caused the symptoms'. Since the body is an internally organising structure, the event prior to the symptoms would generally add to the body/mental limit of pain free function. The final factor to be the only cause would have to be sufficiently great to bring on symptoms by itself. In addition the pre-existing condition of the patient would dictate the rate of recovery, after the event.

During the history the practitioner will ask about the interaction of the patient with certain extrinsic factors. These extrinsic factors will precipitate the contribution of pre-existing structural lesions to the presenting state of the patient. It is always the patient's response to these factors that leads to the vulnerability towards ill health and injury. Some of these extrinsic factors include fatigue; overuse and abuse (chronic or acute use of alcohol, smoking, recreational and prescribed drugs); violence (either severe and sudden, or less severe and applied for a considerable period of time); dietetic errors; exposure to dampness; sudden changes in temperature, draughts and extremes of temperature; and psychological extremes (joy, excitement, depression and anxiety) (Comstock, 1920). The human body does not make a distinction between physical and emotional trauma; the response is the same: defence. The ability to successfully initiate a defence or adjustment is based on the pre-existing structure of the systems and their communications. We are looking at the breakdown of an adapting nervous system. Ill health is the discrepancy between the soma and the viscera. The nervous system is 'off line'. Nothing makes a bigger contribution to your present state than the culmination of the little things in life.

History taking

'There are a thousand hacking at the branches ... to one who is striking at the root.'

Henry David Thoreau (1817–62)

It is through the case history, the patient's narrative, that the complex interaction of the nervous system (as a whole), and the environment, in which it functions, can be brought into focus. An integrative consciousness, in a time frame, should develop within the practitioner as the history is taken. This will lead to further relevant questioning and a reduction in the habit of asking blind questions. It is with the history that you begin to 'put the patient back together again' and form a dynamic patient-centred course of action and empowerment.

To understand the approach of A.T. Still we will have to refer to the words of Arthur Hildreth, cited in Jackson, 1981. It is worth quoting the complete citation:

'Dr Still said to me one time when we were discussing methods of approach to patients, "Do you know, Arthur, when a patient comes to talk to me about symptoms, how she suffers, and what her trouble is, I seldom observe the patient's clothing. I never notice whether she is beautifully dressed and wears silks and diamonds or covered with homespun cloth. I am listening to her story, and while listening, I am seeing in my mind's eye the combination of systems which go to make up the whole of that body structure. I am concentrating on her story, trying to determine through the description given to me the structural alterations which have occurred to produce the symptoms described.

'I am seeing first the bony framework and the joints which hold it together as one system, the foundation upon which all other structures in the human body are built. I am seeing, especially, the positions of those bony parts and their relationships, one with the other. Then I see the ligaments which hold the framework together, connecting and covering the bones at their joints from the toes to the fingers to the base of the brain, marvellous creations of strength that make the bony structure. Then I see the muscles inserting in various ways all over the bony framework, some of them covering the ligaments and others beginning and ending in them. They are placed to give needed protection to the framework and at the same time move the bony parts in such a marvellous way, with such harmony that it is hard for the mind of man to conceive of the perfection of their functions.

'I am also seeing in my mind's eye the nervous system, this system which acts in the same capacity in the human body that the telegraph system acts in the commercial world for the interchange of thought. The difference between the nervous system of the human body and the telegraph system which encircles the globe is that one is man-created and the other is divinely created, God-made, if you will. While listening to a patient's story, I try to visualise the anatomy of the nervous system in all its relationships, in every function of the body. The nervous system is one of the most marvellous mechanisms ever created.

'I see its division into cerebrospinal part and sympathetic part. The first is made up of the brain, the spinal cord, and the spinal nerves and their branches, reaching out to all the muscles, joints and skin, conveying messages to and from the brain of movement, temperature, pain, etc. The second or sympathetic part is composed essentially of chains of nerve ganglia extending from the base of the brain to the tip of the spinal column, controlling the function of body fluids, and nutrition to the various body parts.

'When you stop to consider how these two great systems are joined together, how they communicate one with the other, you have, in my opinion, the most supreme example of the perfection of the work of the Divine Architect. Each is an individual nervous system, yet so created as to enable nerve impulses to pass from one to the other.

'I further see the arterial system, with its great and small avenues for carrying the blood to every portion of the body. All types of nutritional material and oxygen are carried in that blood stream, substances needed to repair worn-out cells, to grow hair on your head and nails on your fingers, the needed materials for vision and hearing, bone building material, etc. The mechanism whereby these materials are transferred from the blood stream into the vital living cells of the body is beyond description, almost beyond understanding.

'Then I visualise the venous system, another great system of vessels which carries away the waste products to the organs of elimination. There is still a third and most important system of vessels which accompanies the arteries and veins throughout the body. This is known as the lymphatic system. It supplies the serous fluid in which the tissue cells are bathed. It has to do with the mechanism of nutrition, absorption and the protection of cells from harmful poisons and bacteria. And last but not least I see the how it brings about its effect in each particular case.

'Such was Dr Still's line of thought as he listened to complaints of the patient.'

The history from the patient is a narrative of their past and present. In addition it will be a reflection of their expectations for the future, their fears and hopes. Initially the collection of information should be a simple process of data collection, and as you become more familiar with the method of history taking it will become an inquiry and conversation. It should never be an interrogation. As the practitioner in attendance during the narrative you will be influencing what the patient deems relevant due to their preconceptions about osteopathic medicine. Like allopathic medicine most patients will not make the connections between their present complaint of low back pain with a history of irritable bowel syndrome. When you ask about a patient's general health, he or she may not mention their irritable bowel syndrome, because they may still be thinking about their low back. They think their irritable bowel may not be relevant because osteopaths deal with backs. In the allopathic practice the patient will surrender all information as the doctor deals with everything (even if they are not making any connection between the two or more complaints).

It is the objective of the osteopathic history to put the patient *back together again* so a diagnosis or dynamic model of dysfunction can be visualised. This then leads to a purposeful physical examination that has direction and form rather than a collection of individual isolated tests. (Although the initial learning of a physical examination has to be a collection of individual isolated tests; we will look at this later.)

Putting the patient back together again

What are we seeing in the patient who is in pain? A simple answer, for now, is a reflection of the nervous system in discomfort due to pain, tissue damage, poor homeostatic shift, or worry. We are seeing the expression of 'feelings'. The case history has two major functions:

(1) to give some degree of order and form to the feelings for the patient. The patient lays it all out on the table and we organise and arrange things for them. This will allow the patient to make some sense of what is happening.
(2) It is for our need to reach a structure or model for our future actions, albeit a dynamic one.

As a result of these two points we can develop and evaluate an ongoing programme of empowerment for the patient and treatment/management in the form of what we say and do.

Making sense for the patient

The interpretation of the patient's symptoms, giving the patient a reason for their pain, is a good starting point. This has the added advantage of releasing some of the patient's anxieties, or not, as the case may be. More often than not the patient will come with four or five symptoms one of which includes, for example, back pain. The patient's expectation is that you only treat the back pain and that the other symptoms have no bearing on the matter. This breaking up of the patient is a disempowerment. With the patient in 'bits' they are unable to understand the reason for their ill health and therefore cannot help themselves. The osteopath has to relate the patient's signs and symptoms to the organisation of the nervous and other systems and help the patient to understand that there is only one problem with many expressions, if this is the case. Any part that is not considered can only tax the potential for recovery; this includes reciprocal emotional and physical states. This is patient empowerment.

Organisation of the injury and illness

The central theme of osteopathy is an attempt to understand the organisation of the illness or injury by the nervous system. We can now go further and describe the osteopathic case history as *a dialogue and narrative with the aim of understanding the interrelationships of health, ill health and injury as a reflection of the myofascioskeletoneuroendocrine-immune systems etc.* This is an example of the unifying approach of the osteopathic history. How do these systems relate to each other for the patient? The true osteopathic history tries hard not to be polyreductionist but integrative and unifying with an organic consciousness. Here it is important to realise that the sums of the allopathic or biomedical parts do not make an osteopathic whole.

As Patterson (1976) reminds us,

'the philosophy utilised by Still in the development of osteopathic medicine was organised around the tenet that the human body, while constructed of identifiable organs and systems, functions not as a collection of semiconnected parts but as a functional unit. Certainly this holistic philosophy of human function was not unique to Still. It had been presented centuries before in the philosophies of Hippocrates in early Greece. Although the concept of total functional capacity was ancient, Still's original contributions lay in his views of the interrelationship between diagnosis and treatment. In these and in the system of functional methods for maintaining or restoring proper function lay the unique germinal events that have led to the insights and methods of current osteopathic philosophy and practice.'

Putting the patient back together again begins with the aforementioned allopathic parts of system interpretation then progresses to a central neuroendocrine system. The autonomic nervous system and its relationship with the endocrine system play a central role in the organisation of our health, ill health and rate of recovery from illness and injury. As a central theme in history taking, it should never be forgotten that a human being is a complete human being at all times.

Integrating the signs and symptoms

Common errors in the taking of a history are the inductive mechanical pre-conceptions of the practitioner and patient. The diagnosis is forced to fit a mechanical biomedical model that is reductionist and disempowering. While not wrong it weakens the osteopathic diagnostic and treatment potential if used without an osteopathic consciousness. There can be a tendency to ignore the relevance of other seemingly minor signs and symptoms in the face of the quick categorisation, naming and overanalysis of the presenting signs and symptoms. It is not realised that the short-term speed of a local diagnosis as a finalisation of the problem leads to a comfort zone for the practitioner and patient, which will be repeated in the long term by a relapse. The short-term difficulty and practice of an osteopathic diagnosis leads to the long-term development of an integrative and dynamic model. This direction is the course of empowerment and treatment of the patient. As we are reminded by Swope (1938) on the point of a 'diagnosis', 'it is convenient, but it can never express the severity of the illness; it does not indicate the former health status of the patient nor does it indicate his condition following the illness. Writing a diagnosis at the completion of a case history is like ending a story "and they lived happily ever after". It is a brief implication of what happened.'

How do we integrate our history? This is a process of visualisation and holding a dialogue with the patient. The visualisation is of the integrative anatomy of the nervous system. For example, we must always be aware of facilitation, general adaptation syndrome and the psychophysiological coping capability of the patient. While listening to the patient talk we can make sense of the seemingly 'separate' signs and symptoms. The patient's injury and illness is *organised* from the inside out and not from the outside in, therefore we must *visualise* the patient from inside out not from the outside in. We must consider where there might be physical patterns or locations that may be the result of past psychophysiological-nutritional events that may be obstructing the body from correcting itself.

Example: 30 year old female patient

Presenting complaint: Recurrent sprain-strain of left ankle over a three-year period.
Past treatment: Osteopath, physiotherapist and GP.

General history
General health: Fine.
Accidents and operations: Nothing abnormal complained of except for ankle injuries.
CVS: Minor headaches just before monthly cycle.
Respiratory: Nothing abnormal complained of.
Orthopaedic: Other than ankle, left hip 'clunks' every now and then. Had mild sciatica in left low back and gluteal region a few years ago.
GI: Has a little irritable bowel every few months.
Gynaecological: Has abdominal bloating, low back ache and aching in the tops of both thighs a day or two before the onset of monthly cycle.

Any discipline can extract the same information from the patient. We can now look at this patient in three basic ways, none of which are wrong:

(1) The analytical orthopaedic considerations of the ankle joint and local tissue. This looks at the damage to the ankle region in relation to the structural and nutritional status.
(2) The broader, and truer, orthopaedic approach of involving the posture, tissue tone and other joint functions into the relationship with the ankle. By looking at the whole posture and tissue tone the body can be easily seen as a machine rather than an organism. Here is an example of poly-reductionism rather than integration of the patient as a whole.
(3) The integrative organisation and restorative capability of the nervous system in relation to the inability of the ankle to heal. Since the nervous system acts as a whole all the time, we will see in this case that it is the choice of the patient to come to you for the ankle rather than the associated problems with her monthly cycle. It is the integrative function of the nervous system that is struggling and the ankle is one of the casualties.

Although the above have their value, only the third is an attempt at Andrew Taylor Still's 'oneness in wholeness', integrating the patient. The other two are orthopaedic models that could have been added to by a gynaecologic and gastrointestinal model.

Name and status

The title, especially in female patients, can set a relationship status. This status is with the spouse and others. For example, and I am trying to be careful here, a female patient who still uses her maiden name while happily married wants, and rightly so, some professional independence in her work, possibly separate from her role as a mother and wife. She may go on to use the title Ms or Miss: this again reflects a sense of how she would like to be perceived by others. Mister may obviously seem a lot easier. Today we are all more correctly aware of homosexual relationships and cultural differences. Never assume a heterosexual or homosexual relationship, they are relationships and should be considered that way until the situation demands greater emphasis on the health of the patient. Sensitivity towards cultural differences should always be apparent. If you are not sure ask.

How did the patient hear about you?

If you are consulted by a friend or a patient who has known you for years they will already have been discussing you. If you were treating a new patient at your school or hospital then they would have already heard about the establishment. The chances are they will feel less apprehensive, they may even have high expectations.

Date of birth

Knowing the age of a patient will immediately allow you to include the common predispositions and vulnerabilities of that age group. From the infant to the elderly, genetic, environmental, habitual, psychological and past health all have an influence on illness and injury predisposition and recovery potential. Mature patients forget things. You may find that when you put events and feelings back together they will remember more. Young patients in the main do not know where you are leading with your questioning, so ask them if they understand. Make analogies for them to be able to create a mental picture.

Occupation

The occupation will indicate social status, income, stresses, etc. Are they happy in their work? Is the organisational behaviour of the working environment conducive to personal development or repression? It should never be forgotten that people spend most of their waking time at work.

Hobbies and pastimes

How does the patient spend their leisure time? They may have a sedentary job six days a week and on the seventh play four hours of squash. At 43 years of age they have come to you with left sided chest pain. Do they train in the evening twice a week? Are they walkers, swimmers or stamp collectors? Depending on the patient, stamp collecting could be more beneficial than swimming, allowing for mental relaxation.

Quantitative and qualitative physical examination

'Don't just do something; stand there.'

Anon.

We can broadly place the osteopathic physical examination into quantitative and qualitative components. Quantitative physical examinations are analytical, procedural, senseless, direct and non-transferring. Qualitative physical examinations are reflective, intuitive, sensitive, indirect and transferring. It is important that we do not interpret these as opposing, but as complementary towards a fuller understanding of the patient's problem.

Quantitative examination

It is important that the patient is examined in relation to him or herself. All examination should be directed at the normal just as much as the abnormal. There should be an unbiased examination of the patient. Too often the examiner is quick to find and become distracted by 'the bit that hurts'. Information collected from the body and communication with the patient must be considered in relation to the signs and symptoms to allow for an evaluation of the patient in relation to himself. We must include the patient in the examination. We should not examine the patient from the one-sided view of just symptom hunting. There is always the risk of the examiner looking to classify the patient's signs and symptoms in relation to a textbook, making the findings a textbook case.

As Swope (1938) goes on to say:

'we are attempting to make a distinction here between examination and diagnosis, and one may say that it is unnecessary. Yet we have a conviction that the therapeutic methods of osteopathy can be improved by making a clear distinction and distinct separation of these terms and practices, i.e., examination is not a procedure directed toward a diagnosis (or naming the disease) but a classification of findings to determine the health status of the patient. Examination should lead to a concise, detailed list of all normal and abnormal findings on the first or second visit. It may be added to, or used as a comparison for, later findings and in this way it becomes more valuable in the study and treatment of the case.'

These findings include things like trophic changes, evidence of vasomotor disturbance and the linking of various findings in the context of the patient. It may be better to get a colleague to talk aloud through the steps. And as an example, it has been established that surface temperature increases due to the inflammation, organ distension or spasms of underlying viscera. This temperature increase is due to the firm establishment of viscerosomatic reflexes (Johnston *et al.*, 1987).

Standing

This may not always be possible as those who are ill and injured may not be able to stand.

(1) Colour and health of skin: face, chest, abdomen, back and limbs; signs of trophic change, pigment distribution, sweating (local and general), rashes, lips
(2) Soft tissue distribution
(3) Hair distribution
(4) Body type: endomorph, mesomorph, ectomorph and combinations
(5) Skull, limb and body size relationship
(6) Posture.

Sitting and lying

Head and face

Stand a little distance from the patient initially then move in closer.

(1) Skull dimensions should be overviewed in relation to the age of the patient. A degree of symmetry, masses, swellings, thickening ridges, fontanelles, pigmentation and vascularity
(2) Face: indicating fullness in the face, acromegaly, cardiac disease, kidney disease, nose, eyes, mouth and neural damage
(3) Craniofacial dimensions indicating flexion, extension, side bending, and torsion lesions
(4) Cranial nerve examination.

Hair and scalp

(1) Hair colour, distribution, thinness, thickness, oiliness etc.
(2) Alopecia, dandruff and inflammation of scalp
(3) Wig, hairpiece or implant – why?

Ears

(1) External appearance; shape, size and position
(2) External canal; shape, colour, obstructions (wax), walls, and lesions
(3) Drum colour and integrity
(4) Hearing test.

Eyes

(1) Orbit size and variation between right and left
(2) Colour of surrounding tissue. Is one side darker? Are both sides appreciably darker than surrounding tissue?
(3) Compare eyebrows and eye lashes
(4) Compare eyelid shape, swelling, texture and function
(5) Compare colour of sclera and conjunctiva (inflammation)
(6) Eyeball pressure and appearance of protruding. Exophthalmos (unilateral or bilateral)
(7) Quick test for peripheral vision
(8) Eye sight: Snellen chart. You also use a magazine or newspaper for general idea of sight acuity
(9) Colour vision test cards
(10) Eye muscle test
(11) Ophthalmic examination: Looking at the optic disc (swelling), blood vessels (tortuosity, A-V nipping), retina (detachment), haemorrhage and oedema.

Nose

(1) External observation (anterior and lateral). Asymmetry, swelling, shape and displacement. The nose in relation to the maxillofacial region
(2) Ventilation and sound during inhalation and exhalation. Is patient mouth breathing?
(3) Internal examination: polyps, thickening of mucus membrane, septal deviation, and inflammation
(4) Discharge: quantity and character

Mouth

(1) External facial observation: overall face shape, symmetry, cheeks, parotid gland swelling, and infections

(2) External lips: colour, width, symmetry, thickness and angle of mouth; dehydration, tumours, cyanosis, herpes, etc.

(3) Internal lips: colour and texture continuity; ulcers, tumours and fungal infections

(4) Gums: colour, structure and texture continuity; inflammation, ulcer, receding line, oedema and bleeding

(5) Teeth: number, distribution, colour, shape, occlusion, inflammation and fillings; false teeth

(6) Tongue: size (in relation to mouth), fissures, symmetry, colour (fungal infection), coating (furry and white), inflammation, bite marks, ulcers and tumours. Any gross deviation on protrusion?

(7) Sublingual (under the tongue and floor of the mouth) region: palpation under the jaw; hard and swollen lumps, lymph nodes and salivary glands. Look under the tongue at frenulum; colour, structure and continuity

(8) Inside cheeks and mucus membranes: colour, structure and continuity of the surface. Ulcers, patches, ridges (bites), and tumours

(9) Soft palate: symmetry, colour and inflammation of soft palate arch; deviation of uvula; continuity with throat.

(10) Hard palate: symmetry, colour, patches, height, and width; ulceration from dentures.

Throat

(1) General colour and surface continuity
(2) Tonsils: presence, size and colour
(3) Tosillar fossae: depth, continuity, tags and scar tissue
(4) Deep throat (pharynx): scar tissue and colour. Inflammation and retro-pharyngeal haematoma (from neck injury).

Neck

(1) Observation in relation to the rest of the body; anterior, lateral and posterior aspects; symmetry, fossae, occipitocervical junction, supra-clavicular and infra-tracheal region

(2) Visible lumps, enlargements, skin and pulsations

(3) Thyroid: fullness and loss of surface contours, enlargement, tightness on neck movements, palpatory and non-palpatory tenderness, texture, and mobility

(4) Tracheal cartilage: pain free swallowing and palpatory mobility

(5) Submandibular region: palpation of submandibular area and omohyoid mobility

(6) Carotid arteries: observation, palpation, and auscultation. Displacement, tenderness, and bruit

(7) Cervical spine: active and passive movements. Any findings should be in relation to additional clinical findings.

Thorax

(1) Observation in relation to the rest of the body. Anterior, lateral and posterior aspects. Symmetry, fossae, skin (tattoos), muscle distribution and breathing rate and depth. Any change in breathing comfort/discomfort from standing to sitting.

(2) Palpation: superior palpation for upper ribs, lateral palpation for middle and lower ribs, and anterioposterior palpation for additional information at all three areas. Rib movement, range of motion and crepitus. Follow up any suspect findings. Apex beat of heart, location, rate and intensity.

(3) Thoracic spine: always examine in relation to the rib cage and thoracic contents. Is there a straight spine (relative lordosis)? Palpate thorax for straight spine syndrome. Is there a kyphosis or scoliosis? Spinous process point tenderness, commonly indicative of poor joint motion with local aberrant reflex activity, oedema and possible trophic change.

(4) Auscultation: usual cardiorespiratory examination. Always examine in relation to the myofascioskeletal findings around rib cage and thoracic spine. This will include bilateral blood pressure and pulses.

Abdomen and Pelvis

(1) Patient supine: observation of gross distribution (visceroptosis), contours, skin discolourations, pulsations, fat distribution, stretch marks (may indicate sudden loss of weight), muscle bulk, distribution of muscles (may indicate hernia), position of umbilicus, swellings (lymph nodes), scars (caesarean section, violence), and pelvic floor tissue distribution and tone.

(2) Palpation of skin, muscle tone, masses, fluid (turgidity), and abdominal contents

(3) Patient prone: observation of lower thoracic, lumbar and gluteal region. Skin tone, texture (trophic changes), redness, stretch marks, horizontal muscle bands, hair, prominent sacro-coccyx and sinuses.

(4) Bony land marks, sacro-iliac mobility, lumbar spine mobility, posterior iliac spine tenderness and gluteal tone.

Shoulder and upper extremities

(1) Observation of length and form in relation to the rest of the body. Soft tissue distribution and fossae from the root of neck to tips of fingers, bilaterally.

Skin colour consistency, scars, scratches, possible needle marks and tattoos. Signs of inflammation and general oedema. Specific lymphatic, cardiovascular, neurological and orthopaedic examination procedures

(2) Palpation: begin at the root of the neck to the fingertips. Palpate for tenderness, oedema fullness, muscle tone, fat depth, joint enlargement, lumps, and warmth

(3) Nails: check for ridges, signs of recent general ill health, thickness, fungal infections, trophic changes and brittleness.

Lower extremities

(1) Observation of the relative length and form of the limbs in relation to each limb, the other limb and the thorax. The skin, hair and soft tissue distribution. Superficial vascular disturbances (varicosities), red lines (inflamed and infected lymphatics), cellulite (sympathetic disturbance), and scars.

(2) Palpation standing and lying. Skin drag, myofascial tone and joint examination.

Back and spine

(1) Observation with regards to the skin: trophic changes, acne, hair, pigmentation, texture, sweating, and scars. Myofascial bulk and distribution, creases in waist and maintained tone while relaxing.

(2) Palpation of the skin: its tonus, drag over the underlying tissue, texture change and oedema over the spinous processes. Myofascial tone and sensitivity and vertebral joint examination.

Qualitative examination

'Organisms only exist in the present.'

Wolfgang Schad

Observation

'Our eye finds it more comfortable to respond to a given stimulus by reproducing once more an image that it has produced many times before, instead of registering what is different and new in an impression.'

Friedrich Nietzsche

On this subject of qualitative observation the author feels that the best book ever written in the last millennium has to be Goethe's *Ferbenlehre* or *Theory of Colours* (1810). Ludwig van Beethoven is quoted as saying 'can you lend me the *Theory of Colours* for a few weeks? It is an important work. His last things are insipid.' The following is an opening account on observation:

'The conclusions of men are very much different according to the mode in which they approach a science or branch of knowledge; from which side, through which door they enter. The literally practical man, the manufacturer, whose attention is constantly and forcibly called to the facts which occur under his eye, who experiences benefit or detriment from the application of his convictions, to whom loss of time and money is not indifferent, who is desirous of advancing, who aims at equalling or surpassing what others have accomplished – such a person feels the unsoundness and erroneousness of a theory much sooner than the man of letters, in whose eyes words consecrated by authority are at last equivalent to solid coin; than the mathematician, whose formula always remains infallible, even although the foundation on which it is constructed may not square with it.'

Andrew Taylor Still was a manufacturer, as shown by his creativity and inventiveness. The osteopath must attempt to master subjective vision to complete his or her range of clinical qualities (Fig. 15). More recently, Crary (1996) comments on Goethe's subjective abilities: 'Goethe insistently cites experiences in which the

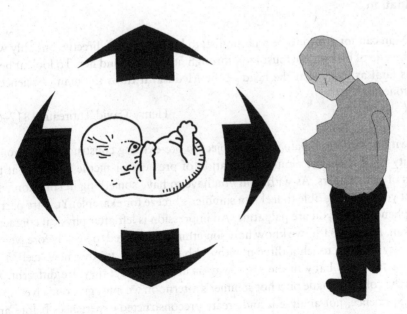

Fig. 15 Subjective (phenomenological) vision. The physician is part of the experience and qualities witnessed.

subjective contents of vision are dissociated from an objective world, in which the body itself produces phenomena that have no external correlate.' Goethe includes closing the eyes. Not to cut us off from what we are observing, on the contrary, he wants us to become the phenomenon we are witnessing. Your physiology is part of and vital for vision. As with all sensory phenomena we only get out of it what we let in. Remember the cold glass of lemonade on a hot summer's afternoon. You did not resist the experience. Subjective observation urges you not to resist the phenomena you are observing; do not dictate to the form in front of you. If it could speak what would it be saying?

On one's physiological presence as a necessary part of observation, Goethe continues

'The impression of coloured objects remains in the eye like that of colourless ones, but in this case the energy of the retina, stimulated as it is to produce the opposite colour, will be more apparent. Let a small piece of bright-coloured paper or silk be held before a moderately lighted white surface; let the observer look steadfastly on the small coloured object, and let it be taken away after a time while his eyes remain unmoved; the spectrum of another colour will then be visible on the white plane. The coloured paper may be also left in its place while the eye is directed to another part of the white plane; the same spectrum will be visible there too, for it arises from an image which now belongs to the eye.'

Palpation

'Man cannot afford to be a naturalist, to look at nature directly, but only with the side of his eye. He must look through her and beyond her. To look at her is as fatal as to look at the head of the Medusa. It turns the man of science to stone.'

Henry David Thoreau (1817–62)

As with observation, palpation is subject to pre-existing constructs. Palpation in reality is far from the simple stimulation of pressure or tactile receptors at the ends of your fingers. As with light you have to have something in common with what you feel to be able to feel it, a summer's breeze for example. You are part of the phenomenon you are palpating. An impression is left after physical contact is broken. As osteopaths we know how something is expected to 'feel' before we feel it. Every time we touch a three-month old baby there is another new 'feel'. You cannot treat this baby in the same way as another baby; they are different. As with the cold lemonade on a hot summer's afternoon we must give ourselves up to the experience, not analyse it and create preconstructed experiences before and during palpation. Osteopathic palpation only occurs in the present, as do all living forms. Its essence is that it 'senses the patient' rather than 'trying to make sense of the patient'.

So called 'objective evaluations' are not wrong but they are a continuation of the Newtonian–Cartesian model of quantification and measurement, squeezing the patient into the symbols and constraints built upon by the historical need for certainty. Palpate with reflection and imagination not with total analytical visualisation. The human form in the shape of the practitioner will be led, with experience, towards and through the structure of the body. What is felt in the hand and what is imagined will meet in the practitioner, leading towards analytical actions known as treatment.

The osteopathic centres

The following is an adaptation of the original work by D.L. Tasker, DO, *The Principles of Osteopathy*, 1925. Consistent with osteopathic understanding of communication within and between systems there are areas on the surface of the body, particularly spinal, that have historically been termed 'centres'. These centres were part of the osteopath's technical vocabulary. Once again terms such as this should not be confused with similar terms used by, for example, physiologists. The original use of the term centre in the physiological sense would refer to a functional area of the central nervous system that governs the function or action of an organ or other structure.

An osteopathic centre is that point on the surface of the body that has been demonstrated to be in closest central connection with a physiological centre, or over the course of a governing nerve bundle.

We must remind ourselves again that the nervous system functions as a whole all of the time. Segmentation of the nervous system is purely academic and artificial and limits our mode of integrative thinking. We must never 'hard wire' the nervous system. Independent functioning of any area of the nervous system is a matter of interpretation with areas of the nervous system having a tendency towards a more dominant influence than other areas. A good example is the individual ganglia lying within the gastrointestinal tract. The enteric or gastrointestinal part of the autonomic nervous system is composed of ganglia and is capable of relative independent function (Appenzeller and Oribe, 1997).

Present knowledge supports earlier osteopathic presumptions of the functioning of the central nervous system that:

- there are individual areas of the central nervous system that show some relative independence and
- that these areas are not only in the brain; the spinal cord is an active processor of neural function and is not a passive relay station.

Segmentation of the central nervous system especially in the spinal cord is a blending of one area in relation to another due to structural and communication links. From a certain segment spinal cord nerve fibres are distributed to the skin, skeletal muscle, involuntary muscles, mucous membranes of the viscera and muscular structures of the arteries. Stimulation of the skin, mucous membrane, muscle, or other structures transmit impulses towards the central nervous system. These impulses are organised within the central nervous system and affect all structures that share that segment of the central nervous system for their own function. We can then talk of two or more structures being in communication at a particular segmental level of the spinal cord.

The examination of the patient brings these areas to the attention of the practitioner but it is the skill and placement of meaning of these findings that makes these centres clinically relevant. The osteopath must relate an area of oversensitivity or hyperaesthesia at any point along the spinal area of the back to all paths and structures related to that area.

Tasker (1925) took the first four cervical nerves as an example of this examination and the integration of the anatomical paths and their relation to clinical findings.

The first cervical nerve leaves the spinal canal between the occiput and atlas. A study of its distribution will inform us what structures are governed by it. Its anterior division forms a part of the cervical plexus. This division communicates with the sympathetic nerves on the vertebral artery, the vagus (pneumogastric), the hypoglossal and superior cervical sympathetic ganglion, innervating the rectus lateralis and anterior recti. The posterior division of the first cervical nerve is the suboccipital. It supplies motor fibres to the posterior recti muscles of the head, the superior, and inferior oblique. Sensory fibres originate from the scalp. This is consistent with Hilton's Law on the supply and distribution of nerves.

Hilton's Law

The anterior division of the first cervical supplies the synovial membrane of the occipital articulation, the muscles which control movements of the joint and the skin over the joint. Of clinical importance is that the muscles controlling the occipito-atlantal articulation will move the joint on the basis of the nerve impulses reaching them from the sensory fibres of the first cervical. These sensory fibres originate from the skin of the back of the head and upper neck and from the synovial membrane. Clinically this can explain the cooling of the skin over the neck and head leading to a stiff neck with 'subluxation' of the occipito-atlantal joint. This basic three-point distribution, and its clinical consequences, is an example of Hilton's law and is apparent at all spinal joint levels.

The involuntary mechanism

All matter has a vibratory frequency. The ganglia of the complete sympathetic chain traverse all cavities, and according to Robinson, function reciprocally with the cardiovascular needs, physically and emotionally. Cranial nervous vibrations, thoracic cardiorespiratory rhythms and abdominopelvic motions all reflect within each cavity. The total steady (i.e. constantly adjusting) state can be referred to as the involuntary mechanism. Even the paramecium shows involuntary motion and there is not a single neurone in sight (Bouratinos, 1999). There tends to be an agreement that anything short of the organism-as-a-whole within the universe and the therapist as a part of the expression of consciousness is abstractive. This may be seen in the palpation of the involuntary mechanism which is thought to be the collective material expression of metabolism, as vibration, rhythm and motion. Once the osteopath palpates the patient the osteopath becomes part of the expressive process of form as a universal expression of life (Bortoft, 1999). Biomedicine teaches us to stand in front of the phenomenon, the patient, and reduce it to its parts and then attempt to put it back together again to explain how it works. Osteopathy teaches us to stand 'behind' the patient and, in Goethean style, palpate the patient *coming into being* as we are at that time in space. This coming into being is not neurological but like Proteus the body may be seen as in the words of Plato,

'... but you are only deceiving me, and so far from displaying the subjects of your skill, you decline even to tell me what they are, for all my entreaties. You are a perfect Proteus in the way you take on every kind of shape, twisting about this way and that...'

Subjective observation and palpation is essential for recognition of this phenomenon. Unfortunately you are part of the phenomenon. These cavity phenomena cannot be separated at a qualitative level only at a quantitative academic level. Once this separation has taken place the patient is seen as a collection of three separate phenomena causing an instant abstraction. Goethe realised the importance of bone in the type of mechanism and Bouratinos (1999) recognised the importance of bone in the expression and form of a living consciousness as movement in higher forms. With the central nervous system encased in bone the rapid frequency can be held in check and contained with additional help by structures such as the falx cerebi allowing an overall motion to be guided. Thoracic rhythm is slower and needs less bone containment, hence the construction of the ribs, sequencing of bone with gaps. The abdomen is free with the omentum and other myofascial structure allowing it to move with a gentle motion.

Diagnosis and prognosis

'I tell the patient his troubles, and what he thinks is his disease, and my explanation is the cure. If I succeed in correcting his errors I change the fluids in the system, and establish the patient in health. The truth is the cure.'

Phineas Parkhurst Quimby

What is a diagnosis? Swope (1938) goes on to say

'diagnosis is the science and art of distinguishing one disease from another, *naming* the disease, if you please – symptomatology classified or grouped to determine the more obvious named disease. Diagnosis is an opinion formulated in the physician's mind as a result of comparing abnormal findings with textbook symptomatology. The osteopathic physician should never be satisfied with a named disease. He should be interested in the total health picture of the patient. It is not the principle of osteopathy primarily to treat the symptoms developing from pathological conditions. We are attempting to find the cause as elicited from these effects. It is *not* [my italics] in our favour, with the health of our patient as our goal, to direct treatment from the actual knowledge of physical findings rather than basing our therapy on an opinion which is a mental picture derived from the combination of several outstanding symptoms.'

Stimpson and Webb (1975) could see ahead to the turn of the century and the fact that we are now seeing the true value and cost of diagnostic procedures that can never be allowed to stand alone 'there is so much room for variability in diagnosis, even with seemingly "hard" information such as x-ray photographs, that diagnosis is not the cut-and-dried scientific exercise that it often made out to be'. The above shows how Swope's reasoning falls short of an organic explanation. The above is not the original meaning of the word diagnosis, for this we have to deconstruct the word. *Dia* from the Greek 'through' and *Gnosis* where the G in Greek is the K in English, leading to *Knosis*, 'knowledge' or 'coming into knowing'. Once we see through the patient then we will know. It is nearly the opposite of the positivist understanding.

The medical conception of diagnosis was to estimate conditions so as to be able to name the disease, so that the appropriate remedy could be administered. If it happened that there were additional ailments existing, these were also recognised and additional remedies were given; hence the gun-shot mixtures of the mid-Victorian era of medical history, before the modern renaissance, in which our particular school has played such a large part.

The osteopathic conception of diagnosis, on the other hand, recognises the obligation to consider each patient as an individual presenting a new problem: a separate disease entity having definite underlying causes which may vary widely in different cases, although the symptoms may seem to classify it as a typical condition. *This is the diversity factor in the unifying of the patient.*

Symptoms, while they are the first things to be brought to our notice, are really the last things to be considered. A thorough and comprehensive study of the structural tissues gives us such an understanding of the strength and weakness of various parts with tendencies towards disease and latent disturbances frequently revealed before they arise as so-called symptoms. One fact to be observed, especially in the progress of acute diseases under osteopathic care, is that the symptoms are masked so that textbook cases are the exceptions.

No definite picture can be formed of a condition, however true it is at the time, that is more than momentary in its existence. A disease is a variation from the normal in a degree only, and the slide under our microscope represents only one phase of that variation, not what came before it or what might come after it.

Diagnosis is not a mathematical problem to be solved at one sitting or by the use of an algorithm (Fig. 16). It frequently involves a continued research and constant weighing of values. However scientific we may be in applying all the various yardsticks in our armamentarium, the x-ray, the chemical laboratory, the microscope, psycho-analysis, the learned opinions of the various specialists, we will find that diagnosis is not only a science but an art (Vaughan, 1918).

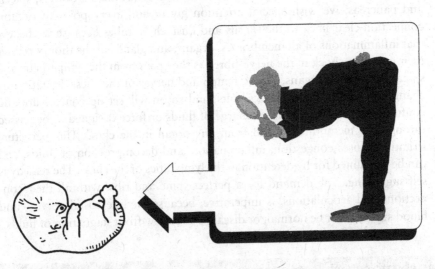

Fig. 16 The objective-algorithmic approach. The physician as the on-looker, objective (without mind) and not involved in the signs and symptoms of the patient!

Louisa Burns, writing in *The Journal of the American Osteopathic Association* in June, 1921, under the title 'Look for lesions' cites Andrew Taylor Still in a demonstration of the integration of anatomy in relation to ill health and diagnosis:

'I have spoken of the membranes that connect the tongue, trachea, oesophagus, lungs, and heart to the spine above the diaphragm; also of the whole list of membranes that hold the liver, spleen, and other organs of the abdomen in place. I have drawn the attention of the student to the blood -, nerve -, and lymph-supplies of the mesenteric systems of both large and small bowels, with the general remarks on the mesentery of all organs of the abdomen and their uses, in order that the student can have a direct method in seeking the causes that produce abnormal conditions of any organ of the chest, abdomen, and pelvis. Explore the spine for bony abnormalities at all points that any organ receives nerve-supply from the spinal nerves. Then pass to the abdomen for twists or folds of the mesentery or any change of position of any of the organs. You may find abnormalities in form and place of the bladder, uterus, bowels, kidneys, liver, spleen, and other organs below the diaphragm, that lead to disease and death by strangulation or suspension of the fluids of the meso-system, all the way from the tongue to the end of the sacrum. It is the connective tissue of the spine that directly connects the omentum and mesentery to the spine and other places of attachment to which we would like to point the attention of the student, because this connecting tissue is the bridge that conducts the nerve-forces to the great omentum and mesentery, generally, with their lymphatic vessels. To the connections with the stomach, bowels, spleen, and pancreas, we wish special attention given, and every point of organic connection clear back to the tonsils and Eustachian tubes because we believe that inflammations of all membranes, organs, and glands of the thorax receive their irritating shock in the nerve-fibres as they pass from the sympathetic and spinal cord to the organs, blood, lymph and nerves of the chest. Irritation by changes of temperature, shocks, jolts, and so on will set up contracture and confusion of the receipt and discharge of fluids or force designed to be passed through the membrane to and from any organ in the chest. This perpetual irritation causes congestion, inflammation, and decompression of fluids, and can be accounted for by detention in the lymphatics of the chest. The remedy is self-suggesting. The demand for a perfect spine and ribs, with all their connections and articulations, is imperative, because the intercostal nerve – and blood supply must be normal, or disease will follow from stagnation of fluids.'

Osteopathic manipulative therapy

'You will find making the bony adjustments to be the easiest part of osteopathy. All you have to do is to carry them through their normal physiological range of motion without force or injury, keeping in mind that in any joint carried, much less forced, beyond its physiological range of motion the ligaments are damaged beyond repair. And injured ligaments are like fractured bones; how long they will be painful to the patient depends on how long the patient lives.... I do not instruct the student to punch or pull a certain bone, nerve or muscle for a certain disease, but by knowledge of the normal and abnormal, I hope to give a specific knowledge for all diseases.'

A.T. Still

The original meaning of the word *therapy* was from the Greek, *therapeuo*, meaning 'I serve, worship or attend to a higher god, master or mistress'. This is significant as the osteopath by his or her action recognises that they are serving whatever is the self-adjusting capability of the body. Coats (1998) translated the works of the Goethean ecologist Viktor Schauberger (1885–1958). Schauberger wrote

'the fundamental proposition that nothing can be created out of nothing was formulated by science. However, it failed to recognise the form of motion through which a densified product of concentration becomes manifest through the agency of the relatively highest-grade expansive motion. From every pore of this cycloidally-moving Earth a new entity ascends and takes its place. It unfolds itself in the ante-chamber of the "hereafter". With the stimulating assistance of oligodynamic, decay-furthering and catalytic recombination-enhancing influences, this negatively charged, dynamite-like formative substance consumes the fertilising precipitates of solar energies.'

Of particular interest is the use of the word *oligodynamics*. Oligodynamics refers to energetic processes or physical products produced or triggered by small or subtle forces, which despite their apparent magnitude may also be extremely powerful.

The following shows an early osteopathic understanding of oligodynamics in the writings of Lawrence (1918):

'Just what takes place in the body as the result of an osteopathic treatment; wherein is the curative value of the treatment? ... Every cell of the body is aquatic in nature. By that we mean that every cell of the body is bathed in a liquid called lymph, from which it takes its nourishment, into which it throws off its waste products, and by which its life processes are influenced, just as is the case with those minute forms of life that live in water. ... The single-celled animal most commonly studied by medical students is the paramecium, found in stagnant water. Under the microscope these tiny animals are seen to possess the ability to respond to certain external stimuli such as light, heat, food etc. These responses to stimuli are called *tropisms*. ... Thigmotropism, or response to touch, is illustrated by a vine twining around a string or twig; geotropism or response to gravity, by trees growing erect against.... It is a well known principle of physics that energy of one kind may be transformed into energy of another kind, as for example, potential heat energy of coal may be changed into electric energy. Likewise there is a degree of interchangeability of the tropisms referred to, which interchange depends upon the kind of stimulus and the nature of the cell receiving the stimulus. . . . In case of a germ disease, the body, in accordance with the tropisms referred to, begins at once to elaborate antibodies in blood to counteract the influence of the germ, thus establishing an immunity. . . . If we place the fingers of both of our hands along the back of a patient in the mid-dorsal area and exert steady, deep pressure, we can soon observe gurgling in the stomach and intestines. What is taking place? The impulse has been not only transmitted from cell through the nervous system, but also changed into peristaltic motion of the intestinal walls: an example of thigmotropism causing muscular action. In like manner glands may be caused to pour out their secretions.'

The body does not segment itself. As I have mentioned before it is us looking in that compartmentalises the body. It adjusts as a whole all the time. The initial remark by Still of not officially teaching techniques will not sit well with some practitioners. But it must be understood that if the conquering of the technique procedure becomes the short-term goal of the practitioner this detracts from the practice of following or reading tissue in the relation to the needs of the patient. Applying techniques imposes the technique on the patient and can lead to a diagnosis to fit your skills rather following abnormal tissue based on palpation. Still would say 'manipulative treatment is not osteopathy. Spinal adjustment is not osteopathy. Each is a part of osteopathy and must be considered only as a part.'

Osteopathic therapy is generally applied on the basis of the sympathetic system. It is important to remember that, generally, the sympathetics inhibit and the parasympathetic activates.

Here are some examples of an autonomic disturbance:

- *Stomach:* ulcers, gastritis and hyperchlorhydria definitely indicate the need for treatment of the sympathetic nervous system. This treatment should be directed to the areas from the fifth to ninth thoracic, the most important segments being the fifth, sixth and seventh. By treating this area one inhibits muscular activity, decreases glandular secretions, and diminishes the production of hydrochloric acid. In treating hypochlorhydria, parasympathetic stimulation by way of the vagus is definitely indicated, because the vagus causes contraction of muscles, increased activity of all glands, and increased output of hydrochloric acid.
- *Heart:* the sympathetic nerve supply to the heart originates from the first to the sixth thoracic. These fibres pass to ganglia, which in turn send fibres directly to the heart wall. The general action of inhibition is reversed to the heart, the action being activation or acceleration. It has been found that the osteopathic manipulative approach applied to the first to the sixth thoracic, increases the heart rate without increasing the blood pressure.

Be aware that absolute diagnostic categorising leads to treatment categorising. Although this is desirable at an academic level it is vital that it does not monopolise the life of the practitioner, otherwise the osteopathic practitioner will only be able to treat the muscles and joints; not being able to 'see' through the myofascioskeletal system. *The myofascioskeletal system will become the Medusa of the osteopath.*

References

Appenzeller, O. and Oribe, E. (1997) *The Autonomic Nervous System. An Introduction to Basic and Clinical Concepts* (Fifth edition). Elsevier, London.

Bortoft, H. (1999) Personal communication. At the presentation of *The Transformation to a Dynamical Mode of Consciousness in Scientific Thinking.* Tenth Mind and Brain Symposium: The Evolution of Consciousness – Consciousness and the Self. Saturday 13th November. Institute of Psychiatry, London, England.

Bouratinos, E. (1999) Personal communication. At the presentation of *Consciousness and the Snare of Civilisation: A Brief Survey of Human Evolution.* Tenth Mind and Brain Symposium: The Evolution of Consciousness – Consciousness and the Self. Saturday 13th November. Institute of Psychiatry, London, England.

Coats, C. (1998) *Nature as Teacher.* (Volume Two of *Eco-Technology.*) Gateway Books, Bath.

Comstock, E.S. (1920) Osteopathic therapeutics in infectious diseases. *The Journal of the American Osteopathic Association,* 20(3) 111–13.

Crary, J. (1996) *Techniques of the Observer: On Vision and Modernity in the Nineteenth Century.* The MIT Press, Cambridge, MA.

Goethe, Johann Wolfgang von (1810) *Theory of Colours.* (Translated by C.L. Eastlake, introduced by D.B. Judd.) MIT Press, London.

Hubbell, P.R. (1921) Adjustment – the last word. *The Journal of the American Osteopathic Association.* June 582–3.

Jackson, P.A. (1981) The Technique of A.T. Still. *1981 Year Book* pp. 15–18. The Osteopathic Institute of Applied Technique, Maidstone.

Johnston, W.L. *et al.* (1987) Somatic manifestations in renal disease: a clinical research study. *The Journal of the American Osteopathic Association,* 87(1) 22–35.

Lawrence, C. (1918) The biological phase of an osteopathic treatment. *The Journal of the American Osteopathic Association.* Dec 170–72.

Patterson, M.M. (1976) A model mechanism for spinal segmental facilitation. *The Journal of the American Osteopathic Association.* 76(1) 62–72.

Pottenger, F.M. (1984) *Symptoms of Visceral Disease.* (Sixth edition) C.V. Mosby Company, St. Louis.

Stimpson, G. and Webb, B. (1975) *Going to see the Doctor – The Consultation Process in General Practice.* Routledge and Kegan Paul, London.

Swope, F.L. (1938) Examination and diagnosis in acute diseases. *The Journal of the American Osteopathic Association,* 37(5) 171–4.

Tasker, D.L. (1925) *Principles of Osteopathy.* (Fifth edition). Birkeley and Elson Printing Co.

Vaughan, F.M. (1918) Physical Diagnosis. *The Journal of the American Osteopathic Association,* 18(4) 172-4.

Waitley, D.D. (1948) The autonomic nervous system in osteopathic therapy. *The Journal of the American Osteopathic Association,* 47(9) 447–50.

White, P.A. (1990) Ideas about causation in philosophy and psychology. *Psychological Bulletin,* 108(1) 3–18.

Index

9 780632 052639